T0091938

FROM WHISPERS
TO SHOUTS

FROM WHISPERS TO SHOUTS

The Ways We Talk About Cancer

ELAINE SCHATTNER

Columbia University Press

New York

Columbia University Press
Publishers Since 1893
New York   Chichester, West Sussex
cup.columbia.edu

Library of Congress Cataloging-in-Publication Data
Names: Schattner, Elaine, author.
Title: From whispers to shouts : the ways we talk about cancer / by Elaine Schattner.
Description: New York : Columbia University Press, [2022] |
    Includes bibliographical references and index.
Identifiers: LCCN 2022015190 | ISBN 9780231192262 (hardback) |
    ISBN 9780231549745 (ebook)
Subjects: LCSH: Cancer—Social aspects—United States—History. |
    Cancer—United States—Public opinion. | Cancer in mass media. |
    Health attitudes—United States.
Classification: LCC RC276 .S328 2022 | DDC 362.19699/4—dc23/eng/20220919
LC record available at https://lccn.loc.gov/2022015190

Columbia University Press books are printed on permanent and
    durable acid-free paper.
Printed in the United States of America

Cover design: Noah Arlow
Cover image: Women's Field Army button (private collection).

CONTENTS

PROLOGUE

I never imagined I'd be writing a book like this. Twenty-five years ago, as an ambitious young oncologist, I devoted myself to research and patient care. In the lab, I studied how immune signals can trigger malignant cells to survive, proliferate, or die. In the clinic, I cared for patients with lymphoma, leukemia, and other blood disorders. My job was both intellectually and emotionally challenging. I loved what I was doing and worked hard, expecting to become a tenured professor of medicine, run a laboratory for a couple of decades, and continue helping patients until I retired. That didn't happen. A series of serious health problems including breast cancer irreparably ruptured my career. It took me years to get over the loss of my lab. As for the loss of my clinical work, that still hurts. Being a doctor remains essential to who I am. It is why I have written this book.

From Whispers to Shouts probes public perceptions of cancer: how ordinary people talk about malignancy outside of doctors' offices, how that's changed, and why this matters. If there's one take-home message—what I've learned in recent years as a journalist and patient advocate—it's that cancer treatments have improved more than many people, including doctors, appreciate. A century of philanthropic, government, and corporate investments and scientists' dedication has yielded actionable knowledge of malignant cells, the immune system, and genomics. In ways that were unfathomable when I became a doctor in 1987, technological advances, ranging from the internet to computational biology, permit doctors to apply molecular details in each case to optimize therapy.

Today many cancers are treatable, and many more will be soon. Yet people remain fatalistic about cancer. Attitudes can be lethal. This happens in two ways. If individuals believe beneficial treatments to be harmful or useless, they will avoid medical care. On a larger scale, if policy-makers view oncology drugs as ineffective or as a luxury, they may limit access to lifesaving treatments for all but the wealthiest patients, who can pay thousands of dollars for diagnostic tests and hundreds of thousands for medicines, year after year. And I should clarify up front, by "attitude" I don't mean having an upbeat mood or "fighting spirit" to combat cancer. Such popular notions appear in stories about cancer, considered later in this book, and should be dispelled. There is no such thing as a tumoricidal mindset.

Cancer patients today enjoy unprecedented access to medical information. On the web, they exchange tips and updates, chat peer-to-peer, and consult experts in real time. Yet cancer facts can be hard to discern from hype, advertisements, and outright fraudulent claims. At the heart of this book is this paradox: as cancer therapy improves, patients' choices become harder because the decisional stakes rise. As more treatments become available, options overwhelm. Even if oncology drugs were affordable and available to all, patients and doctors might not be aware of what's best. Amid a surplus of cancer reports and advice, in traditional news and social media, truth is elusive, data confusing.

I believe that effective cancer care—whether curative or palliative—still depends on effective communication and trust between patients and doctors. If either is lacking, patients suffer.

How I arrived at this topic is a consequence of my curvy career path. That's another story. but not irrelevant. I'll summarize, so that you might know where I'm coming from—what motivates and informs my writing. That would include my education, my work as a researcher and oncologist, and aspects of my medical history, my biases. Initially I approached the subject—cancer—with a physician's mindset, for which I credit my Dad. When I was a teenager on Long Island in the 1970s, he taught me some math and quizzed me about chemistry. He was a demanding, no-nonsense doctor with a compassionate streak. Most evenings after dinner, he would sip tea and return calls, and I would hear him speaking on the phone. He treated people with rare empathy, a word I didn't yet know, and care. Besides being a role model as a physician, always he encouraged me to think independently, to speak my mind, and to value each day of my life.

Unknowingly I became a patient at age six, when a pediatrician noticed my scoliosis. Into adolescence I wore an ungainly contraption called a Milwaukee brace to straighten my spine, but despite my diligence in wearing it, the curvature got worse. After exhaustive consultation with orthopedists, we decided that I should have surgery that involved grafting a fourteen-inch steel Harrington rod to my vertebrae. I have vague memories of brutal traction before the operation, hallucinating in the ICU afterward, and staying in a drab hospital room for most of six weeks. At surgery, I received seven units of blood. Then I developed a blood clot, so I wound up on a blood thinner until the body cast came off nine months later, days before my fifteenth birthday. After that, apart from the long scar down my back, I appeared healthy and moved on.

In college at Yale, I majored in political philosophy. I read utopian theory and decided in my junior year to pursue medicine because I wanted to do something more pragmatic than getting a PhD in philosophy. As a freshman I'd taken math and physics, so I only needed to catch up in basic biology and chemistry. Neither subject interested me much until I took courses in molecular and cell biology. I was turned on by the *lac* operon and whatever else was known, around 1981, about gene transcription—how DNA is converted to protein-encoding RNA, and what controls that. Amazed by the complexity of each cell, I wanted to learn more science. Upon graduating I moved to Manhattan, started working as a technician at Rockefeller University, and applied to medical schools. While in the lab that was elucidating the structure of the neural cell adhesion molecule, N-CAM, I used what must then have been a cutting-edge protein sequencer. As I think back on that year of research—pouring stuff though columns, loading and running gels, analyzing results on graph paper—I realize how primitive were our research methods, not forty years ago.

When I entered medical school at New York University in 1983, I wasn't sure what kind of doctor I wanted to become. During the first two years, I took required courses: anatomy, physiology, pathology, genetics, and that sort of thing. During summers, I worked in a cell biology lab. In July 1985, the start of my third year, Bellevue Hospital was crowded with AIDS patients. There I was assigned rotations in surgery, obstetrics and gynecology, psychiatry, and pediatrics, along with a stint in internal medicine at the university hospital. In my final year I took electives in subjects ranging from cardiology to medical history, traveled to Bolivia where I learned firsthand about parasites by catching one, and completed what we called a "subinternship" at Bellevue. Most of the experiences I recall from medical school took place in that public hospital, and most of the patients I remember were suffering and dying from AIDS.

As an intern and resident at the New York Hospital in the late 1980s, I cared for many AIDS patients. Some were beginning to live longer on antiviral medicines, but that trend was not yet clear. Before completing my residency, I became convinced that "heme-onc"—the combined subspecialty of blood (hematology) and cancer (oncology)—was worthwhile. Each year I'd spent a few months on rotations at Memorial Sloan Kettering Cancer Center, and that influenced me. Oncology seemed a promising field of medicine in which progress—deliverable through science—would happen in my lifetime. I wanted to be a part of that.

Although doctors in training are said to be overworked and sleep deprived, and I was both, this was a very happy period of my life. During my residency, I married the man I love. While a fellow in hematology and oncology, I gave birth to my two sons. But I didn't stay at home much. My thoughts centered on work. I wanted to learn as much as possible, so I could take best care of my patients and accomplish meaningful research.

I was absorbed in my laboratory investigations. During my fellowship and for another year I worked in an HIV lab. I was interested in AIDS-related lymphomas and how, in patients with HIV, the immune system failed to keep some tumors in check. Lymphomas excited me. At a time when many oncologists didn't distinguish between cancer subtypes, I became obsessed with how different kinds of malignant B or T lymphocytes—the cells comprising lymphoma—respond to natural and medicinal immune triggers.

In 1993, I joined the faculty at Cornell as a lowly instructor. If you'd asked me about my research, I might have launched into a lecture explaining how just as cancer is not one disease, lymphoma is not one malignancy. The same applied to other blood cancers, like leukemia. To treat cancer effectively, you have to know the subtype, I insisted. (Nowadays this applies to most cancer types, but scientific knowledge of "solid" tumors—like prostate and lung cancer—was nearly absent in the 1990s.) A few years later, in my own lab, we examined healthy and malignant human lymphocytes to see which stimuli promote malignant cell survival and which induce a healthy form of cell death called *apoptosis*.

While this might seem a digression, in this book about cancer attitudes, it's relevant to current discussions about costs of cancer care and the emerging field of precision oncology. Although some skeptics downplay the role of science in the clinic, I believe that finding the best and least toxic cancer therapy depends on elucidating molecular details in each case. For doctors to advise patients and select optimal care, they need know enough basic science to discern among malignant subtypes, and to distinguish curable or treatable cases from those which cannot be helped.

In October 2002, my life took an unexpected turn. Like many thousands of other women that year, I was diagnosed with breast cancer. By then I was an associate professor, midway up the academic ladder, a blood and cancer specialist with expertise in lymphoma, chronic leukemia, and rare blood disorders. Months before, I'd closed my research laboratory for lack of a second grant and switched to a full-time career path in clinical medicine. Although I was devastated about losing my lab, I thought I'd be OK career-wise, that I was professionally set, because I enjoyed seeing patients and teaching.

My breast cancer diagnosis arrived amid other health problems. Starting around 1998, I'd experienced pain while walking. X-rays showed that my lower vertebrae were crumbling below the old Harrington rod. Fearing surgery, I swam laps in an effort to strengthen my back muscles. But my spine and posture continued to deteriorate. It became clear that if I wanted to keep walking, I'd need have my spine repaired. While planning that risky neurosurgical operation, my internist advised a screening mammogram; at age forty-two, I was overdue. Those images were cloudy and suspicious, so the radiologist ordered an ultrasound and detected a stage 1, invasive ductal breast cancer.

Having early-stage breast cancer didn't scare me. In retrospect, I think it should have. As an oncologist, I understood my tumor was treatable. But I underestimated the emotional and sexual consequences of premature menopause induced by chemotherapy, and the psychological repercussions of mastectomy. I'd seen badly reconstructed breasts in clinic and fretted for my patients, that as "teaching cases" they'd been operated upon by surgeons in-training. I thought mine would come out looking better, but I was mistaken. My appearance was irreversibly damaged. As for the long-term medical toll of treatment—thin bones, elevated risk of heart disease, and more—my doctors and I are still reckoning with those effects.

At the time, I didn't seek additional information about breast cancer. It helped, of course, that I was practicing oncology. I knew my options. Had I searched, I would have found only a narrow selection of patient-oriented resources. I'd heard about *Dr. Susan Love's Breast Book* from patients and affected friends; the third edition of that best-selling "bible" was circulating. Hotlines and support groups existed, but as a physician I didn't consider availing myself of either. Few websites covered breast cancer. Social media—or its predecessors, more accurately—consisted of a few blogs and email listservs. Future platforms like Facebook, Twitter, and YouTube did not enter my imagination.

With less science and fewer drugs back then, oncology decisions were limited and, in some respects, more straightforward. Submitting an individual's cancer for full genomic evaluation was inconceivable. Doctors knew of a few breast cancer–related DNA changes, like *BRCA* mutations, but testing for those was far from routine. Molecular pathology tests like Oncotype DX, to inform prognosis, were not available. Herceptin, an antibody that's now standard treatment for breast cancer with high levels of HER2, a protein in some malignant cells, wasn't approved by the FDA for early-stage patients until 2006, so checking for that didn't make a difference. How I proceeded was to consult with doctors I liked and respected, and let them "drive." I opted for bilateral mastectomy, because reducing weight on my chest would be good for my back. Fearing side effects of chemotherapy, I chose the lowest-dose regimen that would reduce the odds of recurrence.

Since 2002, one thing I've observed is that as more people are surviving longer and speaking up about the toxicity of cancer treatment—including employment and financial problems—doctors are beginning to listen. Oncologists are paying attention not only to survival statistics, but to patient-reported outcomes—patients' actual experiences. It's no longer sufficient to say a cancer patient is "lucky to be alive." Quality of life matters. Another recent advance has been the careful pullback of therapy to avoid overtreatment. This trend should continue, along with better and targeted chemotherapy agents designed to destroy tumor cells rather than healthy body parts.

So much changed for me, personally and professionally, including the nature of my work, what tools I use to find information, and how I communicate about illness. After the spine surgery, my posture improved and my back pain disappeared, but I have difficulty standing. My lower gut became inflamed. I became profoundly depressed and stopped practicing medicine. What helped me in a low period, among other things, was reading and learning from perspectives of other patients. I went on to study journalism, started a blog and joined the online fray, cautiously at first, with an open mind.

∾

This book reflects my immersion into the evolving realm of conversations about cancer that exists apart from doctors. It extends from the 2009 master's thesis I wrote at Columbia University's Graduate School of Journalism, titled "Democracy in the Doctor's Office: The Internet Opens Dialogue and Care Choices for Cancer Patients." Then, as a seasoned oncologist and cancer survivor who'd relied exclusively on textbooks, medical journals, and specialists' advice, I became intrigued by how people who are not doctors find medical information. As we'll see, open chatter about illness has expanded dramatically since 2009, when few patients or doctors used social media.

Why this matters is that public understanding of cancer is at a critical juncture. As treatments improve, some patients gain months and years of life, possible cures. Oncologists—my former colleagues—are thrilled to be seeing patients survive for a long time with conditions that, just ten years ago, they deemed hopeless. Many friends now—people with stage 4, metastatic cancer—are living well beyond the "expiration dates" when doctors and statistics predicted they'd be dead. Which leads me to worry for patients I haven't met, who don't participate in online discussions or attend conferences, who may not be aware of—and whose doctors do not know, or dismiss—clinical advances.

As a practicing physician, I discounted cancer's social side. I didn't consider the possibility that "word on the street"—what journalists, celebrities, patients in support groups (now on social media), and others who are not doctors were saying about cancer—might influence what treatments patients would be offered or choose. To understand the issue, I dove into the history of cancer awareness and found old threads in stories, images, and journalism about malignancy that are woven into modern-day debates. I discovered that amid modern progress against cancer, emotional and social factors that hindered care a hundred years ago—fear, feelings of hopelessness, shame, and ignorance—still determine patients' decisions and outcomes. Attitudes about cancer have an unmeasured but profound impact on what care patients receive. Beliefs nudge individuals toward or away from treatment.

Before researching this book, I didn't fully appreciate the degree to which racist views and other prejudices, the notion that some human lives are "expendable," have contributed to and, in effect, limited medical knowledge across a wide swath of medical fields including oncology, much of what I'd been taught. A long history of medical racism and systemic neglect of people of color, ethnic minorities, Indigenous Americans, and others, has engendered deep distrust of mainstream physicians in some communities, which in turn leads many individuals to avoid appropriate care. A raft of current publications has only begun to acknowledge the extent to which ignorance and disregard of cancer, particularly as it occurs in people of color, cuts survival of those affected.

My book is unfortunately incomplete, not only for the narratives and voices I could not include but for stories unknown to me. As we'll see, cancer awareness campaigns emerged predominantly in well-educated, white communities like mine. Affected individuals who identify as LGBTQ+, those who are poor, of color, and of other marginalized groups were unlikely to enter public conversations about cancer; their perspectives remain underreported. I hope that this work will spark fuller examination of cancer awareness and its ramifications in diverse communities.

At the start of this century, physician-scientists called out the sometimes fatal interval between laboratory and clinical advances; it took twenty years, at least, to translate molecular understanding of cancer into effective, available therapy. This book suggests a "perception gap"—a harmful disconnect between how scientists, doctors who keep up-to-date, educated patients, and other insiders view cancer, and how most people see it.

Let's take a look.

PART I

CANCER AWAKENS

This part of the book tells the story of cancer's emergence into the public sphere. We'll see how and why a charity, aiming to reduce cancer's toll in the early 1900s, targeted fear and ignorance about the disease.

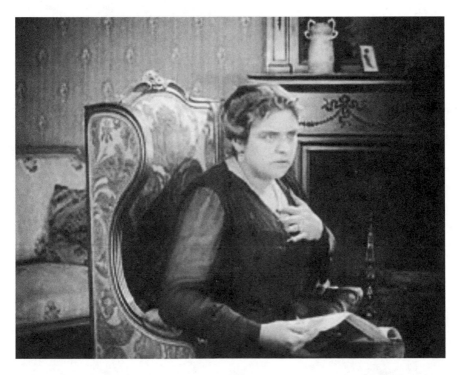

Mrs. Flint feels a breast lump in *The Reward of Courage*, a 1921 film about cancer produced by the Eastern Film Corporation for the ASCC.
(National Library of Medicine)

CHAPTER 1

CANCER, KEPT APART (BEFORE 1900)

I n April 1883, the Ladies' Auxiliary Board of the New-York Skin and Cancer Hospital held a fundraiser at Delmonico's, a famed Manhattan restaurant. Playing on the city's New Amsterdam roots, they called it a *kirmess*,
a Dutch term for a traditional village festival. The event planners, chiefly Mrs.
Richard Irvin Jr., Mrs. B. H. Van Auken, and Mrs. John A. Lowery, scheduled
activities from two o'clock in the afternoon until midnight on a Saturday. During
the daytime, games and magic would entertain children. At night, there would
be dancing. "It is understood that a number of the prettiest girls of the season
are rehearsing the Dutch national dance for the occasion," reported the *New York
Herald*.[1,2]

Buzz for the upcoming gala spread around the country. The *St. Paul Sunday
Globe* ran these words in a "Gossip of Gotham" column: "Charity, in this age, is a
shrewd nymph. She should for her keen business insight, be called a Yankee. Now
what do you think the generous handed dame proposes to do next? Why, have
a jolly dinner, fair, ball, etc., at Delmonico's." The columnist observed, "Charity
will have her fun for her money, and the cash will go to help the new skin and
cancer hospital." Advertisements listed C. Vanderbilt and J. Pierpont Morgan
as patrons. Mrs. W. M. Astor and Mrs. W. K. Vanderbilt—rivals of old and new
wealth—cooperated in this cause. Tickets cost $1, equivalent to around $26 today
(figure 1.1).[3,4]

On Saturday, April 28, hundreds of charitable merrymakers poured into Delmonico's Madison Square branch. "This is the largest crowd that has ever been in
this building," Charles Delmonico, the proprietor, told the *New York Times*. The
restaurant was fitted like a "grove from fairyland" with evergreens, myrtle, ferns
and flowers, and lit with Chinese lanterns. Young and old *kirmess*-goers played

THE KIRMESS.

Brilliant Success of the Charity
Festival at Delmonico's.

CROWDS OF MERRYMAKERS.

A Scene of Sylvan Loveliness—
Kaleidoscopic Costumes.

GRACEFUL DANCES AND GAY PASTIMES

A Large Sum Realized for the Relief of
Sickness and Suffering.

SOME HISTORIC REMINISCENCES.

KIRMESS.

For the benefit of the

SKIN AND CANCER HOSPITAL.

AN OUTDOOR SPRING FESTIVAL

will be given at
DELMONICO'S,
April 28, from 2 P M. until midnight.

AFTERNOON—Children's entertainment and fancy
dress carnival; gypsy encampment and tricks.
EVENING—Dancing, music by Lander; Dutch national
dance; Zither Club and Tyrolienne dance; gypsy divina-
tion, palmistry, &c.
Flowers and refreshments on sale.
Tickets, $1 each, to be had of Delmonico and at 196
Madison av. and of the following ladies and gentlemen:—

PATRONS.
A. WRIGHT SANFORD,
CHAUNCEY M. DEPEW,
CHESTER GRISWOLD,
O. K. KING,
W. H. BRIDGHAM,
C. VANDERBILT,
J. PIERPONT MORGAN,
J. COLEMAN DRAYTON,
A. B. HOLLINS,
L. VON HOFFMAN.

PATRONESSES.
Mrs. WM. ASTOR,
Mrs. JOHN SHERWOOD,
Mrs. JAMES WATERBURY,
Mrs. LEWIS JONES,
Mrs. AUGUST BELMONT,
Mrs. BAYARD CUTTING,
Mrs. ROBERT HOE, Jr.,
Mrs. J. B. POTTER,
Mrs. W. K. VANDERBILT,
Mrs. JAMES A. BURDEN,
Mrs. M. O. ROBERTS.

Mrs. R. IRWIN, Jr., President,
Mrs. VAN AUKEN, Vice President,
Mrs. J. A. LOWRY, secretary,
Miss M. L. WALKER, Treasurer.

of Auxiliary
Board of Hospital.

COMMITTEE ON WAYS AND MEANS.
Mrs. WM. C. SCHERMERHORN, Mrs. JULIUS CAT-
LIN, Jr., Mrs. R. P. LOUNSBURY, Mrs. J. O'CONNOR,
Miss M. L. WALKER.

Mirth and mercy combined to weave a chaplet of
success to crown the ladies under whose management the Kirmess festival took place yesterday
afternoon and evening at Delmonico's. Fortune
smiled on them; their friends rallied to their aid,
and they succeeded in accomplishing a result for
which the poor and the suffering will long continue to bless them. Their purpose throughout
several weeks of careful planning and devoted
effort has been the establishment of a fund whereby
the benefits of the Skin and Cancer Hospital may be
extended to such of the stricken as are too poor to
pay for them. This end has been to a great extent
accomplished. For obvious reasons it cannot yet
be told just what the amount realized may be, but
it is confidently hoped that it will reach several
thousand dollars.

1.1   (left) An advertisement for the upcoming *kirmess* in the April 22, 1883 *New York Herald*; (right) news of the event in the April 29, 1883 *New York Herald*.

games and sipped lemonade. Some bought flowers at the auction, offering high bids: $200 for a single rose and $100 for a boutonniere. "The ghosts of the old Knickerbockers must have groaned at the prodigality of their representatives," observed the *San Antonio Light*.[5,6]

Women arrived at Delmonico's in "flaming petticoats of scarlet, orange and other hues, waists or bodices of black velvet." Their attire "defied the pencil of a news man." In a parlor overlooking Fifth Avenue, Mrs. Julius Catlin and Mrs. F. Hopkinson Smith supervised a "gypsy encampment" offering "divinations, palmistry, etc." Mr. Montefiore Isaacs, said to be the Gypsy King, gave tidings "so very good that his fame speedily spread around the rooms, and he had more custom-ers willing to 'cross his hand with silver' than he could take care of." That eve-ning, young New Yorkers performed European folk dances in the ballroom; their costumed renditions of the *Ländler* and *Tyrolienne* generated so much applause that they gave encore performances for all to see. The philanthropists drank *sangaree* and danced until midnight.[7,8]

Before 1900, most people with cancer died at home. If a wealthy person became sick, a doctor might be solicited for a house call and what treatments he prescribed taken privately. Surgery might be performed in the kitchen. Non-operative treatments were mainly palliative: alcohol or opiates for pain, enemas or laxatives for constipation. In a few large institutions, like Boston's Massachusetts General Hospital and Philadelphia General Hospital, some patients underwent surgery. Paupers' services, like those on Blackwell Island in New York City, accepted those suffering with cancer, but those were places of last resort. The poor avoided hospitals, too.

Many afflicted succumbed without knowing of their condition. People with symptoms hesitated before seeking medical evaluation. Even if they had the means—and will—to consult a physician, the disease was often missed. Doctors lacked knowledge or tools to distinguish cancer from other ailments. Diagnostic failures didn't matter much, however, because there were no effective cancer treatments other than surgery, which was brutal and often futile. Disclosure of a serious diagnosis, especially to women, was unusual. Without a therapy to give or procedure to try, telling a person they had cancer could seem pointless or even cruel. Many physicians preferred not to inform patients of bad news, believing that it would only add to their suffering.

The picture began to change toward the nineteenth century's end. With development of crude anesthesia, unthinkably painful operations became, at some institutions, treatments to consider. Knowledge of bacteria and antiseptic methods reduced risks of infection from surgery. Yet many practitioners questioned the "germ theory" and resisted adopting basic hygienic practices like handwashing. Even in the best hospitals, surgery remained an ordeal. Medical progress lagged in the United States relative to Europe, where some American physicians traveled to study science and surgical methods. Patients crossed the ocean, too, if they had means.

By the 1880s, Europe's lead in countering cancer spurred efforts to establish specialized hospitals in America. Surgeons needed facilities with operating rooms, stocked with supplies and staffed by trained nurses, to render procedures safer and more likely to yield favorable results. U.S. citizens wanted their doctors to provide the latest techniques. They sought better care and chances of relief.[9–12]

Physicians credited Dr. James Marion Sims with spearheading America's first cancer hospital. Together with Mrs. General George (Elizabeth) Cullum, a grand-daughter of Alexander Hamilton, he led early efforts to establish the New York Cancer Hospital—what eventually became Memorial Sloan Kettering Cancer Center.[13–15] Sims's legacy is compromised, however, because he performed surgery on enslaved persons. His story exemplifies how some respected medical practi-tioners gained experience by operating on people who could not give consent, and foreshadows how cancer knowledge has been acquired, in part, through experimentation on people of color and others who were vulnerable, desperate, and without means to pay for their care.[16,17]

Born in Lancaster County, South Carolina, in 1813, Sims studied medicine in Philadelphia and settled near Montgomery, Alabama. In a chilling 1830s account, he describes visiting a woman with a high fever and rapid pulse, likely from consumption (tuberculosis). After a senior colleague performed blood-letting, the patient died. Sims weighed on the futility of medical practice: "I knew nothing about medicine, but I had sense enough to see that doctors were killing their patients; that medicine was not an exact science," he wrote. "It would be better to trust entirely to Nature than to the hazardous skill of the doctors." More than a hundred years before clinical trials became routine, doctors had little evidence to guide their prescriptions. Medicines consisted of blended natural compounds and homeopathic solutions. Giving a drug to an ailing person was a matter of trial and error, or plain guesswork. Sims decided to focus on surgery.[18]

Sims built a small structure in a corner of his property, "a little hospital," to house and treat ailing Black people. Some enslaved women had vaginal tears and fistulas involving the rectum. (These complications of childbirth cause pain, incontinence, and foul odors, leading to abandonment of some women.) In Alabama, Sims carried out hundreds of operations. In his autobiography, he called some of those procedures "experiments." The women and their owners approached him in desperation, he wrote. Some neighbors and colleagues com-plained about the facility in his yard and provision of care to "negroes."[18]

Sims also operated on men. In the 1847 *American Journal of the Medical Sciences*, he reported excising an orange-sized tumor from the jaw of an eighteen-year-old enslaved man named George (figure 1.2). Initially, the young man did well after surgery. But two months later the cancer reappeared; it grew rapidly near George's eye and caused terrible pain. Sims administered morphine. The young man endured a lengthy second procedure during which he repeatedly cried, "oh!" The operation proved futile. The tumor came back, taking away George's sight and filling his throat so he could no longer speak or breathe. By contrast, in a more successful operation, Sims removed a jaw tumor from a sixty-eight-year-old man, Jack, "property of John M. Sanders, Esq., of Macon Co., Ala." The next day, Jack was chewing tobacco. "In two weeks he was out chopping wood," Sims noted, adding: "He went home perfectly well."[19,20]

In Alabama, Sims didn't earn much. He incurred debts. In 1853 he moved to New York, and his practice flourished. Soon he founded the Woman's Hospital. The four-story building at 83 Madison Avenue opened in 1855 with a few dozen

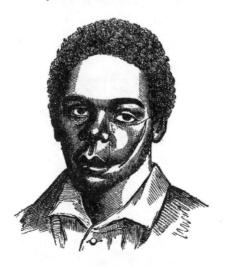

312   Sims, *Removal of the Superior Maxilla.*   [April

spongy bones of the nose. The orbitar edge of the maxilla was transformed into a sort of *spiculated* osteo-fibrous structure.

The tumour is almost perfectly round. That segment of it extending

1.2 Woodcut depiction of a man's face after cancer surgery, J. Marion Sims, *Amer. J. Med Sci.*, 1847

beds. It was chartered to provide care not only for wealthy women, but for those of middle class and modest means: "wives and daughters of clergymen, lawyers, doctors, merchants' clerks, merchants who have been unfortunate in business, college professors, teachers, druggists, artists, farmers, [and] mechanics."

The Woman's Hospital fussed over its reputation, with reason. Providing—or receiving—gynecological care could cause a stir. Undergoing physical examination by a male practitioner outside the home, with vaginal inspection no less, risked a woman's dignity. Many ladies avoided gynecological examination until they experienced terrible symptoms and, even then, demurred. Some families wouldn't permit it. "No lady is degraded by entering the Woman's Hospital as a patient," Sims wrote. The hospital was often full.[21,22]

During the Civil War, Sims left the United States for Europe. He worked with some of the world's most eminent doctors, and his reputation grew. Sims became a physician to the empress Eugénie of France, the duchess of Hamilton, and the empress of Austria. When he returned to New York, well-to-do women sought Sims's expertise. By the early 1870s, doctors from around the country came to the Woman's Hospital to observe his surgical techniques and so frequently crowded the operating theater that the institution hired a guard to limit onlookers.

The Woman's Hospital received complaints about Sims admitting women with cancer, "thereby causing great discomfort and danger to the other patients in the ward." In 1874, its Board of Lady Managers, followed by its Board of Governors, voted to deny admission of women with cancer. People worried that tumors might be infectious and spread from one patient to the next. Many considered cancer a divine punishment for ill behavior. Others simply didn't want to be near the dreaded disease.[15,23,24]

Sims left the Woman's Hospital amid those accusations.[14,25] He moved on, becoming president of the American Medical Association and, later, president of the American Gynecological Society. Shortly before his death in November 1883, Sims wrote a widely circulated letter to the lawyer John E. Parsons about the need for a cancer hospital in New York: "We are now making great progress in every department of medicine. Why should not cancer derive some benefit from this general onward movement?" Sims questioned. He was influential; newspapers and physicians quoted these words.[13,26,27] A decade later, his former colleagues, "loving patients and many admirers" presented a statue to the City of New York recognizing his "brilliant achievements" in surgery. Initially set in Bryant Park, it was relocated to Fifth Avenue opposite the New York Academy of Medicine in 1934 and, amid criticism of Sims's having operated on enslaved persons, to Brooklyn's Green-Wood Cemetery in 2018.[28–31]

Still, cancer patients had few places to turn.

One little-known Manhattan hospital did offer care to people with cancer. In November 1882, a group led by Dr. L. Duncan Bulkley, a dermatologist, chartered the New-York Skin and Cancer Hospital. They purchased an "ordinary dwelling house" at 243 East Thirty-Fourth Street. Before they could admit "inmates," as hospitalized patients were called then, the brick building needed an overhaul of its plumbing and heating. Years later, Bulkley credited one woman, Ellin Lowery, with establishing the institution. "We had practically no money," he recalled. Her pragmatic, serious nature set her apart from others involved in the project.[32]

Mrs. John (Ellin) A. Lowery was thirty-three years old when she helped found the Skin and Cancer Hospital. Her efforts typified those of countless women who, later on, volunteered to help people affected by cancer. Through financial ups and downs, many friendships, and two marriages, Ellin proved a constant philanthropist. Three decades later—as a very wealthy Mrs. James Speyer by her second marriage, and with plenty of experience—she helped found the organization that became the American Cancer Society.[33]

Ellin "Nellie" Lowery was born in October 1849 in Lowell, Massachusetts. At midcentury, the bustling mill city on the Merrimack River drew workers from New England, Canada, Ireland, and beyond. It was, in some ways, a progressive place in Ellin's day. Many employees—single women living apart from families—resided in company-owned dormitories. In the decade before her birth, Lowell corporations built an industry hospital for laborers, the first of its kind in the United States. When Charles Dickens visited in 1842, he commented favorably on conditions in the factories, dormitories, and hospital. Workers published the *Voice of Industry*, a printed weekly.[34,35]

After her father's death, Ellin came to live in Manhattan with a wealthy uncle, William Travers. Travers provided his niece with private tutoring, exposure to the arts, and social connections. He and his wife had nine children; Ellin received little inheritance. But through her vibrant personality, she garnered friends and influence. Years later, a 1932 *New Yorker* profile of her second husband, James Speyer, said of her, "Not exactly beautiful, she had unusual charm, dressed in the

height of fashion, and as one of New York's most successful hostesses was identified with the higher theatrical as well as social circles."[36-38]

Ellin married John Lowery in 1871. The couple was childless. He, a Princeton
graduate and grandson of New York's former mayor Stephen Allen, was a man
of leisure. John frequented the Union Club, an exclusive Manhattan society, and
the South Side Sportsmen's Club, an enclave on the Connetquot River near Long
Island's Great South Bay. At the lodge, men and their companions would drink,
picnic, and spend the night before an early hunting expedition or after a day
spent fishing for trout.[39,40]

While her husband played, Ellin engaged with charity. When Mrs. Richard
(Mary) Irvin Jr., a neighbor and banker's wife, invited her to assist with the
Hospital Saturday and Sunday Association, Ellin signed on as secretary of the
Woman's Auxiliary and soon became its treasurer. Over decades of Ellin's involvement with this organization—which later became the United Hospital Fund—
donations escalated from hundreds, to thousands, to tens of thousands of dollars. The *New York Times* reported on gifts to the association. A telling example
from January 1891 foreshadows modern cause marketing: the newspaper listed
$100 from "Lord & Taylor" and $50 from "Bloomingdale Brothers." These donations from stores served both the charity and companies' reputations.[41]

In 1882, Ellin joined Bulkley in establishing the New-York Skin and Cancer Hospital. She got right to work as secretary of the Ladies' Auxiliary,
arranging for renovations of the building. Within two months, the hospital
offered a dispensary and outpatient clinic. By February 1883, it opened a
first-floor ward with five beds. After an infusion of cash from the *kirmess*
that spring, the institution expanded to accommodate twenty-nine patients
in separate wards for men, women, and children. Typical daily expenses at
the Skin and Cancer Hospital, largely for drugs and food, were $1.93 per
patient. The hospital was run in "the most economical basis possible," the
auxiliary reported. The women hired a matron, Mrs. Carswell, to keep the
facility orderly and clean.[42]

It was no accident that the idea of building a U.S. cancer hospital came to fruition at the peak of the Gilded Age. Between the economic panics of 1873 and
1893, railroad tycoons, industrialists, and investors made fortunes. A new class

of wealthy citizens, comfortable in commerce but less accepted among old New York families, wanted to display their wealth—and good will—through charitable contributions.

Intellectual shifts factored in, too. After Charles Darwin had published *On the Origin of Species* in 1859, it took a while for his ideas to catch on. By the 1880s, educated Americans spoke of heredity, breeding, and other concepts related to Darwinism; later, these ideas fed the American eugenics movement and, much later, cancer knowledge. *Popular Science* magazine provided subscribers with updates in chemistry, engineering, and biology. Thinking based in empiricism—that cancer was rooted in abnormal growth of cells, and not some sort of punishment for misbehavior or consequence of divine will—paved the way for research and effective treatments. Confidence in science bolstered enthusiasm for building specialized cancer institutions where experts could perform investigations and provide better care.

The need for a cancer hospital was becoming evident. As fewer people died from infections in childhood, more lived long enough to develop malignancy. Cases numbers were rising. As reported in the April 1883 *New York Herald*, "The percentage of deaths caused by cancer, it is said, has trebled in the last twelve years. During that time no less than 5,405 persons have died from it in this city alone."[1]

In late 1884, General Ulysses S. Grant learned he had incurable cancer. At age sixty-two, the former U.S. president and Civil War hero felt a lump in his throat and winced from pain upon eating. He was broke, and delayed consultation. Eventually Dr. John H. Douglas, a Manhattan throat specialist, used a small mirror to identify a mass at the base of Grant's tongue and cancerous spots on the palate. Douglas submitted a biopsy to Dr. George F. Shrady, a cancer maven, for pathological examination. Shrady told Douglas the cancer diagnosis was clear: "General Grant is doomed," he said.[43–46]

Although doctors cloaked Grant's diagnosis in medical jargon, the general understood his illness to be malignant and fatal. Douglas told him of an "epithelial" condition; his problem had a "cancerous tendency." Grant's wife was unwilling to believe the ailment was incurable. The general accepted treatments, mainly palliative, for nine months. He gargled herbal elixirs and "cocaine water" to soothe his mouth pain, besides taking brandy and morphine.

Grant soon became the world's most famous cancer patient. Journalists paced by his East Sixty-Sixth Street home, trying to glimpse the goings-on. Editors spared no words. The *New York Times* ran this headline in March 1885: "Sinking Into the Grave. Gen. Grant's Friends Give Up Hope." Weeks before he died, Grant traveled to a friend's cottage in upstate New York. Curious onlookers surrounded the place. Reporters took photographs. Some had the audacity to enter and converse with the stricken general. "They will talk me to death," Grant said.[46–49]

Grant penned an autobiography (figure 1.3). Securing income for his family— and regaining a favorable public reputation before death—motivated this final endeavor. He scribbled obsessively, composing as many as ten thousand words a day, according to his friend Mark Twain, who stayed with Grant at times during the illness. Anxious to finish the manuscript before dying, he worked through pain. Near the end, he resorted to dictation. Grant completed the two-volume project days before his death in July 1885. The *Personal Memoirs of U.S. Grant* sold over three hundred thousand copies, earning nearly a half-million dollars for his family.[50]

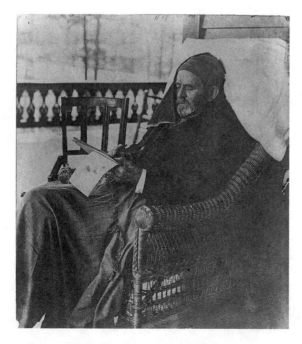

1.3 General Ulysses S. Grant writing his memoirs, Mount McGregor, NY, June 27, 1885 (Library of Congress)

It's hard to say to what extent having cancer elevated Grant's platform as an author. Shortly before his death, Grant wrote a letter to his son in which he reflected on what sympathy he'd received:

My ~~supposed~~ [sic] expected death called forth expressions of the sincerest kindness from all the people of all sections of the country. The Confederate soldier vied with the Union soldier in sounding my praise. The protestant, the Catholic and the Jew appointed days for universal prayer in my behalf. . . . It looks as if my sickness had had something to do to bring about harmony between the sections.

As told in this rare firsthand account, Grant's cancer brought people together; it unified Americans.[51]

Grant's case contributed a sense of urgency to establishing cancer hospitals in America. The New-York Skin and Cancer Hospital embraced research as an aim from its start. The founding president, G. Hilton Scribner, wrote that the hospital would investigate "the disease, its causes and cure, in every possible manner." It welcomed cancer patients from other U.S. regions and particularly sought those with early-stage disease for admission, a strategy that bears on modern debates about the benefits of early detection. With "greater publicity given to the subject of cancer, a very much larger proportion of cases than now will come in the early stages of the disease, at which time alone science can, at the present day, afford a reasonable hope of cure," Scribner wrote.

To encourage investigations, Scribner requested contributions for a cash award to anyone introducing a cure for "well authenticated" cases. Mrs. Esther Herrman, a Jewish immigrant who led the philanthropy committee of Sorosis, a professional women's club, gave repeatedly from 1884 until she died in 1911, but the prize lay untouched. The Skin and Cancer Hospital acknowledged her legacy as late as 1918, when it reported $3,023.90 in the fund for a cancer cure "accumulated through the efforts and contributions of Mrs. Esther Herrman."[42,52,53]

Surgeons, pathologists, and other doctors at the Skin and Cancer Hospital provided services without charge. "Hopeless" patients, however, were not welcome. Severe cases were rejected for admission. Consensus held that patients with advanced cancer should be kept apart, for their sake as well as for those who might be cured. The hospital's first annual report addressed disappointment of patients with tumors deemed incurable who were denied entry: "Some were in such a condition that to place them in the small wards of such a building as is now used would be to pollute the atmosphere to such a degree that the other beds could not be occupied," it stated. "To fill up the comparatively few beds with hopeless, chronic, distressing, and offensive cases would, in the end, be to wrong a very much larger number of individuals who could with some certainty receive benefit."

The hospital's 1884 message—separating curable from incurable patients—anticipated current rifts among cancer charities and advocates. For instance, some people with metastatic cancer today say they're overlooked and even shunned at brightly themed events and survivorship programs. Debates arise over priorities—whether to fund studies of preventing cancer, improve treatment of early-stage forms, or develop remedies for advanced cases. Philanthropists—and insurers, perhaps—question if they can afford to help all affected.

The *kirmess* at Delmonico's raked in over $7,000, netting $3,297 above expenses for the New-York Skin and Cancer Hospital. Already that institution's leadership was seeking funds for a country pavilion to house "incurables." To raise more money in 1884, the Ladies' Auxiliary moved the event to a bigger place: the new Metropolitan Opera House, an ornate Broadway building with three thousand seats.

In May 1884, the *New York Herald* reported, "The Metropolitan Opera House was never too small till yesterday, when the revised edition of the Kirmess established itself within the vast enclosure and New York out-Hollanded Holland." Inside the colossal music hall, a kaleidoscopic spectrum of flags and botanical greens dazzled entrants. "Good looking American girls dressed in the national costumes of Turkey, Spain, Sweden, France," and other countries "mingled" with patrons amid a "picnic of many nations." At one booth decorated with a star and crescent, Mrs. H. A. W. Post and her assistants dispensed "Turkish tobacco, candy and rugs." Mary Irvin took charge of an area designated "America," where, among other amusements, "live canaries sang songs to a frisky monkey." The outlandish affair generated $7,000 for the hospital.[54-56]

In a nineteenth-century prelude to extreme cancer fundraising, which we'll examine in later chapters, philanthropic *kirmesses* became fashionable and spread to other places and causes. From 1883 to 1887, charity *kirmesses* took place in New Haven, Cleveland, Chicago, and elsewhere.[57-59]

In New York, the Ladies' Auxiliary tweaked the theme each year, delivering thousands of dollars for the Skin and Cancer Hospital. They *had fun* with it. In 1886 they held the *kirmess* out-of-doors "in true Dutch style" over two days in a Manhattan lot outfitted with a giant maypole and "farmyard" replete with a donkey, a goat wagon, a prize-winning cow, and roosters "with pedigrees longer than their tail feathers." Children attending were amused by a merry-go-round, Punch and Judy (puppetry) show, and soda-water fountain. *Kirmess*-goers were shielded from sun or rain by large awnings while they shopped for imported Dutch ceramics, flowers, and novelties. A *café chantant* added European flair to the occasion. The temporary hut enclosed a stage and space for participants' sitting, drinking, and mirth. Privacy and security concerned the partying philanthropists. For this outdoor *kirmess*, the ladies ordered construction of a thick fence. And reassured ticket-buyers, "Nothing can be seen from the surrounding streets, and electric lights will make things brilliant in the evening."[60-65]

At a superficial level, the *kirmesses* broached the subject of cancer. But there was no pretense of education at these festivals, as happens at contemporary awareness events. The ladies didn't distribute information about malignancy. They didn't include cancer patients, but how could they have? Few survived. Then, as today, cancer fundraisers adopted a strategy of mood inversion; the women cloaked the topic in pleasantries. Their goal was plainly to raise money for the hospital to provide care, including experimental care.

Journalists didn't fail to pick up on the paradoxical aspect of celebrating for a cancer-related cause. Headlines like "In the Cause of Charity" hint of Gilded Age snark. After the first *kirmess*, the *New York Herald* reported,

> This festival has a two-fold aspect. On the one hand, as a work of charity it suggests scenes of anguish and misfortune, wherein the needy groan in neglect under the affliction of the most terrible forms of disease. On the other hand, the Kirmess demands consideration as an entertainment, a matter of pleasure. . . . But the two views overlap and blend into each other, for the anguish of the former is softened in the light of a coming alleviation, while the beauty

and the joy of the second gain a freshness and a zest from the noble motive that animates them.

A *Boston Herald* correspondent, "Miss Lookabout," had a similar take: "Nobody could have the heart, however, to condemn the kirmess . . . although it was an imitation of a Dutch village fair, and was in effect a glorification of Knickerbockerism. The good interest served was a deserving charity, and that fact covered all of the vanity incidental to the occasion."[7,54,66]

Back indoors at the Metropolitan Opera House in 1887, the ladies went all out. An elaborate calendar theme featured booths for each month. "January" contained a full-size cotton snowman and a model toboggan. By donating a few cents, a child could send the sled, loaded with winter-clad dolls, down a slide. "April" presented a spectrum of umbrellas, parasols, and walking canes. "August," with its yacht, mast, and semaphore flags signaling "danger" to those in-the-know, was a highlight for many visitors; there, women in sailing outfits sold cigars and lottery tickets for toy boats. The October booth offered equipment for sports like tennis, besides fishing and hunting gear including guns and pistols. December's station displayed a chimneyed house, Santa Claus, and "every toy that could charm and delight a child's heart."[67–69]

The final *kirmess* for the New-York Skin and Cancer Hospital was marred by the death of Mrs. Daniel T. (Annie) Worden a few weeks after the big event. Annie, whose husband belonged to the New York Stock Exchange, was only thirty-eight when she died.[70,71] In prior *kirmesses*, she'd supervised the all-important Dutch station. In 1887, she took charge of "June," where flowers were sold.

In June 1887, the Springfield, Massachusetts, *Republican* published these cautionary words:

> On Monday died one of the most beautiful and interesting women of the city, Anna Augusta Worden, wife of Daniel T. Worden. . . . Mrs. Worden had been for several years secretary for the managers of the skin and cancer hospital, and overexertion at the recent kirmess in the Metropolitan opera-house was the cause of her death.

The festivals came to a halt. But thanks to the efforts of Ellin Lowery, Annie Worden, and others, the New-York Skin and Cancer Hospital opened a branch in Fordham Heights, near the city's northern edge.[72] Despite sugarcoating the cause at hand—or perhaps as a consequence of its sugarcoating—crucial money was raised to advance cancer research and treatment.

Elizabeth Cullum, Hamilton's granddaughter, had neither time nor inclination to participate in *kirmess* fundraisers. At fifty-two, she was suffering from cancer of the womb.[73] In February 1884, she invited a group of acquaintances to her home to discuss the pressing need for a cancer hospital in New York. Elizabeth's cousin, Mrs. John Jacob (Charlotte Augusta Gibbes) Astor III, attended, along with other Woman's Hospital board members who objected to its "no cancer" policy. Recently Charlotte's husband, John Jacob Astor III, had offered $185,000 to the Woman's Hospital to build a separate wing for cancer patients, but his enormous offer had been declined.[23,74]

Elizabeth, often described as a charitable and Christian woman, enjoyed a life of leisure. She lived with her husband on Fifth Avenue, summered in Newport, Rhode Island, and socialized with New York's elite. Elizabeth founded a literary society, the *Causeries du Lundi*, attended by women of prominent families—her sister, Mrs. (Maria Eliza Hamilton) Peabody, Mrs. Parsons, Mrs. Drexel, and others. The "Monday chats" provided an acceptable way for adult women to meet and learn. In salons, the ladies took turns presenting papers on topics such as ancient art, music, and architecture, with occasional digressions into plant biology.[75,76]

Establishing a cancer hospital in New York became Elizabeth's end-of-life mission. For this cause, she donated a plot of land she'd inherited from her mother, Maria Eliza Van den Heuvel Hamilton, in the Bloomingdale section of Manhattan. Old maps and photographs from around that time depict the hospital site on Eighth Avenue (now Central Park West), between 105th and 106th Streets, in a desolate area with scattered shacks near an orphanage and a brewery, not far from an insane asylum. The group hired an architect, Charles C. Haight, who designed a chateaulike structure with rounded stone walls to deter accumulation of germs and windows in each room for ventilation (figure 1.4).[74,77–79]

In May 1884, weak with illness, Elizabeth joined in laying the institution's cornerstone.[77] She did not live to see the hospital erected, however. She died that September at age fifty-five. Obituaries stated that she had suffered from cancer.[80,81] How exceptional was her frankness, in an era about which it's said people were secretive about the disease, and if Elizabeth explicitly wished to reveal her condition, are unknown.

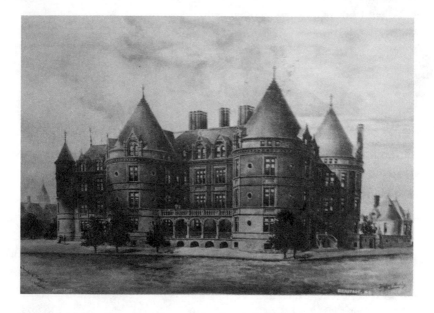

1.4 The New York Cancer Hospital opened in 1887 on Eighth Avenue between 105th and 106th Streets. This 1885 rendering appeared in the First Annual Report of the New York Cancer Hospital.

Scan, courtesy of the Patricia D. Klingenstein Library, New-York Historical Society

When the New York Cancer Hospital finally opened in December 1887, its Astor Pavilion for women contained seventy beds. The first admitted patient, a Romanian "houseworker" with nine children, was discharged after surgery. Around half of the patients received care for free. Many were European emigrants. The most common diagnosis was uterine cancer. Among its prominent staff were Grant's surgeon, Dr. George Shrady, and Dr. Clement Cleveland, who in 1913 would found the first nationwide cancer society.[82–84]

In the summer of 1890, Ellin Lowery's husband died unexpectedly. In the twenty years before his death, she had developed an eclectic group of friends with whom she volunteered her time and talents. This was not unusual. Decades before they could vote, forward-thinking ladies stepped out of their homes to address domestic concerns like sanitation, parks, health, and education. After the financial crisis of 1893, Ellin's fortunes wavered. Needing money, she and a longtime friend, Miss Margaret Wilmerding, opened a tearoom on Fifth Avenue. Their dainty establishment yielded some income, newspaper reviews, and gossip about their circumstances. In 1897 she married James Speyer, a Jewish banker twelve years younger than she.[85,86]

Upon her engagement, the *New York Times* suggested the wedding would help charitable causes Ellin espoused: "Through her marriage with Mr. Speyer she will assume a position at the head of a wealthy household which will enable her to largely increase her sphere of usefulness."[87] As Mrs. Speyer, Ellin continued her charity efforts non-stop. Among her accomplishments, she established a league for the prevention of cruelty to animals, cofounded what became Teachers College at Columbia University, and helped start the cancer society. For years she led the Irene Club, an organization providing social and educational programs for "working girls"—employed, single women living in cities apart from their families. Her dedication was such that upon her taking ill in 1919, Irene Club members gave Ellin a "loving cup," filled with roses, to honor their benefactress.

When Ellin died in 1921, the *Times* ran a full obituary emphasizing her philanthropy. Through her volunteerism, she'd earned respect of many.[34,88]

In the summer of 1893, a time of economic duress, President Grover Cleveland had a malignant tumor removed in a covert operation. The surgery took place on a yacht in Long Island Sound. Doctors removed a sarcoma, several teeth, and part of the president's upper jaw. The boat departed from New York's Battery Park and arrived, days later, at Gray Gables, Cleveland's place on Buzzards Bay in Cape Cod. When the president arrived in Massachusetts, he was said to be taking a vacation. Although word of Cleveland's surgery appeared in a few newspapers, his staff refuted the account. The president had had a toothache for which teeth and bone were removed, officials stated.[89–92]

Cleveland's story highlights the perceived need for keeping cancer a secret, particularly for a political leader. Yet Cleveland's apparent cure indicates progress. In 1917, years after he died from another cause, one of his doctors, Dr. William Keen, wrote to Cleveland's widow for permission to publish details. She consented. After a twenty-five-year delay, Keen reported on the successful treatment of the president's malignant sarcoma.[93]

The New York Cancer Hospital's imposing towers and, presumably, screams and deaths within, led to its nickname, "The Bastille." Contributions dwindled; the institution failed to attract enough paying patients. A published list of gifts to the hospital reveals a hodgepodge of items resembling a thrift shop's inventory: books, a paperweight, plants, a footstool. People donated fruit, ice cream, and bundles of religious papers. Mrs. D. W. Bishop paid for "Central Park Drives" for patients weekly in summer.[78] Boarding charges for "ward" patients were $7 per week, $15 for patients occupying double private rooms, or $20 for private rooms. The hospital ran a deficit. The men's building did not open until 1898, for lack of funds.[79,84,94,95]

In 1899, the New York Cancer Hospital neared bankruptcy. To encourage entry of patients with nonmalignant conditions who might pay for treatments, the institution's board changed its name to "General Memorial Hospital for the Treatment of Cancer and Allied Diseases." Three years later, a gift from Mrs. Collis P. Huntington, wife of the railroad tycoon, would help the hospital to survive. Four decades later, the hospital moved to Manhattan's east side and, eventually, became Memorial Sloan Kettering Cancer Center.[96]

A few specialized cancer institutions arose elsewhere. In 1898, *Buffalo Evening News* publisher Edward Butler used his editorial influence and political connections to persuade the state legislature to fund a cancer laboratory at the University at Buffalo (later, Roswell Park Cancer Institute). In Massachusetts, a gift of $100,000 from the estate of Caroline Abigail Brewer Croft to Harvard University resulted in a Harvard commission for research into cancer cures. After the Johns Hopkins Hospital opened in 1889 in Baltimore, it emerged as a leading center for cancer surgery. But Hopkins remained a general hospital. In the decade ahead, Philadelphia's American Oncologic Hospital and St. Louis's Barnard Free Skin and Cancer Hospital would open.[11,97,98]

Meanwhile, hospitals advertising fraudulent remedies proliferated. Legitimate oncology care was not yet lucrative, and few affected patients sought cancer treatment.

CHAPTER 2

CANCER'S SPRING (1900–1920)

"Rich Women Begin a War on Cancer," announced the *New York Times* on April 23, 1913. A group of concerned women, businessmen, and philanthropists had met at the New York residence of Dr. Clement Cleveland, a gynecologist. The ladies were a powerful bunch: Mrs. Frederick W. Vanderbilt enjoyed unusual wealth. Mrs. E. R. Hewitt, a university graduate, belonged to a prominent New York family and headed the Woman's Municipal League. Mrs. James (Ellin) Speyer, a banker's wife, knew all about fundraising; she'd helped found the New-York Skin and Cancer Hospital and served as treasurer for several health charities.[1]

Together with physicians at the gathering, the socialites heard from cancer experts. They listened to Frederick L. Hoffman, a leading statistician employed by the Prudential Life Insurance Company, who spoke of climbing cancer death rates. Dr. Livingston Farrand, who led efforts against tuberculosis, gave tips on public health campaigns. Dr. Le Roy Broun, chair of the American Gynecological Society's lay education committee, explained how and why his organization sought to inform women about malignancy.

What drove the Progressive Era ladies, bankers, and doctors to the meeting was an emerging confidence—or naive optimism—that cancer could be controlled. In their lifetimes, they'd witnessed how knowledge of germs had reduced the toll of infectious scourges like cholera and typhoid. They considered that malignancies could be tackled by education, too. At the time, cancer patients with symptoms rarely came to medical attention until after the disease had spread—when surgery, if feasible, would be unlikely to help. The experts believed that tumors could be cured if caught early. Yet most people, including doctors, deemed cancer hopeless.

They formed the first nationwide U.S. cancer charity, the American Society for the Control of Cancer (ASCC). The society's goal was, first, to counter ignorance about cancer. To achieve its mission, the organization sponsored lectures, distributed bulletins, and invited journalists to write about malignancy. The ASCC founders believed that cancer's ravaging effects could be ameliorated by rendering the disease familiar. They involved women, who helped spread the word, raise money, and distribute "propaganda"—informational pamphlets, flyers, and posters—on cancer symptoms and treatments.

Through World War II, the ASCC worked almost singularly, through a network of regional chapters and women's clubs, to change public opinion about cancer and its curability. Three decades later, this organization would become the American Cancer Society. The ASCC delivered cancer as a subject of conversation—a matter of health, about which the facts should be plainly discussed—into the public domain.

At the start of the twentieth century, a malignant diagnosis portended doom. Physicians knew little about cancer, and what they observed was grim. Surgery was the only established remedy, but results were dismal: 90 percent of cancer patients died within three years. People feared "the knife." Cancer specialists, mainly surgeons in large cities east of the Mississippi, were scarce. Many afflicted fell prey to hucksters selling painless salves and bogus "cures." Myths and stigma prevailed.[2–4]

A few purported nonsurgical remedies gained traction. John Beard, an embryologist at the University of Edinburgh, published a book on the power of digestive enzymes, purified from animal pancreases, to shrink tumors. Hype over Beard's "trypsin treatment," as it became known, led physicians to denounce his claims as false. Elsewhere, doctors reported beneficial effects of inoculating patients with infectious germs like *Streptococcus* bacteria and even malaria. Yet expert consensus held against nonoperative cancer treatments.[5–7]

In a telling episode, a Massachusetts man opted to have frogs applied to his neck to treat a recurrent malignancy. Reports of the "frog cure" spread rapidly. The *New York Times* ran this headline: "Frogs Fail to Cure Cancer: Animals Were

Applied to Patient's Neck, but He Is Dead Now." The paper took the unusual step of naming the patient, William L. Davis, a druggist who died in July 1908. That a man of means and, by his profession, knowledge of pharmaceuticals, chose such a strange and unlikely remedy reflected patients' overwhelming desperation.[8]

Cancer research was in its infancy. Physicians had only an inkling about the origin of a few cancer types and plenty of false notions. Some thought cancer might be caused by a parasite. Others connected tumors with sexually trans-mitted diseases. Doctors wrote that cancers arise at sites of persistent irritation. They knew, for example, that lip cancer was more frequent in men who smoked pipes. Physicians recognized that chimney sweeps were prone to bladder cancer, but they weren't sure why. They described tumors that cropped up on the bel-lies of people in Kurdistan and Tibet. In medical journals, they attributed those exotic malignancies to the regional custom of strapping hot coals to the torso for warmth while traversing cold mountain passes.[9–14]

One of the more peculiar theories surfaced in upstate New York, where sci-entists implicated diseased fish in human cancers. Dr. Harvey R. Gaylord, of the New York State Institute for the Study of Malignant Disease in Buffalo, noted a spike in thyroid tumors in trout of nearby rivers. Gaylord superimposed maps of cancerous fish and people. As those revealed similar patterns, he speculated that river trout might somehow transmit cancer to humans, perhaps by people consuming diseased fish. Alarmed by Gaylord's report, in 1910 President William Howard Taft requested that Congress appropriate $50,000 for animal research into cancer's causes. At the time, Buffalo was a hub of industry. Rochester, another upstate city, housed the young Eastman Kodak Company on banks of the Genesee River. But Gaylord didn't mention the possibility that pollutants in water might cause malignancy. Few physicians linked industrial chemicals with illness. People did worry about contracting cancer by eating diseased fish or being near afflicted people. Such fears contributed to cancer stigma.[15–19]

Newspapers reported rising case numbers. Then as now, doctors debated statistics, questioning if the upward rate stemmed from more cancer diagnoses rather than a true spike in disease. People worried that cancer might be conta-gious. Many considered that it could be inherited. A malignant diagnosis could compromise marriage prospects for someone with an affected parent or sibling. Unlike infections, against which wealth and better living conditions appeared protective, there was no prophylaxis for malignancy, no apparent way to reduce one's odds of getting it. Cancer affected rich and poor. Experts wrote that cancer takes its victims at random. In the words of journalist Burton J. Hendrick, writing for *McClure's Magazine* in July 1909, "It is the anarchist of the body."[20–22]

Dr. Cleveland arranged for the preliminary meeting of the nascent cancer organization in his Park Avenue home. The backdrop was wealth. In 1913, he lived in a palazzo-styled building with high-ceilinged duplex and triplex apartments. Cleveland's daughter, Mrs. Robert (Elizabeth) Mead, attended and soon assumed a central role in fundraising.[23,24]

Then thirty-six, Elizabeth (Elsie) Mead had enjoyed lifelong privileges. As a child, she'd swum and played tennis with some of America's richest children in Newport, Rhode Island, where the Cleveland family summered and her father maintained a seasonal practice. Elsie's elaborate 1898 wedding, detailed in newspapers, involved flower girls, ten bridesmaids, and ten ushers. The couple had a daughter, Theodora. Over thirty years, Elsie's personal connections—Madame Curie, John D. Rockefeller Jr., and many of her "ordinary" neighbors who volunteered and gave to the society—would benefit the ASCC and later the New York City Cancer Committee (NYC Cancer Committee), which she steered.[25–27]

Clement Cleveland led a comfortable life, yet he worked hard. During the Civil War, he'd left his Baltimore home for boarding school in New Hampshire. After attending Harvard College, he moved to New York and, in 1871, received a medical degree from Columbia University's College of Physicians and Surgeons. Cleveland interned at Charity Hospital on Blackwell's Island (now Roosevelt Island) in New York, a rough place housing people deemed insane and the poorest with illness. Soon he earned staff positions at private institutions including the Woman's Hospital. Cleveland joined the New York Cancer Hospital as one of few surgeons on staff when it opened in 1887.[23,28,29]

From Cleveland's publications, it's evident he took a hands-on approach to treating cancer. He reported on palliative care of women with uterine (womb) tumors. His 1889 paper, based on his experiences at the New York Cancer Hospital, reveals deep expertise. He detailed surgical instruments and gave advice about how to manage bleeding, wounds, odors, and pain. Opium is the "only reliable remedy" for pain, he wrote. Presciently, he cautioned practitioners about the narcotic's potential: "Its use should be deferred and should be as sparing as possible." For advanced cancer, Cleveland advised palliative care that might be considered holistic, attending to patients' general condition, nutrition, and bowel movements. "Beef-juice, beef-tea, and milk make the best form of diet," he specified. "Healthful surroundings are a necessity. Fresh air, and an abundance of it, is also of the greatest importance."[30]

Like other physicians of his time, Cleveland kept a private practice while volunteering at hospitals where he operated on destitute patients. An 1894 sketch in the *New York Journal of Gynaecology and Obstetrics* refers to Cleveland having "an immense and distinctly fashionable *clientèle*." His motives for working at the cancer hospital can't be known and were likely complex. Many doctors considered it their Christian or moral duty to provide care to the poor. In addition, non-paying patients provided bodies and illnesses for doctors to learn and teach, often without consent.

Cleveland bridged two worlds. His work with cancer patients served as a counterpoint to his rich social life. After performing a long cancer operation, he might have stopped by the University Club, Century Association, or Harvard Club and chatted up the "cancer menace." His professional and personal associations—and his daughter Elsie's enthusiasm for the cause—favored the ASCC's future success.

As reported in the *Boston Medical and Surgical Journal*, the National Anti-Cancer Association was formally organized at the Harvard Club in New York on May 22, 1913. Experts came from as far as Chicago, Denver, and New Orleans to join. Besides physicians, leaders included George C. Clark, a prominent banker, Thomas W. Lamont, a partner at J. P. Morgan, and V. Everit Macy, a philanthropist. James Speyer of New York, whose wife, Ellin, was involved with health causes and women's organizations, led a "laymen's committee." In June, the nascent organization was renamed the ASCC.[24,31,32]

Doctors involved with the ASCC perceived that the outlook for cancer patients was brightening. But they represented a well-traveled and educated minority of U.S. physicians. These men read and believed reports from Germany that women with tumors of the uterus were living longer. European doctors attributed this favorable survival trend to an educational campaign informing women of cancer's signs and symptoms. They described a spiraling positive effect: as women sought care for minor cervical bleeding, surgeons learned to recognize smaller tumors and adjusted their methods to remove tiny abnormalities with fewer complications and better results. The American group aimed to extend those results in the United States.

The ASCC did not explicitly state the aim of helping white, upper- and middle-class citizens, but that was clearly the demographic group its leaders had in mind. As we will see, at least until the 1960s, most anticancer and early detection campaigns were directed to affluent white Americans. The ASCC founders built on programs conceived by like-minded physicians in several U.S. cities.

In Baltimore, Dr. Thomas S. Cullen had been tallying outcomes of women with gynecological tumors at the Johns Hopkins Hospital. Only 27 percent of women survived five years after uterine cancer surgery, he observed. This figure unsettled Cullen, not because it was so low, but because it was too high! He realized that this bleak statistic didn't include the hardest cases: women with cancer who entered the clinic too late, when surgery was futile or impossible. Cullen became convinced that if women were cautioned about cancer's early signs and symptoms and understood that surgery could be curative, they'd seek care readily and be more likely to survive.[33,34]

When the American Gynecological Society met in Baltimore in May 1912, the gynecological surgeons discussed the need to educate women about cancer's curability so that they would seek prompt attention upon noticing symptoms. Cervical and uterine cancers were then leading malignant killers. "These extremely advanced cases, no matter what you do for them, die . . . or, at any rate, they wish they could die. I believe, as has been said here, the only hope lies in education of the laity and early removal of the disease," said Dr. Seth C. Gordon of Maine. "There is no question in my mind but that we can cure cancer of the uterus, the same as we can cure cancer of the lip."

Dr. Frederick J. Taussig of St. Louis piped up during the Baltimore session. He told of an ongoing cancer educational program in Missouri. Doctors affiliated with his institution, the Barnard Skin and Cancer Hospital, were giving talks to medical societies in nearby counties, Taussig said. But it wasn't only doctors spreading the word. In St. Louis, nurses were handing out information to women. "Concerning uterine cancer I have had printed a small leaflet which is so worded that it can be safely distributed," he said. "The visiting nurses particularly are distributing among the women of the city literature concerning tuberculosis, and, at the same time, leaflets concerning cancer may be distributed with propriety."[35,36]

The gynecologists agreed it was sensible to educate women about malignancy. But they didn't agree on the best approach. The specialists—all men—formed a committee to address how best to instruct women about cancer. Cullen sought a coast-to-coast informational campaign: "There is absolutely no reason why the majority of the women in the United States should not be made aware of the dangers of allowing cancer to advance to the inoperable stage." Publishing carefully written and well-illustrated lay articles, without "creating alarm," would do more good than giving medical lectures, Cullen said, noting: "We have in this country weekly magazines that have tremendous circulations, magazines whose editors are aiming to do all they can for the welfare of the country."

General surgeons took up the subject of cancer education. "The public was anxious to know the truth about cancer, and the profession had reached the conclusion that unless the public knew the truth progress in the cure of cancer would continue to be slow, as it has been in the past," said Dr. Joseph C. Bloodgood of Johns Hopkins before the Medical Society of the Missouri Valley at a cancer symposium in Kansas City, in March 1913. "The truth must be presented to the people in such a way that it will not create fear but confidence." Bloodgood was concerned not only with countering the public's fear and fatalism about cancer; he realized the need to persuade his colleagues of cancer's curability: "In the control of cancer . . . we shall have to combat this skepticism both in the ranks of the profession and among the people," he wrote in the *Journal of the American Medical Association (JAMA)*. "We have the evidence that cancer can be cured and we must bring it before the profession and the public in such a way that they will believe it."[37,38]

Meanwhile Cullen had written an article on cancer intended for a lay audience and submitted it to the *Ladies' Home Journal*. The managing editor, Karl Harriman, said it was "too damn clear." If published, "half our women readers would grab their hats and rush for the closest doctor," Harriman told him. But he and Edward Bok, the *Journal*'s editor-in-chief, were keen on the idea of running a feature on cancer. They told Cullen that he should ask a journalist to write the story, so that the subject would be rendered palatable to their readers.

Cullen arranged to meet a popular writer, Samuel Hopkins Adams. After Adams penned a 1905–06 series for *Collier's Weekly* exposing fraudulent advertisements for patent medicines, physicians trusted him. Over dinner in Baltimore, Cullen persuaded Adams of the importance of educating people about cancer.[3,33,39]

In May 1913, the gynecologists' efforts came to fruition with publication of "What Can We Do About Cancer?" in the May 1913 *Ladies' Home Journal*. At a time when many people relied on newspapers and circulars for health information, the influential magazine had over two million subscribers. The *Journal* then covered treatments for a range of maladies, interspersing medical advice with recipes and homemaking columns. It touched on mental health with stories on anxiety and depression. But the *Journal* had not previously published a feature on cancer, a subject considered distasteful.

Adams's article—visually softened by a lattice floral border framing the first page—guided readers in plain language and blunt terms. Cancer is increasingly common, he wrote. "Latest comprehensive reports from England show that out of every eight women who attain the age of thirty-five years, one is slain by it; one out of every eleven men." While there is no agreement on its cause, and limited consensus about cancer treatment, as to what the public might do about it, doctors are unanimous, he wrote: "Educate the people to save themselves" (figure 2.1).

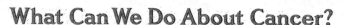

What Can We Do About Cancer?

The Most Vital and Insistent Question in the Medical World

By Samuel Hopkins Adams

AUTHOR OF "THE GREAT AMERICAN FRAUD," ETC.

WHAT is to be done about cancer? No other question is so insistently demanding of medical science a definite reply. For some unascertained reason this dreaded scourge seems to be increasing in a startling ratio. A generation ago it was far down the list among the causes of death, not higher than tenth or twelfth. Today it ranks fifth or sixth: in some localities even as high as third, being exceeded in its number of victims only by tuberculosis and pneumonia. Latest comprehensive reports from England show that out of every eight women who attain the age of thirty-five years, one is slain by it; one out of every eleven men. In the year 1908 forty thousand Americans are known to have succumbed to it. General figures for the years since are not yet available, but local figures almost without exception indicate a startling growth. The next census may well show an appalling increase.

Notwithstanding this threatening condition no general movement has been, until recently, organized against the spread of the malady. Science has been face to face with a blank wall. Frankly and sadly it admits its fundamental ignorance.

Some fifteen years since I interviewed a number of physicians and surgeons on the question, "What causes cancer?" I received a wide variety of brilliant and conclusive answers, all of them wrong. In this year of enlightenment, 1913, I put the same query to a tableful of specialists, each with a nation-wide reputation. One after another they made the same reply: "I do not know." Yet when, from the science of the closing Nineteenth Century, the responses had been assured and direct I got no satisfactory reply to the logically sequent question: "What is to be done about it?". But from the science of 1913, grown in wisdom to the point of recognizing its own limitations, the answer to the second query came, sharp, positive and unanimous: "Educate the people to save themselves."

Medicines are Useless: Delay in Operating Is Deadly

TO SAVE themselves from an uncomprehended peril? At first thought any education from those who are themselves ignorant of the fundamentals of the disease would seem absurd. "How," says the layman, "can

---

AN AUTHORITATIVE INDORSEMENT OF THIS ARTICLE

I HAVE read Mr. Adams's article on "What Can We Do About Cancer?" with the greatest interest. It gives in a most readable form the essence of our present knowledge on this subject. Surgeons are heartsick to see the many cancer patients begging for operations when the disease is so far advanced that nothing can be done.

Cancer is in the beginning a local process and not a blood disease, and in its early stages can be completely removed. When the cancer is small the surgeon can, with one-fourth the amount of labor, accomplish ten times the amount of good.

If the many readers of THE LADIES' HOME JOURNAL will profit by the advice given by Mr. Adams this article will be the means of saving thousands of lives.

THOMAS S. CULLEN, M.D.
Chairman of the Cancer Campaign Committee of the Congress of Surgeons of North America.

---

the mysteriously invading cell. It is known that no skin cancer ever develops except at a spot where there has been some previous and persistent irritation. There are curious proofs of this. Men who smoke clay pipes are peculiarly liable to cancer of the lip. This form is rare in women; where it occurs it usually develops that the woman is a smoker. Cancer of the tongue often arises from the slight chafing of a jagged tooth, the corollary to which is that a visit to the dentist may well be a life-saving move. In India the rough betel nut is carried all day in the hollow of the cheek by the natives. Cancer in India is most commonly found in the cheek; in Occidental countries it is almost unknown. Natives of Kurdistan, who go up into the cold mountain passes, wear a pan filled with live charcoal across the stomach. Among these people the prevalent location of cancer is on the skin of the abdomen, a spot practically exempt elsewhere in the world. "Chimney-sweep's cancer" is a well-recognized form. The sweep swings, while at his occupation, on a hard, narrow saddle, and the falling soot, trickling down his neck, irritates the skin at the point of pressure. Hence cancer of the groin is typical of the sooty brotherhood.

Any Irritation Should be Investigated at Once

BY ANALOGY it is inferred that internal cancers develop only after some prolonged irritation. Without this irritation they would not develop. Obviously, then, the warning is plain: Permit no irritation, internal or external, to be of long continuance. Better the appeal to surgery at once than the risk. Once the cancer develops the knife is inevitable and the chances are less favorable.

In the mind of the woman who, having developed cancer, faces the knife, this question inevitably and poignantly arises: "What chance have I?" The indirect but primarily logical answer is grim enough: "Other than the knife, no chance whatsoever." Cancer never relinquishes its hold. It never remains quiescent. No medicine cures it. Steadily and surely it saps out the life. The cancer must be eradicated or the case is hopeless.

"But it is hopeless anyway. Why suffer the added torture of surgery?" That is the cry of fatalism. For generations the scourge has destroyed

---

2.1 Start of cancer article by Samuel Hopkins Adams, approved by Dr. Thomas S. Cullen, in the May 1913 *Ladies' Home Journal*.

After surveying "a tableful of specialists, each with a nation-wide reputation," Adams offered "the best" medical advice and opinion. "No cancer is hopeless when discovered early," he wrote. "The only cure is the knife." Writing for the *Ladies' Home Journal*, Adams annotated this statement with an asterisk; the footnote mentions an exceptional effect of toxins in sarcoma, a rare malignancy, and reflects an uncommon attention to detail in news of cancer. Almost no specialists then believed that chemicals benefited cancer patients. "Medicines are worse than useless," he emphasized. "Delay is more than dangerous; it is deadly."

Adams implored readers to consider cancer in light of progress against tuberculosis, once deemed lethal: "Fatalism is as misplaced in cancer as it would be in tuberculosis. Yet only a generation or so ago the consumptive was regarded as doomed. Nobody now believes that consumption is sure death." He wrote this about stomach cancer: "Only a generation since this was generally regarded as inoperable; or, if operation were decided upon as a measure of desperation, it was only a means of alleviating pain and prolonging a forlorn life for a few months." And considered: "There are today plenty of men and women walking the streets, bending over their books or typewriters in offices, selling goods behind the counter or on the road, plowing a straight furrow or cooking a good farm dinner, with one-third of a stomach apiece."

His statements in the *Ladies' Home Journal* foreshadow modern debates on cancer treatments and statistics. For instance, in cases of "absolutely hopeless" stomach cancer at a leading hospital, "nearly a third of the 'doomed victims' who come to [the operating table] go forth, literally, as good as new," Adams reported. "A very considerable proportion of the subjects from which the figures are compiled come to the operating table in the late stages of the disease, when there is perhaps only one chance in a hundred." Nonetheless, some people with advanced stomach cancers chose surgery because the alternative was sure death. "If the surgeon were intent solely on showing favorable figures he could, by excluding the desperate cases, perhaps double his thirty per cent." Adams concluded, "To paraphrase a current word play, these are the figures which put the 'hope' in 'hopeless.'"

While many cancer facts of 1913 are now obsolete, the message of the *Ladies' Home Journal* article is surprisingly modern. Adams's piece is devoid of paternalism. He placed responsibility for health squarely with his readers. People ought to learn about cancer's early signs and take charge of their health, he pleaded. But he took the mantra of awareness and early detection to a point of harsh blame.

Consider the section on breast cancer: "Here the outlook is most encouraging," Adams wrote. "In the reasonably early stages—excluding those in which, through fear, stupidity or ignorance, the victim has let the malignant growth involve the whole breast—a good half of the afflicted are permanently cured." In other words, women were culpable for letting breast cancer grow beyond a certain stage. If women sought treatment promptly, their chances were excellent: "The ratio of cures is at least seventy-five per cent and not improbably ninety per cent," he wrote. "Waiting to see is what kills three fourths of the women who die of cancer."

Adams flagged alarmist language that could scare women. "There is a quack who advertises, in such newspapers as will accept his falsehoods: 'Any lump in a woman's breast is cancer.' This is absurd and vicious. Many such lumps are non-malignant growths," he explained. "It would be quite true, however, to say that any lump in a woman's breast is suspicious." He gave advice. A woman with a breast lump should be checked. "Immediately upon her discovery of it she should go to her physician. If he says 'We'll wait and see,' let her consult some other physician." He described how breast cancer surgery should be performed, "preferably at a well-equipped hospital."

He encouraged patients to seek expert care and get second opinions. In a parable-like section, "If Your Doctor Is Doubtful Get Another Doctor," Adams describes a friend whose wife was stricken with breast cancer. The surgeon favored a small operation, but her husband knew better; he had read about cancer and insisted that his wife undergo a full mastectomy. She did extremely well and remained "sound as a bell" years later. However, her unmarried younger sister was not so fortunate when she, too, developed breast cancer. The sibling didn't agree to radical excision of the breast and died "after cruel suffering." Adams told of another friend, a lawyer, whose wife had stomach cancer. Luckily, she had visited a young and open-minded physician with the courage to say, "I don't know." That doctor referred the woman to an experienced surgeon. An early-stage malignancy was found. "It was cut out and today she is as good as new."

Historians regard Adams as a muckraking journalist. Yet in reporting on cancer he cooperated with experts. The magazine printed the endorsement of "Thomas S. Cullen, M.D., Chairman of the Cancer Campaign Committee of the Congress of Surgeons of North America" at the article's top and center, like a stamp of approval. At its June 1913 meeting, the American Medical Association honored Adams with associate AMA membership, an unusual award for a writer.

The *Ladies' Home Journal* story marked the start of the first U.S. cancer aware-ness campaign. Adams published two related pieces: "The Saving Hope in Can-cer" in *Collier's* and "The New Hope in Cancer" in *McClure's Magazine*. Many newspapers printed excerpts. A year later, the articles were said to have reached between eight and ten million readers.[40–43]

Anticancer momentum was building. Although the awareness campaign didn't achieve mainstream popularity until much later, it gained traction before World War I and again during the interwar period. The ASCC involved a selective, small roster of specialists. Most doctors remained skeptical about public education. Many didn't believe that cancer was curable by surgery or by any other means.

In June 1913, physicians from around the United States gathered for the AMA's sixty-fourth annual meeting in Minneapolis. Dr. J. Henry Carstens, a public health maven, said this:

> We must talk cancer day in and day out. . . . I have been advocating for several
> years that we set aside one day in the year as cancer day; that all the newspa-
> pers write about cancer, that all the ministers preach about cancer and that
> all the lay press write and print "Cancer, cancer, cancer," so that the people
> will be aroused and the profession will be aroused and these cases will have
> early attention.

Prominent doctors heard Carstens speak. In the same AMA session at the Uni-versity of Minnesota's Institute of Anatomy, Dr. William J. Mayo of Roches-ter, Minnesota, presented a paper on stomach cancer. By then, William and his younger brother, Dr. Charles H. Mayo, were cementing reputations as outstand-ing surgeons; their family-run operation would become the Mayo Clinic.[44]

Carstens's perspective stemmed from practicing medicine in Detroit. Surgical advances were useless if patients couldn't be persuaded to seek prompt evaluation, he considered. Women were reluctant to seek care for early-stage, treatable prob-lems, especially when those involved reproductive organs. That's why he pleaded for more talk about cancer. Like Cullen, his contemporary in Baltimore, he empha-sized vigilance about cancer. Both doctors encouraged women to be assertive, insist on thorough evaluation, and not let practitioners dismiss their symptoms.[45]

At the AMA meeting, Carstens mentioned that he had proposed holding an educational "cancer day" in Detroit. But his idea had been rejected by local colleagues. Perhaps they didn't agree that a cancer informational campaign would be helpful. Before persuading the public about the benefits of early detection and surgery, the cancer specialists needed to convince their physician peers.

By early 1914, Elsie Mead had rented a Manhattan office space and hired a secretary for the ASCC. That February, she traveled to Pittsburgh for a public meeting about cancer at Soldiers' Memorial Hall sponsored by the ASCC, the Twentieth Century Club, and the Pittsburgh Academy of Medicine. It featured Hoffman, the Prudential statistician, who spoke on cancer's rising threat. Community leaders including Jewish, Catholic, and Presbyterian clergymen also spoke at the event. A photograph shows Mead in Pittsburgh sitting with "Dr." Frederick Hoffman and Rabbi J. Leonard Levy, among others (figure 2.2).[46]

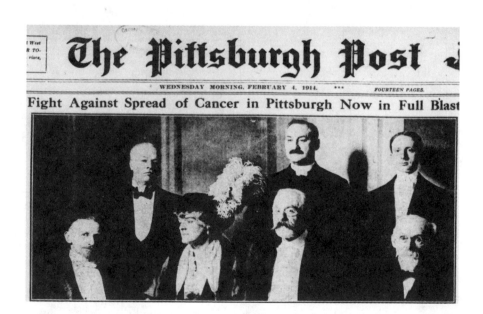

2.2 Elsie Mead and other ASCC leaders in Pittsburgh for public meetings on cancer, *Pittsburgh Post*, February 4, 1914.

Left to right, seated: "Dr." Frederick Hoffman, Elsie Mead, Dr. Edward Reynolds, Dr. John A. Brashear; standing: Edward Woods, Rabbi J. Leonard Levy, Curtis E. Lakeman

In New York City, the ASCC sponsored a series of three public programs on cancer including a March 1914 meeting at the women's Cosmopolitan Club. As reported in the *New York Times*, the meeting at the women's club—moderated by Mrs. Richard Aldrich, featuring Dr. James Ewing, a Cornell professor of pathology, and Hoffman—got heated. "Experts Disagree on Treating Cancer: Dr. Ewing Upholds Radium as a Cure, but Thinks an Overdose Killed Bremner," the *Times* headlined. Weeks before the Cosmopolitan Club event, U.S. Representative Robert G. Bremner of New Jersey had died at age thirty-nine after receiving radium treatments for cancer. The congressman's case had gained national attention, so much so that Henry Phipps Jr., the multimillionaire of Pittsburgh whose fortune came from Carnegie Steel, informed Congress that he might donate $15 million to obtain radium and build institutes where it would be administered.[47–50]

In 1914, radium was expensive, scarce, and controversial as a cancer remedy. Newspapers reported on the "wonderful effects" of radium in some cases. But most of the cancer experts, surgeons, disagreed with its use in operable tumors. At the women's club, representatives of the New-York Skin and Cancer Hospital appealed for help in procuring radium. Controversy aside, doctors at their institution wanted to offer it to their patients.

Some doctors considered that public cancer education could be harmful. At a 1914 meeting of the Academy of Medicine of Northern New Jersey, Cullen tried to address their concerns: "It has been intimated that people may be frightened by being enlightened as to the symptoms of the various forms of cancer and further that those with vivid imaginations will think they have cancer," he acknowledged. "These objections are valid ones but are soon dissipated. In either case the individual will seek medical advice, and if after careful examination nothing be detected the patient's mind will be set at rest," he countered. "All of you will agree with me that it is better to unnecessarily alarm a person now and then than to allow others through ignorance to drift along with a cancer until it is too late—until all chance of a cure is past."

Cullen recounted anecdotes of patients with early, curable cases who presented in response to Adams's magazine article. "Within a week after the appearance of Mr. Adams' publication a colleague of mine told me that he had just operated upon a patient for cancer of the breast," Cullen relayed. "The nodule was not larger than a pea, and when asked why she had come so early the patient said she had just read the article in the *Ladies' Home Journal* and thought that it would be unwise for her to delay." He added, "The outlook in this case is excellent."[43]

Not all women were sold on cancer education, either. Mrs. Russell (Olivia) Sage was an eager philanthropist. After her husband, an infamous railroad tycoon and financier, died in 1906, Olivia inherited over $75 million; she controlled a fortune. Newspapers reported her participation in the meeting at Dr. Cleveland's home, but it's unlikely she attended.[51] After contributing a small amount to the cancer group, Olivia avoided Elsie Mead and declined to give more. Her reasons for snubbing the ASCC are unknown. In her will, Sage donated generously to agencies for women, Presbyterian charities, the Children's Aid Society, educational institutions and museums, but she left out the ASCC.[52,53]

As cancer awareness took off, the American eugenics movement was gaining steam. Hoffman and Bloodgood were among the ASCC leaders with eugenics leanings. Hoffman, a self-educated immigrant from Germany, authored an authoritative text on cancer's incidence and dozens of papers on cancer statistics and epidemiology. His racist views were well known.[54] He traveled constantly, lecturing and receiving honors throughout North America and in Europe. In 1912, Hoffman spoke at the first international eugenics conference in London; in 1918, he was elected to the executive council of the Eugenics Research Association based in Cold Spring Harbor, New York. In the late 1920s, Hoffman participated in Eugenics Research Association meetings at the American Museum of Natural History.[55-57]

Dr. Bloodgood, a Johns Hopkins general surgeon, penned literature for the society. His wife, Edith Holt Bloodgood of New York, was a daughter of publisher Henry Holt and friend to women in Mead's circle. Bloodgood peppered an early pamphlet distributed by the AMA, "What Every One Should Know About Cancer," with eugenic language and concepts. The health of workers is crucial to a prosperous, industrial society, he wrote. In a section on "the economic value of public health," he stated,

> The majority of the 75,000 and more who die annually of cancer are adults, vigorous, healthy bread earners and family rearers of this country. . . . On the whole cancer is more apt to attack the healthy and robust. This information,

about which there is no disagreement, shows the economic value of the control of cancer, as we are protecting the strongest and more essential members of the race.

Bloodgood emphasized that cancer is not hereditary.[58] In general, the ASCC sought to dispel perception that cancer tends to occur more often in some families. Fear of a malignant diagnosis marking relatives and generating stigma led some people to skip evaluation. "There is no shame in having cancer," the society stated in pamphlets and later in films.

These statements were compatible with a eugenicist's *weltanschauung* (worldview). As long as the ASCC leaders maintained that cancer is not hereditary, and that it could be treated effectively if caught early, they avoided contradiction. Rather, by lessening the burden of illness on society, financial and physical, the informational campaign would improve the well-being of prosperous U.S. citizens.

In April 1917, the United States entered World War I. Physicians served in field hospitals; nurses aided wounded soldiers; women who'd been active in local charities volunteered for relief agencies and took men's jobs. For most of a year, the society continued its education efforts. During wartime, women constituted the audiences at many lectures: In Detroit, Dr. W. P. Manton addressed nurses at Henry Ford Hospital. In New York, Dr. James Ewing spoke at the Bellevue Training School for Nurses. In North Carolina, Dr. Hubert A. Royster drew two hundred people to the Woman's Club of Raleigh for his lecture, "What Every Woman Should Know About Cancer."[59,60]

Dr. William J. Mayo, then a major in the U.S. Army Medical Corps, spoke to civilian employees of the War Department. In a 1918 lecture arranged by the surgeon general, given inside the Department of the Interior building in Washington, DC, he said,

> One of the great difficulties in the treatment of cancer is the popular attitude towards it. . . . Many persons believe that cancer is hereditary and carries a stigma with it. Hence many who have been operated upon and cured of cancer conceal the fact, and only those cases who die become known. This has resulted in an unjustified pessimism with regard to the possibility of curing the disease.

The auditorium was "packed" with listeners, many standing for lack of seats, the ASCC reported.[61,62]

Cancer was deemed a public health concern. In Texas, the State Council of Defense issued flyers titled, "Help Win the War by Preventing Unnecessary Sickness: Learn the Danger Signals of Cancer" (figure 2.3). The National Safety Council sponsored a flyer for posting on bulletin boards in factories and men's workshops. A 1918 bulletin claimed, "6,000,000 Workmen Read Warning Signs of Cancer." The ASCC planned a poster on cancers of the breast and uterus for display in places where women worked. The posters for women were delayed, however, likely by the 1918 pandemic.[63,64]

Over a quarter of the U.S. population was affected by the flu in 1918; an estimated 675,000 Americans died. The cancer society, strapped for dollars, workers, and speakers, published old lectures and made efforts to link its mission to the war in Europe. The ASCC newsletter, dubbed *Campaign Notes*, mixed announcements of cancer lectures and medical progress with notices from agency directors serving at army bases and field hospitals abroad. Elsie Mead, among others, had left for France. She'd been appointed to the War Personnel Board of the YMCA.[65]

No. 16
(Please release during week beginning Monday, March 11, 1918)

TEXAS STATE COUNCIL OF DEFENSE
COMMITTEE ON SANITATION AND MEDICINE

Help Win the War by Preventing Unnecessary Sickness

Learn the Danger Signals of Cancer

Do you know that Cancer is a very common as well as a very serious disease? In some Texas cities Cancer kills nearly twice as many people as typhoid fever and malaria combined.

But with early detection and operation, the chances of cure are very good. They decrease with every day of delay. Remember that the early and hopeful stages of this disease are usually painless. If you suspect Cancer, don't wait until there is pain, be examined at once.

Cancer is at first a local disease. In external Cancer,—for example, on the face, lip, or tongue—there is usually something to be seen or felt, such as a lump or scab, or an unhealed wound or sore. Lumps in the breast may be of special significance. Cancer inside the body is often recognized by symptoms before a lump can be seen or felt. Persistent indigestion with loss of weight and change of color, as well as other abnormal body conditions, should be thoroughly investigated.

Beware of advertised "Cancer Cures." Do not waste time and money by using valueless medicines.

The Best Preventive is a Thorough Physical Examination At Least Once a Year. In China, doctors are paid to Keep People Well, not to cure them after they get sick.

Don't Wait Until It's Too Late

WHAT ARE YOU DOING TO MAKE YOUR CITY A HEALTHIER AND A BETTER PLACE TO LIVE IN?

(Please publish in this form as nearly as possible.)

2.3 1918 Texas public health notice about cancer.

(*ASCC Campaign Notes*, March 15, 1918)

In its *Campaign Notes*, the ASCC picked up on a *Cleveland Plain Dealer* column, which in its 1918 pages offered cancer as a twisted metaphor for the nation at war. It quoted Dr. R. H. Bishop Jr., Cleveland's commissioner of health:

> To have a better understanding of the dread thing we know as cancer just compare it with the war. . . . Prussianism might well be called the cancerous growth that is trying to kill the other nations of Europe, for cancer, of itself, is a lawless growth of body cells which destroys life if allowed to run its course.[66]

When the Great War ended in November 1918, the ASCC's anticancer campaign had nearly stopped. Elsie Mead and others had witnessed devastation. Hundreds of doctors and thousands of nurses served; their views on the relative importance of cancer control may have changed. The epidemic highlighted the need to manage infectious illnesses. Malaria and other tropical diseases persisted in large pockets of the United States.

For many Americans, cancer was not a priority. Yet the ASCC kept on with its efforts and, in some regions, did so successfully. On April 15, 1919, for instance, the Georgia Federation of Women's Clubs held a meeting on cancer. The president of the Medical Association of Georgia presided; Hoffman and Dr. Francis Carter Wood, of Columbia University, spoke before an audience of nearly one thousand in the Wesley Memorial Church, the ASCC reported. The event was well attended despite a thunderstorm and competition for the crowd from Billy Sunday, a popular evangelist, speaking that day in a nearby auditorium. The following day in Atlanta, Dr. Wood "addressed a group of young negro women and teachers at the Spellman [sic] Institution," the ASCC reported.[67]

The ASCC printed new flyers. Some listed "Fourteen Points About Cancer," a reference to President Wilson's Fourteen Points plan to achieve world peace. When these ASCC circulars, distributed by the United States Public Health Service, sold out in September 1919, the agency printed a second run of one hundred thousand copies. Despite dramatic and deadly changes in the world, war, and disease, public interest in cancer persisted and grew.[68]

Cancer had sprung! In the next decade, the awareness campaign would involve thousands of Americans. Unfortunately, treatments were not yet adequate; most afflicted patients would not be helped. A disconnect—between publicity and the reality of cancer care—would emerge.

CHAPTER 3

EDUCATIONAL CAMPAIGNS (1920–1930)

When Marie Curie stepped onto a New York City pier in May 1921, she was greeted by a flock of admirers and press. The frail physicist embraced women from the U.S. anticancer campaign and accepted bouquets of flowers from Polish leaders. Five Camp Fire Girls presented the plainly clad professor a red leather bag decorated with a beaded fleur-de-lis and a Camp Fire symbol. The flame was said to represent "the light" Curie gave to the world.

Mme Curie came to America on a mission to cure cancer. At fifty-three, the Polish-born Sorbonne scientist, who'd won two Nobel Prizes for studies of radioactive elements, was a reluctant traveler. She was accompanied in her transatlantic journey by Mrs. William B. (Marie) Meloney, an American journalist, and by her daughters, Irène and Ève, ages twenty-three and sixteen. On arrival, Curie appeared "motherly," pale, and confident, newspapers reported. An automobile sent by Mrs. Andrew Carnegie delivered the group to Meloney's West Twelfth Street home where the family stayed overnight (figure 3.1).[1,2]

Meloney led a committee of U.S. women who'd raised over $100,000 to purchase a gram of radium for Curie. The gift of this precious substance would permit the world's "greatest woman" to continue her anticancer investigations. Around the country, doctors supported the Marie Curie Radium Fund by encouraging contributions to the committee. Mrs. Robert (Elsie) Mead, of the American Society for the Control of Cancer (ASCC), arranged a welcoming tea.[3–6]

Curie's schedule was packed. Soon after arrival she headed north to Smith College in Northampton, Massachusetts, and received an honorary degree. From there she traveled to Vassar College in Poughkeepsie, New York; while en route by automobile, at Mt. Holyoke College in the Berkshire Hills, "the student body

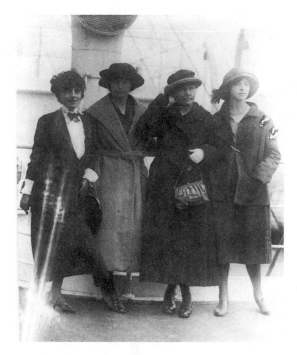

3.1 Marie Curie (holding hat), flanked by her daughters, Ève and Irène, with Marie Meloney (at left) upon arrival in New York Harbor, May 12, 1921. (Library of Congress)

had gathered to give her a welcome as she passed through." Back in New York, she was honored by chemists at a luncheon at the Waldorf Hotel, by the New York Academy of Sciences at a reception at the American Museum of Natural History, by the American Association of University Women at Carnegie Hall, and more— all within the first week. She was escorted by private car with Vice President and Mrs. Coolidge to Washington, DC. Later in Philadelphia and Pittsburgh, Curie visited laboratories, lectured, and received prizes. She became so fatigued that doctors expressed concern; she rested and canceled plans to visit California. She did reach the Grand Canyon, where Irène and Ève trekked down to the river and Marie toured the rim by automobile. Additional stops included Chicago, Buffalo, and Niagara Falls, where Curie inspected power plants, Boston, and New Haven, Connecticut. Most everywhere she traveled, she spoke with scientists and women who'd contributed to the radium fund. It was an exhausting six-week tour of the United States.[7–15]

At a White House ceremony, President Warren Harding spoke of Americans' appreciation for Curie's "genius and energy" and hope that she'd continue her efforts to conquer cancer. Harding handed Curie a key to a miniature mahogany cabinet, draped with ribbons and equipped with ten cylinders for tubes of the precious element. At the National Bureau of Standards, the radium was packaged for Curie's return trip to France. Several hundred guests—scientists, philanthropists, French and Polish diplomats, and U.S. leaders—attended a reception in the East Room.[9,16,17]

President Harding did not use the word "cancer" in his remarks that day. But the attention he drew to the cause was significant. Finding a cure for the most dreaded disease was a goal that unified Americans and people of other nations. Curie's trip, and the women's gift, reflected a cooperative spirit in fighting malignancy.

Curie's American tour kicked off a decade of anticancer activism. The ASCC stepped up its educational programs by orchestrating early "cancer weeks." These informational blitzes—filled with cancer-themed lectures, sermons, radio programs, and newspaper stories—prefigured modern disease awareness months such as October for breast cancer. The ASCC produced exhibits, films, and booklets.

The society fanned out, establishing chapters in most U.S. states. Around the country, regional leaders arranged for specialists to instruct doctors and nurses about cancer; they supplied lay speakers to labor unions, women's clubs, religious groups, schools, and fraternal orders.[18,19] Yet the ASCC was a tiny organization. In 1920, it listed only seven hundred dues-paying members; in 1923, it claimed 2,443 members and a mailing list approaching six thousand.[20-22]

The society took advantage of new technology—telephone, radio, and film—along with magazines, newspapers, and lectures to spread the word. It distributed simple messages: there is no shame in having cancer; the disease is neither contagious nor hereditary; prompt surgery can be curative.[19,23]

The cancer society did not yet invest in research. The value of laboratory studies was not appreciated by many physicians or the public. In the 1920s, scientists knew little about proteins such as receptors that stimulate cells to grow and divide, survive or die. The structure of genes was essentially unknown; DNA sequencing was inconceivable. Investigators could look at malignant bits under a microscope, but not much more. Biology was so poorly understood at the molecular and cellular levels that its current applications in cancer therapy could not have been imagined even by the most forward-thinking scientists.

Doctors' understanding of malignant disease was primitive. Dr. A. C. Strachauer, a Minneapolis surgeon on faculty at the University of Minnesota, articulated this perception: "Cancer cells are but altered normal cells, normal cells 'gone crazy,' normal cells which have lost their ability to live a community existence, normal cells which have become lawless—Bolshevistic."[24]

Scranton, Pennsylvania, was one of the first cities to hold a "cancer day." The earliest events targeted physicians. On a Tuesday in June 1920, three hospitals sponsored surgical demonstrations and diagnostic cancer clinics. Experts came from around Pennsylvania and from New York City. The ASCC encouraged local physicians to bring patients with possible malignancy for evaluation. The event would be instructive for doctors who were uncertain about a cancer diagnosis or best treatment. And it would help the afflicted: "Your patient will have the benefit of the advice of a distinguished specialist without cost, provided he will submit to demonstration at the clinic."

The ASCC called Scranton's cancer day an experiment in public health and a success. The next year, Pennsylvania's cancer day program expanded to Bethlehem and Allentown with public lectures. School superintendents received letters about cancer education. In some Pennsylvania schools, "teachers made a short talk to their pupils in the hygiene classes and required the students to write a short composition on cancer to be taken home and read to their parents."[25,26]

Denver, Colorado, was a hotbed of early anticancer activity. That's where surgeon and ASCC president U.S. Major Dr. Charles Powers lived. When Powers returned from his war service leading American surgical services in Europe, he became enthusiastic about the potential of deploying technology and education to fight cancer. Under his direction the Colorado ASCC arranged a series of public events coinciding with a November 1920 meeting of surgeons in Denver. They called it "Cancer Week."

Powers opened Denver's first cancer week with a speech before seven hundred "representative lay people." Religious organizations—ranging from the Council of Jewish Women at Temple Emanuel, to the Central Presbyterian and Plymouth

Churches, to the Parish Aid Society of St. John's Cathedral—coordinated meetings about cancer. The Elks and Shriners fraternities held discussions, as did the South Side Women's Club and Ladies' Aid Society. Telephone operators needed to know about cancer because they might field inquiries, so Denver's Southern, Main, and York Exchanges held workplace talks for employees.

Before many people had radios in their homes, attending lectures was a popular way to hear about science, politics, and ideas. Yet churchgoers, workers, and social club members may have felt obliged to attend these cancer talks; perhaps they didn't really want to hear about it. ASCC *Campaign Notes* suggest that social pressure to participate was indeed an issue. After two hundred people showed up for a cancer presentation in the drawing room of Denver's Brown Hotel, it reported, "This was a purely voluntary attendance, the meeting not being under the auspices of any regular organization." The strong turnout suggested "the statement so often heard that people are not interested in the subject of cancer and will not come out to meetings is not true."[27–29]

The ASCC promoted upbeat messages about cancer. The *Delineator*, a women's magazine edited by Meloney, published "Good News of a Bad Subject" by Frank J. Osborne, the ASCC executive secretary. In contrast to Samuel Hopkins Adams's *Ladies' Home Journal* piece of 1913, approved by Dr. Cullen, the *Delineator* story was introduced by Carolyn Conant Van Blarcom, a nurse and prolific writer.[30,31]

The society produced lantern slides for teaching. These information-loaded visual aids, typically of glass, revealed images through projected light. After World War I, the ASCC office in New York couldn't mail out these slides fast enough to meet demand for rentals. In Denver and some other cities, movie theaters projected ASCC images before feature films were shown. The pairing of lantern slides with popular films made practical sense; theaters were equipped with large screens on which images could be displayed and waiting audiences.[28,32,33]

Numerous ASCC events took place in New York City, where the society's national office was located. In June 1920, Broadway producer William F. Brady donated his playhouse for a Thursday evening performance of *The Merchant of Venice* to benefit the ASCC. It was reported that when actors heard about the anticancer organization from Elsie Mead's brother, they were eager to contribute.[34,35]

In the spring and summer of 1920, the society organized "shop talks" at workplaces—Pratt Oil Works, Greenpoint Metallic Bed Co. (in Italian), and Acme Foundry among sites in Brooklyn—as well as lectures at political clubs (Democratic and Republican) and the Greenpoint YMCA. The American Museum of Natural History held an exhibit about cancer in its Hall of Public Health curated by Dr. C. E. A. Winslow, a Yale professor and ASCC officer. Museum visitors viewed lantern slides and received "Fourteen Points" flyers.[36,37]

The ASCC's executive secretary, Frank Osborne, was an MIT-educated public health maven. Film is a powerful tool for convincing people to accept proper medical care, he considered. Because emotions influence decisions, a movie about cancer might save more lives than printed words. But to produce a film, the society needed money.[38]

In 1921, Mead landed a gift of $8,000 from the Laura Spelman Rockefeller Memorial fund to produce films about cancer. Laura, wife of the oil magnate John, had died in 1915. Mead and the couple's son, John D. Rockefeller Jr., and his wife, Abby (Aldrich) Rockefeller, were on friendly terms. Abby, who is remembered for founding New York's Museum of Modern Art, was an early ASCC supporter. This gift to create films only hinted at the enormity of the Rockefeller family's future donations for cancer research and clinical care.[39,40]

The first nationwide cancer week took place from October 30 through November 5, 1921. In a letter from the White House, President Harding endorsed the event. He offered "hearty sympathy" and wrote, "It seems to me that in recent times no single misfortune of the race has so sharply challenged science."[41]

The ASCC coordinated release of its first movie, *The Reward of Courage*, with cancer week. The silent film folds several cancer lessons into a thirty-minute drama. First, it's a love story: in a town named Pleasantville, a handsome plant manager woos the boss's daughter, Dorothy Flint; the amorous feelings are mutual. In an early scene, Dorothy's father and beau stop by the firm's on-site clinic for employees. After the company physician, Dr. Dale, casually shares patients' records with the boss, Mr. Flint expresses surprise about an employee's lip cancer diagnosis. Flint asks, "How do you suppose he caught it?" This question prompts Dale to explain that cancer is not contagious, and to review diagrams of the skin, lymph channels, and veins. He points out how cancerous cells can spread inside the body (figure 3.2).

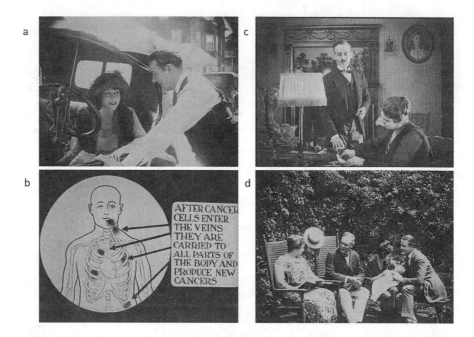

3.2 Composite of screenshots from the *Reward of Courage* 1921: (a) Dorothy Flint, the company owner's daughter, and Gene Barnes, the office manager, fall in love; (b) Dr. Dale explains that cancer is not contagious and is curable if caught early; he uses images like those of contemporary lantern slides; (c) Mrs. Flint, Dorothy's mother, is almost swindled; she writes a check for $200 to a fraudulent salesman for a painless "cure"; (d) Six years after summoning courage for cancer surgery, Mrs. Flint sits in a garden with her husband, Dorothy, Gene, and grandchild.

The young couple's romance is nearly thwarted by cancer when Dorothy's mother, Anna Flint, feels a breast mass. Dorothy worries for her mother's health and, because she's heard that cancer is hereditary, feels she shouldn't marry; Dorothy sends her would-be husband away and becomes despondent. Meanwhile, Anna fears surgery and nearly gets swindled by a patent medicine salesman. She writes a check for $200 for a bogus remedy said to be manufactured by the "Scientific Cancer Cure Institute" in New York. The camera zooms in on the jar labels: "NO KNIFE," "NO PAIN," and "No Failure Recorded." After Dorothy's father and Dale learn of the scam and rush to the family's home, a postal inspector, Brady, arrests the salesman for fraud.

The story ends with the happy family—grandparents, young married couple, and baby—sitting in a garden, six years later. By summoning the courage to undergo surgery, Anna lived to see her grandchild. The movie informed viewers that cancer is curable and that a cancer disposition is not hereditary (a disputable point then and more so today). It cautioned viewers not to be fooled by quacks selling "cures."

Whether audiences were moved, entertained, or turned off by the movie can't be known. "The reports received are all commendatory," the ASCC stated. Around cancer week of 1921, it was shown in scattered states including Maine, West Virginia, Indiana, Michigan, and Oregon. Society records support that initial viewership exceeded ten thousand. The ASCC printed additional copies of the two-reel film and sold those for $85. *The Reward of Courage* circulated into the late 1920s. The total audience likely surpassed one hundred thousand Americans.

The ASCC recognized that a cancer movie could have undesirable negative effects; it might frighten people such that they wouldn't seek care. For this reason, *The Reward of Courage* lacks graphic images. The surgeon stays out of sight. The patient reveals no scars or deformity. "There is absolutely nothing repulsive or objectionable in the picture," ASCC leaders emphasized. The society arranged for physicians to be present during screenings. In Denver, ASCC president Dr. Charles Powers spoke before theater audiences and displayed slides with titles such as "A Message of Hope" and "Danger Signals That May Mean CANCER."[38,42–47]

The cancer society tried impressing the public and physicians with technology. During Denver's 1921 cancer week, it reported, Dr. Powers delivered a fifteen-minute speech into "the transmitting apparatus of a great wireless telephone plant." Thousands of people in western states, gathered in groups of twenty or thirty at wireless receiving stations, could hear his words. Powers pondered "if the day may not soon be here when the speaker will sit at his ease in an arm chair and watch the smoke curl upward from his after dinner cigar, while he discourses on the evils of the tobacco habit to audiences scattered over the continent." And in Nebraska, an airplane "swiftly delivered one of the speakers to his engagements before one audience after another." Dr. Palmer Findley of Omaha reported on the telephone's potential to convey information, as told by the society:

> Through the cooperation of the telephone officials what is known as the S. O. S. call was put out early in the evening, just as the house wife was sure to be washing the supper dishes, and in three minutes time every farm house within a radius of thirty miles had received word of the time and place of a free lecture on cancer.

Findley's "twentieth century adaption of Paul Revere represented by the S.O.S. party line telephone system was a new way of sounding the call for a cancer meeting."[48,49]

In St. Louis, department store windows featured cancer week displays. One contained two electric trains heading in opposite directions: one passed through places named "Ignorance" and "Fear" en route to a cemetery; the other went by "Knowledge," "Early Recognition," and "Prompt Treatment" before arriving at a place called "Cure." A sign cautioned, "Be Sure to Take the Right Train." In another store window, a model house released real smoke from its roof; two engines, "Surgery" and "Radium," rushed toward the miniature building. A notice explained that just as fires should be put out early, cancer should be eliminated before it spreads. "Crowds were standing two deep in front of these windows," the ASCC reported.[50]

Religious groups got into the cancer week spirit. Archbishop Patrick J. Hayes sent a letter to all priests in the New York diocese to be read on Sunday, October 30, about the anticancer movement underway. Catholic people should "take advantage of the literature." Hayes wrote,

> It appears that this terrible scourge is a menace to all and is on the increase, whereas simple knowledge and timely precaution will save lives without number from this deadly affliction of the human family. Remember Christ's mission was one of healing both of soul and body.

Letters about the cancer society appeared in Georgia's *Christian Index* and *Wesleyan Christian Advocate*. At the ASCC's request, the Baltimore journalist H. L. Mencken prepared a letter for ministers, priests, and rabbis to read in churches and synagogues. Mencken's piece began, "The object of Cancer Week is not to spread alarm about cancer, but to bring hope."[51–53]

Some ASCC members invoked religious memes such as the "Ten Commandments of Cancer." In 1917, the Massachusetts Medical Society had published a "Cancer Decalogue" with ten points such as "Early cancer is usually curable by radical operation" and "Late cancer is incurable, though not always unrelievable." Around the country, doctors republished the decalogue; in Arkansas and Detroit, they tweaked it. By 1922, an Indiana surgeon iterated the "commandments" in public health terms. Number six referred to cancer's talkability: "Cancer, unlike venereal diseases, is not a disgrace and may be discussed openly."[54–57]

After producing the film and the 1921 cancer week, the ASCC needed funds. A 1922 gift of $50,000 from Mrs. Morris (Nettie) Lasker, in memory of her son Harry M. Lasker, helped keep the society afloat while it planned a second cancer week. One of Harry's surviving brothers, the businessman Albert D. Lasker, offered another $25,000. (Albert would later marry Mary Woodward; as Mary Lasker, in the 1940s, she and Albert overhauled the cancer society.) With the Lasker Fund, the ASCC produced cancer-themed lithographs.[58]

The DuPont chemical company, based in Wilmington, Delaware, contributed at least indirectly: after DuPont's medical director, Dr. A. K. Smith, took charge of that state's ASCC chapter, "the work went forward with remarkable speed."[59] Insurance companies chipped in, too. The Metropolitan Life Insurance Company sent out 250,000 society-approved circulars titled "Cancer, A Message of Hope." MetLife instructed its insurance agents to leave a copy of the ASCC material with policyholders "during the 'week.'" Frederick Hoffman, the statistician whose analyses helped spark the cancer control movement in 1913, stayed active in the ASCC. Hoffman coauthored the ASCC cancer handbook for lay readers. The Prudential Insurance Company, for which Hoffman was then a consultant, published some of his work as pamphlets including *Some Cancer Facts and Fallacies*.[60,61]

Some physicians objected to the ASCC's informational campaigns. In October 1921, the *Journal of the American Medical Association* (*JAMA*) published two pertinent letters. One begins like this: "Next week we shall be in the throes of another drive." The author acknowledged that publicity was prompting earlier cancer evaluations and concluded: "the campaign of education should be steady and continuous, and not a 'flash in the pan.'" A second letter, titled "Cancer Phobia," cites "phobias almost as terrifying as the diseases feared" as an inevitable outcome of so much attention to malignancy. It states, "The condition itself is sufficiently serious and needs no elaboration as to its terrifying aspects. Give the public all facts—but facts only."[62,63]

Doctors argued about the benefits of public cancer education. In 1922, a prominent surgeon unaffiliated with the society, Dr. Byron B. Davis of Omaha, Nebraska, published an article about breast cancer in *JAMA*. He commented favorably on the ASCC campaigns: "The persistent propaganda carried on by the American Society for the Control of Cancer during the last few years, culminating in cancer week, so recently celebrated, is bearing some fruit." Yet Davis doubted the message; he wasn't confident of breast cancer's long-term curability by surgery. Davis concluded the paper, and would conclude his career, by focusing on cancer's causes and prevention, a goal he considered preferable to its treatment.[64]

"Awareness" entered the cancer society's lexicon. In 1922, Dr. J. Shelton Horsley, who chaired the ASCC's publicity committee, used the term to refer to public knowledge of cancer. In a letter prepared for newspapers in Virginia, Horsley admitted doctors' lack of understanding of cancer, a baffling disease. "Nobody in the world knows why a particular individual contracts cancer and another one does not," he wrote. "Yet enough is known about it in the way of treatment and cure to make the difference between life and death for thousands of individuals if this knowledge is widely spread."[65]

Horsley outlined the society's essential messages: "In the first place, it is believed that cancer is probably not hereditary, and certainly not contagious." Second, "the most effective cure . . . is surgery [, and] radium is helpful in some cases, but the quack remedies sometimes advertised are a deadly danger to the ignorant and gullible," he wrote. "In the third place, cancer is far more often cured than is usually believed." He elaborated on perception of cancer and its curability:

> Many persons go to the hospitals, to be operated on for cancer, who, because of their dread of the disease, do not let it be known, even among their friends,

what the trouble is. They are operated on and cured, and the public generally never knows that this was a case of cancer.

While:

Those cases which turn out to be fatal, by the long and lingering character of the illnesses, advertise themselves so that people in general have the impression that cancer practically always means inevitable doom.

Such imbalance in disclosures of cancer diagnoses results in a mistakenly fatalistic view.

The ASCC timed cancer publicity with availability of physical examinations for screening. In the first week of November, free clinics were held throughout Virginia and other states. "All persons who have any suspicious growth or unusual internal symptom should be able to find out the truth about themselves," Horsley wrote. "Between two mistakes . . . the lack of careful attention and awareness which may let dangerous conditions develop until it is too late, and on the other hand, the credulity which plays into the hands of charlatans, the campaign for education is trying to steer." This was a prescient concern. Today, watching for early signs of cancer—awareness—carries possibility of overdiagnosis, unnecessary treatment, and costs, while fatalistic attitudes lead to avoidance of care.

In Taylorville, Illinois, Mr. Harry M. Hoxsey set up a cancer treatment institute. It was only a few years after Hoxsey's father John, a "quack" who "seems to have dabbled in veterinary medicine, faith healing and cancer curing" died from "Cancer!," *JAMA*'s Bureau of Investigation reported in 1926. Harry, with an eighth-grade education, began by selling a caustic paste containing plant roots and arsenic dubbed the "Hoxide cure." In decades ahead, Harry Hoxsey battled *JAMA* editor Dr. Morris Fishbein and the law, becoming the most infamous U.S. cancer treatment fraudster. He skipped around within Illinois—moving from Chicago to Taylorville to Girard, crossed state lines into Iowa, Texas, West Virginia, Pennsylvania, and New Jersey. Eventually he set up shop in Mexico. Occasionally he was jailed.[66–69]

The Hoxide Cancer Sanitarium lasted for several years in Illinois; "curing" cancer was a profitable business and, evidently, a good fit for Taylorville. The cover of a 1925 brochure issued by the Chamber of Commerce promoted: "Information concerning the successful Treatment of Cancer by the Hoxide Method at Taylorville." The "cured patients whose testimonials appear in this pamphlet are all personally known to some or all of our members," it states. "The Taylorville Chamber of Commerce guarantees the bona fides of every one of these testimonials. They are selected for inclusion in this pamphlet because they refer to cancer cases of widely different types." The pamphlet depicts Taylorville, the capital of Christian County, Illinois, as a pleasant small city, "a mining and manufacturing center" situated 175 miles south of Chicago and eighty-five miles northeast of St. Louis, Missouri. It advertised "attractive residences, churches, schools, lodges," an "excellent hotel," and a park with shade.

Hoxsey succeeded by convincing people that he was successful in treating cancer. He adopted ASCC strategies like cancer day and turned them upside down. For instance, in July 1929 the *Girard Gazette* put a "Hoxsey Day" story on its front page and reported that five hundred people in Girard, Illinois, attended the event. In staged testimonials before an audience, individuals described having terrible cancer, undergoing surgery and radiation to no avail, and then being cured by Hoxsey. (figure 3.3)[70]

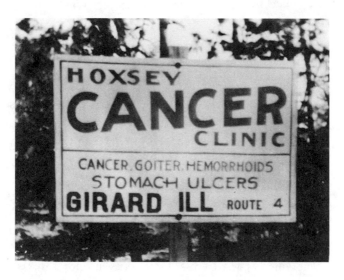

3.3 Undated roadside sign for a Hoxsey cancer clinic in Girard, Illinois.
Courtesy of the American Medical Association, Health Fraud Collection

When ASCC leaders spoke out about cancer and benefits of early surgery, their listeners were predominantly white and prosperous. As noted by historian Kirsten E. Gardner, "throughout most of the twentieth century, cancer education targeted a white and middle-class audience." In the 1920s, most Americans lived in segregated communities; people of color typically received medical care in separate facilities—if they received care at all. The eugenics movement was growing. Membership in the Ku Klux Klan peaked around this time. Many doctors thought, mistakenly, that Black people were less prone to developing cancer than white people.[71-73]

By 1925, the society asserted that cancer weeks had delivered "knowledge of the vital facts of cancer control either directly or indirectly" to over ten million Americans.[74] Even if this were true, however, most people remained in the dark. The U.S. population numbered around 115 million. For those who did get the ASCC's message, however, having information about cancer probably wouldn't have made a difference. For people with breast or skin cancer, caught early, long-term survival was feasible. But for those with hard-to-treat and internal malignancies less amenable to surgery in that era, it's unlikely that education would have helped.

By the late 1920s, cancer hospitals were operating in Massachusetts, New York, Philadelphia, St. Louis, and Rochester, Minnesota. Radium had gained acceptance and was being given to patients at some centers, but surgery remained the mainstay of treatment and the ASCC's first recommendation. The society's view against chemical approaches—as in chemotherapy—for treating cancer was so dominant that L. Duncan Bulkley, the doctor who'd founded the New York Skin and Cancer Hospital, was forced to resign his position for prescribing drugs in cases for which surgery should have been advised.[75,76]

International cancer conferences outside of Europe were unusual. A September 1926 meeting organized by the ASCC at Lake Mohonk, New York, stands out for its scope and news coverage. More than a hundred experts from around the world—including physicians and surgeons, statisticians, radiologists, lab researchers, and public health specialists—gathered to discuss cancer control. Cancer patients didn't participate, of course. Yet word got out. Updates from the Mohonk meeting were published in New York and by newspapers around the country such as Montana's *Great Falls Tribune* and Washington, DC's *Evening Star*.[77–79]

The lodge at Lake Mohonk, with its rambling Victorian frame, porches, and walking paths, was a well-established vacation spot midway between New York City and Albany. Getting there wasn't trivial. Travel to the conference was aided by philanthropy, police, and military officers: In the morning of September 20, ASCC executive committee members escorted their European guests from New York City to Mohonk. As told, "through the courtesy of Mr. Vincent Astor, the yacht *Nourmahal* was used to go up the Hudson from New York City to Bear Mountain, a distance of 45 miles." After a luncheon at Bear Mountain, New York State Police in automobiles escorted the scientists to West Point. "Cadets were paraded" under command of generals and colonels before the cancer experts resumed their motorcade to the hotel.[77]

The meeting's roster reads like a *Who's Who* of early cancer research, ASCC leaders and affiliated doctors. Experts included Dr. James Ewing of New York's Memorial Hospital and Dr. Charles Mayo of Rochester, Minnesota. A handful of women attended including Dr. Elise S. L'Esperance, a pathologist who later established the Strang Clinic for cancer prevention in New York (which still exists); Dr. Anna C. Palmer, a Massachusetts physician and breast cancer survivor who later founded the Cured Cancer Club; and Miss Maud Slye, a Chicago pathologist known for her contested studies of cancer's heritability.

Dr. William H. Welch of Baltimore welcomed international travelers "on behalf of the American medical profession." As dean of the Johns Hopkins School of Medicine, Welch was a research enthusiast who then chaired the Rockefeller Institute for Medical Research.[80] He raved about the ASCC's educational programs, stating they were of "far-reaching significance." Welch noted that public cancer discussions elevate concern, which leads to research donations. Dr. Ewing lectured on the importance and feasibility of cancer prevention, gaining journalists' attention.[81,82]

Dr. Harry Saltzstein, a Detroit surgeon, weighed in on different ways to inform the public about cancer. "Speaking before audiences—luncheon clubs, women's societies, etc.,—is of course more direct: nothing can take the place of the word-of-mouth appeal." However, attention spans are limited, and modern technology can be distracting: "There is a tendency toward the falling off of lecture attendance; the radio and automobiles are responsible," he said. "Billboards, motion pictures, magazine articles and advertising are effective, but may be very costly." Saltzstein favored print: "Everybody reads the newspaper." He noted, "A busy metropolitan newspaper may have a circulation from 100,000 to 1,000,000 and a brief, well-written article has the possibility of reaching that many readers." He graphed cancer publicity in printed newspaper columns in a manner resembling how modern PR firms analyze social media traffic, tweets, and website clicks today. During a January cancer week held in Detroit, for instance, the city's three daily papers carried "831 column inches" of cancer news, he reported.

"Cancer news must be made interesting. Otherwise, editors wouldn't publish it because they need to turn a profit, Saltzstein said. "The public tires. . . . The [cancer] publicity must lead up to a week of considerable activity, and then must stop." Keep messages crisp, he advised. And check the calendar: "The time of the main drive must be carefully chosen not to compete with any national or local campaigns, community drives, Christmas news, etc." His 1926 advice—about timing cancer publicity—explains why cancer awareness months occur in the spring and fall, not in December. People don't appreciate complicated statistics or nuanced debate, Saltzstein noted: "Long discussions about conflicting theories of etiology, specialists' arguments about treatment, conflicts about heredity, or descriptions of the terminal ravages of the disease will not help anyone."[83]

Discussion after Saltzstein's talk confirmed that enthusiasm for the ASCC's informational campaigns had fallen: "It was easier a dozen years ago, when the American Society for the Control of Cancer was organized, to manage a cancer week, than it is today," said George A. Soper, PhD. "People are tired of 'weeks' and 'drives.' The idea, adopted in many fields of health work, has been 'done to death.'" Soper, the ASCC managing director, expounded on attitudes: "Misstatement, either on the side of too much optimism or on that of pessimism, is capable of doing the subject of cancer control serious harm." He defended the use of emotion—namely fear—as a motivating force for health: "It may be worth considering whether it is not desirable to tell people not only the hope which lies in prompt and proper action but the fatal consequences of delay."

Cancer weeks petered out. But people's willingness to give to the cause—when giving was combined with pleasant social activities—did not. A year after the

Mohonk meeting, in September 1927, Mrs. Henry P. Davison sponsored an anti-cancer "circus" at Peacock Point in Glen Cove on Long Island. Two thousand people attended the three-day affair which was so elaborate that Mrs. Davison and others arranged for yachts to ferry socialites between Long Island and Greenwich, Connecticut.[84]

To encourage fundraising, an ASCC pamphlet on "cancer as a subject of popular entertainment" detailed two New York area events. At a concert held in the garden of a Park Avenue building, "tea was served on tables flanked with beds of flowers beneath tall cedar trees. Debutantes in bright spring frocks sold cigarettes, bouquets and programs." A pair of "Scotch bagpipers in gay costume" opened the musical program. A choir of Russian singers and the Metropolitan Opera's tenor, Rafaelo Diaz, followed. The pamphlet does not disclose the amount raised for the ASCC.

A surviving cancer patient, Mr. Swan Abramson, organized an "entertainment" in the town of Central Park (now Bethpage), a middle-class community on Long Island. A few years after surgery for stomach cancer, he was well but suffered from anemia and needed blood transfusions he couldn't afford. Abramson rented a hall, advertised, and charged one dollar for admission. His two children, ages twelve and fourteen, played piano at this personal fundraising event. The society lent Abramson a copy of *The Reward of Courage*, which was shown, and Abramson lectured. He "had made some study of the cancer question and was not without dramatic ability." More than one hundred people attended and no one left early, the ASCC reported.

"Each of these meetings in its own way reflects the changing attitude of the public toward cancer and affords encouragement," the ASCC concluded. "Neither meeting could have taken place a few years ago, for among fashionable people, as among farmers, the word 'cancer' has been taboo."[85]

Soon after the Mohonk meeting, Elsie Mead and her friends established the New York City (NYC) Cancer Committee. The Manhattan-based group served as a local ASCC unit and, at times, competed with the national organization for donations. A later report published by the American Association for Cancer Research justified the split—which resulted in there being two ASCC offices in Manhattan, each with its own publicity department and staff—by stating that both were necessary to serve the city's population of seven million. Evidently, the national ASCC wasn't meeting local needs. This rift anticipated modern splintering of American cancer charities, which number in the hundreds and compete for donors' money.

Seeking an emblem to symbolize the cancer group's mission, the NYC Cancer Committee sponsored a poster contest in 1928. Judges included the popular *Boys' Life* illustrator Francis J. Rigney and *Vogue*'s publisher Condé Nast. The committee selected a poster by George E. Durant with a "radiant sword" emerging from the caduceus, an ancient medical symbol with two snakes entwining a rod and words: "Fight Cancer with Knowledge" (figure 3.4).[86,87]

The NYC Cancer Committee publicized its telephone number (figure 3.5). By this time, women were volunteering in its office to help their neighbors navigate possible cancer diagnoses and treatment. While the committee involved physicians from the city's leading hospitals, it was women who answered the phone and fielded questions. In 1927, the office received 615 requests "by letter, telephone, or personal visit, for definite help or advice." That statistic, representing "outreach," rose to 1,905 in 1928, surpassed two thousand in 1929, and then plateaued for some years.[86]

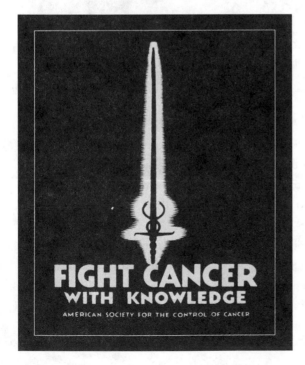

3.4 1928 poster for the ASCC, designed by George E. Durant, selected by the NYC Cancer Committee.

Courtesy of the American Cancer Society

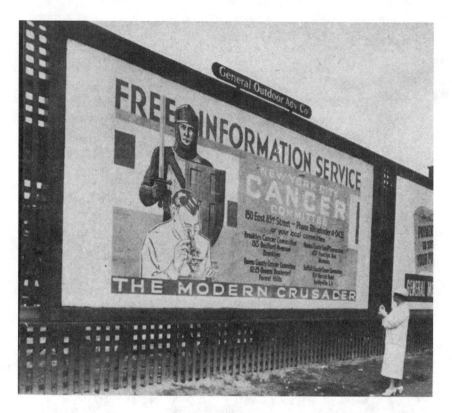

3.5 Billboard advertising the NYC Cancer Committee's cancer information service, c. 1930 (*There Shall Be Light! For All Women: Presented by the Women's Field Army of the American Society for the Control of Cancer*; New York: NYC Cancer Committee, 1936)
Courtesy of the American Cancer Society and New York Academy of Medicine Library

In Massachusetts, the state-run Pondville Hospital opened in Norfolk on the site of an old mental hospital twenty-two miles south of Boston (figure 3.6). The institution offered the "best and most up-to-date treatment for cases of cancer in all stages," Dr. Robert B. Greenough reported in 1927. "There was some question whether its 90 beds could be filled, but within a year the hospital was filled to capacity and had a large waiting list," the superintendent, Dr. George L. Parker, later reported. Need for a cancer hospital was such that in 1928, the Massachusetts legislature restricted admission at Pondville to residents of the Commonwealth who'd lived in the state for at least twenty-four of the previous thirty-six months. For patients who couldn't afford to pay the weekly charge of $10.50, Pondville billed their home city or town $17.50 weekly. Cancer patients were referred through a statewide network of clinics.[88,89,90]

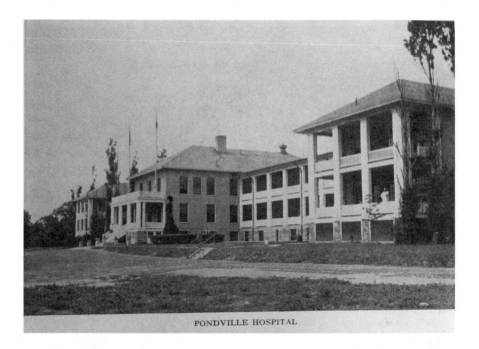

PONDVILLE HOSPITAL

3.6 Early photograph of Pondville Hospital in Norfolk, Massachusetts (George H. Bigelow and Herbert L. Lombard, *Cancer and Other Chronic Diseases in Massachusetts* by George H. Bigelow and Herbert L. Lombard; (Cambridge, MA: Houghton Mifflin, 1933).

ASCC programs expanded until 1930. Membership rose as did the organization's budget. Its mailing list reportedly numbered forty-five thousand. In rural Washington County, Maryland, library wagons delivered ASCC information about cancer; in Baltimore, public school teachers gave cancer leaflets to schoolchildren for their parents to read. ASCC materials circulated in French, Italian, Polish, Russian, Slovak, and Yiddish.[91]

But the ASCC could not crush the public's fear of malignancy. People continued to avoid diagnosis and treatment. In 1928, Senator Matthew Neely of West Virginia called cancer a "loathsome, deadly, and insatiate monster." Speaking in the U.S. Capitol, he pushed for federal funding of cancer research but his proposed legislation failed. It wasn't until 1937, in the midst of the Great Depression, that Neely and others introduced to Congress the law that would gain support and establish the National Cancer Institute.[92]

CHAPTER 4

FIGHTING WORDS (1930–1945)

OCTOBER 16, 1934

DEAR HEALTH CHAIRMEN:

To all of you who are just joining our ranks and to all of you who are continuing with us in our HEALTHWARD-HO campaign—CHEERIO!

Here we are a UNITED HEALTH ARMY with but one objective—a HEALTHIER UNITED STATES. The contribution that the clubwomen can make to the cause of GOOD HEALTH is inestimable if their strength is directed into the most effective channels . . .

Around the nation, General Federation of Women's Clubs (GFWC) leaders received this missive signed by Marjorie B. Illig, chairman of its public health division. Illig spent the decade crisscrossing the country to fight disease. On official stationery, her name appeared as Mrs. Carl W. Illig, Jr. of Onset, Massachusetts.[1]

The GFWC constituted a formidable network in 1934, encompassing thousands of women's groups and claiming around two million members. Illig's task was enormous. In a depressed economy, cuts to essential programs like municipal sanitation threatened Americans' well-being. "Cancer education" appeared second or third on Illig's early agendas; other GFWC public health projects included "social hygiene" to combat venereal disease, "sterilization of defectives" (a eugenics tactic), and provision eyeglasses to poor children.[2-4]

The cancer society's managing director, Clarence Cook (C. C., or "Pete") Little—a Harvard-educated geneticist and eugenicist—realized that the women's organization could help his group spread its message and raise money.[5-7] In 1933, Little met with Illig and others at GFWC headquarters in Washington, DC, and persuaded them to join the cause. The federation adopted the slogan "Cancer Thrives on Ignorance, Fight It with Knowledge."[8,9]

In memos, Illig introduced the subject by reminding readers that "cancer is the outstanding menace to women in the prime of life." She outlined the three-part "duty of every club woman" in combating cancer. First, each must learn to "protect herself" by maintaining careful skin and mouth hygiene, examining body parts regularly, and knowing cancer's danger signs. A woman could improve the chances of successful treatment by recognizing cancer's signs and promptly reporting those to a physician. Second, each GFWC club member had a responsibility to educate her family and friends about "the nature, incidence, and treatment of cancer." Instruction could be accomplished by conversing about cancer, holding annual meetings about cancer, distributing information about cancer, showing films about cancer, etc., at every club. Third, each club woman should give a "voluntary" contribution of ten cents per year to the GFWC Cancer Control Fund.[10,11]

The ASCC was struggling for money, members, and enthusiasm. It published slender monthly bulletins, and that was about it. Few doctors supported its educational mission. In most places cancer weeks had fizzled out. In 1935, the cancer society joined forces with Illig's division and announced formation of the Women's Field Army (WFA) of the American Society for the Control of Cancer. Under Illig's leadership, the WFA grew. It adopted a military style. By 1939, an army of commanders, captains, and lieutenants supervised a few hundred thousand "recruits" who each paid $1 in dues. Unlike the ASCC, led by experts, the field army relied on ordinary women's knowledge and effort (figure 4.1).[12]

The WFA constituted the first major U.S. grassroots organization to distribute information about cancer. Through the end of World War II, the WFA carried out the cancer society's mission. The volunteer army proved so effective that its messages about early cancer detection percolated through communities for many years ahead.

Progress against cancer stalled during the Great Depression. The pace of research was slow. Treatment did not advance beyond surgery, radium or radiation, and palliative care. There were no "oncologists" yet; the idea of treating cancer with

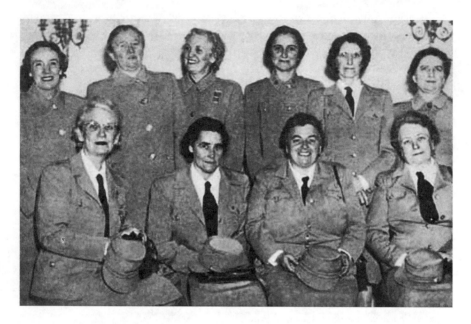

4.1 Women's Field Army regional commanders, 1942 left to right, seated: Mrs. H. C. Peterson, Montana; Mrs. J. C. Carmack, Rhode Island; Mrs. Marjorie Illig, national commander; Mrs. H. B. Ritchie, Georgia. left to right, standing: Mrs. Volney Taylor, Texas; Mrs. Harry W. Smith, New Hampshire; Mrs. David S. Long, Missouri; Mrs. Hobart Herbert, Tennessee; Mrs. Emily G. Bogert, Colorado; Mrs. John S. Harvey, West Virginia.
Courtesy of the American Cancer Society

medicines was verboten. Specialized U.S. cancer hospitals numbered in single digits, and results emanating from those few institutions were miserable. Patients shied away from specialists. Many preferred to take their chances on care from homeopaths or frank charlatans, or chose no care at all, rather than submit to operations. Physicians, for their part, doubted the benefits of surgery; many remained unconvinced of cancer's curability.

The paucity of legitimate experts—along with a lack of available information—rendered cancer patients vulnerable to quacks. Through the AMA's Bureau of Investigation, based in Chicago, *JAMA* editor Dr. Morris Fishbein relentlessly pursued hucksters. Fishbein's authority was limited, however, by state lines protecting Harry Hoxsey and his ilk who upon being charged with practicing medicine without a license or other crimes moved from one place to the next and, even more so, by public support for people selling "cures."[13–16]

American physicians were reckoning with a proposal for national health insurance. While the AMA led opposition to "socialized medicine," some ASCC leaders favored establishing state-funded facilities where cancer experts would perform research and provide free care. Dr. Robert B. Greenough, a Harvard surgeon, advocated for government-sponsored clinics and a registry of all cases. He and Dr. George H. Bigelow, the Massachusetts Public Health commissioner, spoke enthusiastically about Pondville, the state's cancer hospital. There, Massachusetts doctors learned, practiced surgery, and performed clinical research; patients were said to receive "up-to-date" care regardless of their finances. In the 1930s, Greenough and Bigelow each took a turn as ASCC president.[17–19]

Costs of cancer treatment drew physicians' attention. A Los Angeles radiologist, Dr. Albert Soiland, spoke on "Some Economic Aspects of the Cancer Problem" at an international medical conference. Eighty percent of cancer patients couldn't afford curative therapy, he said. Medical fees could deplete a family's savings: "We are confronted here with the stubborn fact that treatment is both long and expensive," he said. "The average patient is unable to pay his doctor even a reasonable fee." Under duress, the patient "must use the little fund which he may have been fortunate enough to accumulate after many years of toil," Soiland stated.[20]

Yet the issue didn't generate much publicity. As few believed cancer treatment to be beneficial, people didn't worry so much about the expense.

Hucksters prospered. In 1930, Hoxsey left Illinois for Iowa, joining forces with Mr. Norman Baker—a businessman later dubbed the "King of the Quacks." In Muscatine, Baker ran a lucrative enterprise including a hospital. Baker advertised that "cancer is curable"—the same slogan pushed by the ASCC—and people flocked to him. Reportedly, he pocketed about $100,000 monthly. Using an "infowar" strategy, Baker promoted his business promoted his business in *TNT* (*The Naked Truth*) magazine, which he published, and on KTNT radio, which he owned. Baker broadcast theories that defied science, such as the notion that testing cattle for a tuberculosis-like bacteria, as required by state law, caused cows to abort. At one horrifying event a crowd of thousands, including children, gathered in a park to watch Baker remove part of the skull of a man said to be suffering from brain cancer. Amid multiple lawsuits, Hoxsey and Baker separated ways. The Federal Radio Commission shut down KTNT in 1931.[21–23]

Hoxsey moved on, setting up clinics in Wheeling, West Virginia; Atlantic City, New Jersey; and western Pennsylvania. Eventually he settled near Dallas, Texas, where he directed a large facility until 1960. He claimed fabulous results in cancer cases previously deemed hopeless. Each year, his crew "treated" hundreds of cancer patients; his clinical experience surpassed that of most physicians. To a desperate public, confusion about whom to believe was understandable.[24,25]

Baker resurfaced in the Ozarks. A 1939 brochure for his "Castle in the Air" in Eureka Springs, Arkansas, advertised a lodge-like hospital "where sick folks get well without operation, radium or X-ray." The pamphlet depicts "a friendly place" atop a mountain, offering therapy for ailments other than contagious diseases. What treatments Baker gave to cancer patients isn't clear. The deceptive brochure spun Baker's Iowa past and move to Mexico, where he'd set up another radio station, triumphantly; it bemoaned his legal battles and persecution by the AMA and listed individuals he'd allegedly cured (figure 4.2).[26]

Some of the most absurd claims reaching the AMAs fraud bureau concerned Mr. Royal Rife's "cancer-killing" ray machines. Rife had begun tinkering with

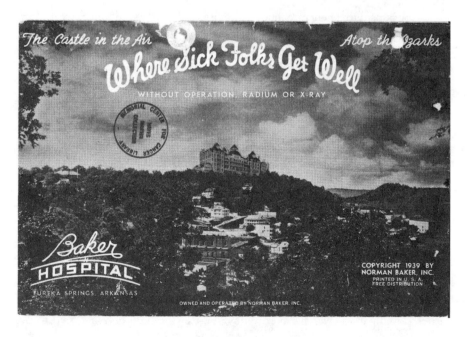

4.2 Cover, 1939 brochure for Norman Baker's hospital in Eureka Springs, Arkansas
Courtesy of Memorial Sloan Kettering Cancer Center Archives (Hayes Martin collection)

medical equipment while employed as a physician's chauffeur. After *Popular Science* ran a 1931 feature about him, with a published photograph of Rife in a white coat sitting by a "powerful microscope," he gained credibility. Rife's "electromagnetic rays" were said to kill the tiniest of germs. When many people thought cancer infectious, the idea of using "Rife rays" against disease caught on. Newspapers called the pseudoscientist "Dr. Rife." In 1940, the *Los Angeles Times* published: "Dr. Arthur W. Yale . . . reported that with the aid of the Rife ray he has succeeded in curing a number of cases of malignant cancer in which patients had been told they had only a limited time in which to live."[27–30]

None of these men were physicians. Each played victim, charging the AMA and medical establishment with conspiring to suppress favorable reports of their methods. Baker and Hoxsey used populist rhetoric to lure patients, appealing to widespread distrust of academic physicians and big-city experts. Hoxsey named Fishbein repeatedly in statements; with antisemitic overtone, he asserted that the AMA editor's motivation was to protect the income of doctors who treated cancer patients with surgery and radiation. Their legacies persist today in fraudulent claims—ranging from Goop to stem cell cures—and in fake health news disparaging expertise.

The United States lacked a big-picture cancer research plan. A scattered pattern of philanthropy depended on private donors' resources and whims. In Pennsylvania, an anonymous donation of $210,000 supported investigations at the American Oncologic Hospital in Philadelphia. In Illinois, the Chicago Woman's Club ambitiously set out to raise $300,000 for a cancer research institute. In Oakland, a gift from Mr. and Mrs. George Roos to the University of California funded a clinic. One of the largest contributions, a multi-million-dollar fund supporting research at Yale University, came from Starling W. Childs after his wife, Jane Coffin Childs, died from cancer. In Indiana, Mr. Edwin L. Patrick, president of the C. B. Cones manufacturing company, gave $100,000 to the Indianapolis City Hospital for a facility in his wife's memory. And so on. There was no coordinated effort.[31–39]

With support from the Chemical Foundation—a philanthropic arm of the American Chemical Society—the American Association for Cancer Research (AACR) began publishing *The American Journal of Cancer*. The foundation was funded by industry; DuPont and other chemical companies—polluters and manufacturers of carcinogens—were, in effect, financing the AACR's journal. Yet few scientists linked cancer to toxic chemicals. The Chemical Foundation's sponsorship of this and other anticancer programs such as NYC Cancer Committee publications, appears to have been accepted, no questions asked.[40–42]

When doctors identified possible cures, philanthropic and commercial offers ensued. An extreme episode surrounded reports by two California physicians, Drs. Walter B. Coffey and John D. Humber, of cancer patients' responses to injections of suprarenal extracts.* Some tumors shrank, and some pain was relieved. By standards of the time, Coffey and Humber were careful to emphasize their treatment's experimental nature. They detailed their methods, collected questionnaires about patients' symptoms including pain, and performed autopsies on those who died. Yet word of the Coffey–Humber "cure" quickly spiraled out of control.

Publicity surrounding the Coffey–Humber treatment was such that a dying woman was flown by airplane from Washington State to San Francisco, hoping to receive life-saving therapy, but she died. Her "vain" effort was detailed in newspapers across the country. The *Brooklyn Daily Eagle* reported that Mrs. Grace Hammond Conners, a wealthy widow, resolved to bring the treatment—or at least a trial of it—to the East Coast. Conners offered her Long Island mansion as a sanatorium for patients receiving injections. On her dime, Coffey and Humber traveled to persuade health officials and cancer experts in New York. But those physicians and a local board of health said no. In Oregon, businessmen spotted opportunity in the Coffey–Humber extracts. The Portland Chamber of Commerce proposed offering the treatments in that city. The local medical society intervened, however, stating that the University of Oregon Medical School should supervise any experimentation.[43–47]

Dr. Fishbein of the AMA weighed in against the injections. But of course he did; the anticancer mantra was all about surgery and radium or radiation. The *ASCC Bulletin* noted the hoopla: "What can we tell the laity about cancer?" asked Dr. William J. Mayo, rhetorically.[48] The society advised doctors to remind the public that medicines are ineffective against cancer—a message that, within twenty years, proved to be untrue.

---

* Suprarenal extracts likely contained cortisol, a steroid hormone produced in the adrenal (suprarenal) gland; this hormone, like prednisone and related steroids now used in cancer treatment, can powerfully shrink many tumors and relieve symptoms, but its effect when given as a single agent would be temporary.

California did permit a trial of the Coffey–Humber treatment, sponsored by the W. K. Kellogg Foundation of Battle Creek, Michigan. When the AMA's journal published disappointing results, the *New York Times* rushed to report, "Coast Cancer 'Cure' Held of Little Use." Among 415 "cancer sufferers" in the study, nearly two-thirds died within thirteen months. Cancerous extensions and new metastases (tumors arising from cancer's spread) developed in some patients after they'd received injections. Some of their tumors grew so large and quickly, the extracts might be stimulating cancer's growth, the *Times* reported, putting the kibosh on enthusiasm for this treatment.[49,50]

Cancer's causes mystified Americans. The *ASCC Bulletin* attempted to dispel misconceptions. One 1933 article, "Cause and Effect in Cancer Research," addressed the "pernicious type of unscientific and faulty reasoning" exemplified by the idea, circulating, that refrigerators cause cancer. Use of electrical refrigeration had increased in recent decades, it noted. "So has, apparently, the incidence of cancer. So has the use of automobiles and airplanes, of cosmetics, of football tickets, of moving pictures and of ocean liners," it continued. "The intelligent public can and does, at once, see the fallacy involved." Rather, "the wise individual" does not assume cause and effect but invokes that relationship "with great caution and only after they have been proved by unassailable evidence."[51]

By 1935, cancer had ascended to second place in U.S. mortality charts. Only heart disease took more American lives. Louis Dublin, a statistician of the Metropolitan Life Insurance Company who, unlike Frederick Hoffman, had a PhD, insisted there was no cause for alarm. Cancer deaths were more common because people were living longer and because doctors had become better at diagnosing it. Cancer deaths were higher among "colored" than white women, Dublin noted. This observation is remarkable because some doctors mistakenly thought that cancer didn't occur in Blacks as often as in whites. Dublin was one of the first experts to clarify that cancer strikes people of all races and socioeconomic classes.[52]

There was a silver lining in the latest statistics. Some twenty-five thousand cancer patients were living without recurring symptoms five years or longer after treatment, Dublin noted. A half-century before doctors applied the term "survivor" to people who survived a cancer diagnosis, he remarked on this favorable trend. Dublin called this landmark indicator of survivorship "encouraging."

Recognizing the importance of media for promoting its message, the cancer society hired its first publicity director, Clifton R. Read. It cultivated relationships with the National Association of Science Writers, medical reporters, and editors. The ASCC invited journalists to meet researchers, visit laboratories, and attend dinners.[53–56]

Radio was crucial for cancer publicity because it reached millions. The ASCC encouraged doctors to embrace this medium as an instrument for public health. Dr. William A. O'Brien of Minnesota filled a 1936 piece, "The Use of the Radio in Cancer Education," with tips for attracting an audience when speaking about cancer. "The finesse in handling such a subject consists of making the potential patient want to reassure herself that everything is all right," O'Brien said. "The average person does not care to hear talks on cancer. . . . This does not mean that we should deliberately bury our ideas so deeply in soft words" that truth can't be told, he advised. Speakers "should use common sense" to avoid "frightening or disgusting" listeners.[57] In Louisiana, the State Medical Society's Cancer Committee conducted numerous broadcasts. "Other states are rapidly following suit," the ASCC reported. Expert talks on cancer, given at New York City's Town Hall Club and the Chicago Woman's Club in November 1936, were broadcast over WJZ in New York and WMAQ in Chicago.[58,59]

Radio did have a downside, though. Some words could be printed in magazines but not said on air. The ASCC's managing director, C. C. Little, later commented, "One still encounters a taboo against the use of certain words such as 'uterus' or 'womb' in some of the more provincial broadcasting stations."[60]

In the months leading up to Congress's vote to establish the National Cancer Institute, magazine articles highlighted cancer treatments and research. *Time* put a photo of Little, pipe to his lip, on a March 1937 cover. The "Cancer Army" feature explained how surgery was performed. It offered statistics and called breast and womb cancers "curable." *Time* avoided offending readers by focusing on Little, Illig and other people leading the war on cancer, rather than disease.[61]

Life presented an entirely different and scarier picture. An image of research mice appeared on the cover. Inside were graphic images of patients' bodies, organs, and x-rays. One photograph revealed the nipple of a woman's cancerous breast as needle on a syringe pokes nearby skin during an aspirational biopsy. Another displayed the brain of a five-year-old girl who had died from metastatic kidney cancer (figure 4.3). Another exposed a cancerous heart at autopsy. Side-by-side images exhibited a man's face with a tumor growing over his eye, before and after treatment. *Life* also showed cancerous cells growing in a Johns Hopkins research laboratory and a scary-looking radiation handler clad in a protective mask and gown. "Radium can cause cancer as well as cure it," the caption noted.[62]

Journalists and doctors collaborated to inform the public about cancer. After editors of *Fortune* magazine wrote *Cancer: The Great Darkness*, pitching research, Doubleday, Duran & Company republished it as a short book with an introduction by *JAMA* editor Morris Fishbein. The *New York Times* advised subscribers not to fear reading *The Great Darkness*: "This is not a sensational or terrifying book, but one which is clear, direct and informative." The *Fortune* editors estimated

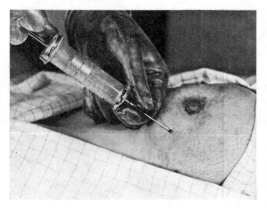 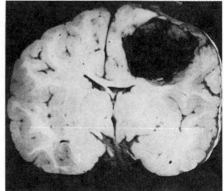

4.3 Cancer images in *Life* magazine, March 1, 1937: (left) aspirational biopsy of a cancerous breast with needle inserted; (right) autopsy photo of the brain of a five-year-old girl who died from metastatic cancer.
(*LIFE* Picture Collection)

that only around $700,000 was spent annually on cancer research in the United States. This was a paltry amount, they considered, while "the public willingly spends a third of that sum in an afternoon to watch a major football game."[63]

The ASCC honored journalists who helped distribute their message. In 1937, Time Inc. president, Henry R. Luce, received the Clement Cleveland Medal from Elsie Mead, Cleveland's daughter, on behalf of the NYC Cancer Committee of the ASCC. The award recognized a "March of Time" film, *Conquering Cancer*, as an "outstanding contribution to the cause of cancer education." At a gala dinner, Mead thanked the cadre of reporters present for helping "to break down old fears and to build up a public appreciation that cancer is curable." Luce responded in kind: "Tonight, you have generously chosen to honor a journalist. In that greater day, you will be inevitably honoring a scientist." Their reciprocity of gratitude appears to have been genuine; few reporters then challenged the ASCC or cancer specialists.[64,65]

Legislation for the National Cancer Institute (NCI) passed through Congress in the summer of 1937. On August 5, President Franklin D. Roosevelt signed the law without fanfare. As told by historian James T. Patterson in *The Dread Disease*, support was not uniform; earlier legislation for a federal cancer program had failed. The AMA and some independent physicians warned of "danger" in putting the government in charge of medical research. Among the officials who voiced strong support was the U.S. surgeon general, Thomas Parran, who'd lost his wife to cancer. Senator Homer T. Bone, of Washington State, emphasized that malignancy affects people of all social classes but hits the poor hardest. Bone had lost his wife, journalist Blanche Sly, to the disease. "Never before had so many medical leaders appeared to plead in behalf of any legislative measure," the *Washington Post* reported.[66–69]

Passage of the National Cancer Act of 1937 reflected changing attitudes: growing concern over cancer death rates, sympathy, and, perhaps, a shred of optimism that research and treatment could improve patients' lives. The *Post* headline, "'Conquer Cancer' Adopted as Battle Cry of the Public Health Service" reflected the prevailing sentiment that defeating cancer warranted a warlike effort. The newest Public Health Service branch would fight cancer on two fronts: While investigators at the institute hunted for cancer's origin, doctors practicing around the country would extend established therapy to regions where knowledge and facilities were "woefully" limited.

That cancer fell within the realm of public health might surprise a modern reader. Since the 1930s, the larger and more lucrative field of oncology practice has diverged from its roots in cancer control, which encompasses cancer prevention and screening. "Approximately 25,000 lives can be saved annually by application of 'the information already available,'" Parran estimated in 1937. Even if research scientists failed to identify cancer's causes, "which is the big hope," efforts to deliver current information and treatment "will more than repay the Nation," the *Post* reported.

The National Cancer Act appropriated $750,000 for building construction and $700,000 annually—the equivalent of nearly $13 million today—for federal cancer research. A plot of land in Bethesda, Maryland, was donated by the family of Luke Wilson, a businessman who died from cancer. The cornerstone was placed a year later.[70,71]

Recruitment to the WFA surged before World War II (figure 4.4). Interest and confidence in the mission rose in 1938, buoyed by support from First Lady Eleanor Roosevelt, and, later, AMA leadership and the Federal Council of Churches of Christ in America. Physicians became more tolerant, if not enthusiastic, about the ASCC's women-led educational arm. Illig's network distributed millions of informational flyers and collected six-figure amounts for the cancer society. By 1939, the WFA involved forty-eight state commanders, squads of deputy commanders, adjutants, vice and city commanders, and majors supervising thousands of captains (1,872), lieutenants (5,574), and sergeants (6,495), along with hundreds of corporals and directors, and several hundred thousand troops.[53,72,73]

Dr. Mary F. Waring, a Chicago physician and president of the National Association of Colored Women's Clubs, signed on as a national WFA adviser. On paper, the ASCC welcomed the association's involvement. In the ASCC's bulletin, Illig referred to separate Black and white WFA units in Washington, DC, where a "negro" division proceeded under the "able leadership" of Mrs. Julia West Hamilton assisted by four vice-commanders and a "committee of six negro women doctors." That and a "colored division" in Kentucky were exceptions, however (figure 4.5). The WFA became most rooted in white, rural communities.[8,53,74]

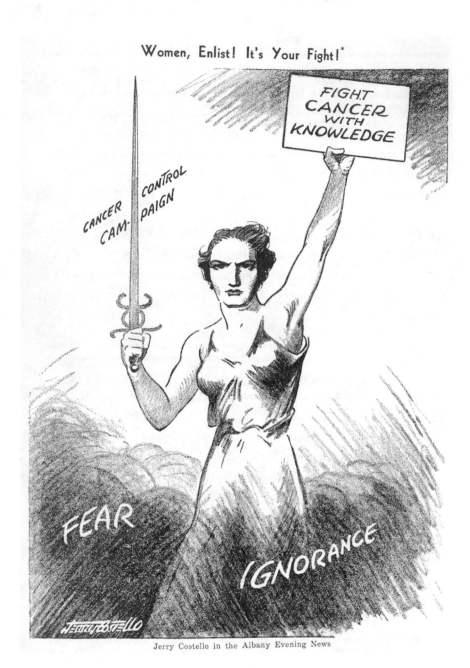

4.4 Illustration by Jerry Costello (*Albany Evening News*, republished in June 1937 *ASCC Bulletin*)

Reproduced with permission of Tom Costello, scan courtesy of the New York Academy of Medicine Library

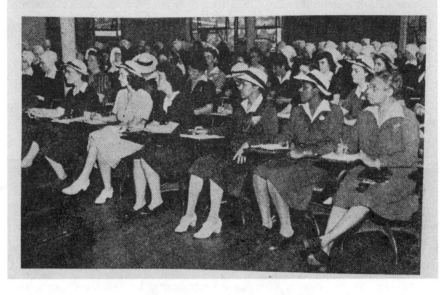

SUMMER COURSE IN CANCER EDUCATION HELD IN KENTUCKY PROVES POPULAR

4.5 Program on cancer for teachers and nurses, Kentucky Division of the Field Army (*Field Army News*, vol. 5; New York: ACS, 1946)
Courtesy of the American Cancer Society and Ebling Library, UW-Madison

The Field Army thrived in areas where contemporary information about disease was otherwise absent and where doctors didn't feel threatened by women's involvement in health education. The Maine division became an early anticancer stronghold under Commander Mrs. William (Marjorie) Scribner Holt. At a meeting in Lewiston, Maine, Dr. Howard Clute of Boston offered comments on doctors' emerging openness to women's involvement in cancer education: "In the past, as you know, it was quite unethical for physicians to discuss the management of disease in public," Clute said. "It is encouraging to note that the education of lay people in medical matters has progressed sufficiently so that *they* are now *demanding* information." Against "cancer phobia," he cautioned, "Do not be scared by our talk today," he stated. "You should not fear the surgery—you should fear the chance of having a cancer unremoved."[75]

A sad cancer story, "Pattern for Three," was then circulating in *Redbook* magazine. This novel by Mary Hastings Bradley tells of an Illinois woman whose comfortable life is upended by her son's death in a storm on Lake Michigan and her husband's affair with his secretary. Soon after divorcing, she notices a breast lump. After surgery by one of "the best doctors" in Rochester, Minnesota (the Mayo Clinic is not named), she's told she'll be fine. Months later, her cancer returns. The protagonist, disfigured, suffers pain, becomes gaunt, and asks her ex-husband to ensure she'll have morphine until death. The grim ending countered the ASCC's positive message about cancer and surgery. When Dr. Clute spoke before the Maine women, he may have been responding to this popular tale.[76,77]

In early 1938, cancer fighter Congressperson Edith Nourse Rogers, Republican of Lowell, Massachusetts, proposed that the president designate April as "Cancer Control Month." This would periodically galvanize doctors, journalists, and women about cancer, she considered. That February, Rogers and national WFA commander Illig spoke on NBC radio in a segment called "Women, Enlist, This Is Your War." In a scripted on-air conversation, Illig addressed the appropriateness of battling cancer amid a threatened world order. She referred to ongoing conflicts in Spain and China, and then stated:

> But our war is of a very different kind. It is a war to save human life, a war for health and happiness. We are not using bayonets or tanks or machine guns: our weapons are leaflets and lectures. We are fighting with facts and our military objectives are the putting [sic] to rout of fear and ignorance. This war is against one of the greatest enemies of health. It is against cancer.

Rogers, in turn, implored all women to enlist in the WFA: "Whether we like it or not we are all involved. . . . We all are potential victims."

Education, what we'd call "awareness," was prized by both women: "Your war is an educational one?" Rogers asked. "Yes," Illig replied. "We shall build a continually enlarging body of our citizens who are interested in cancer, who know a few simple facts . . . and who will be guided by this knowledge in protecting themselves." On radio, she reviewed cancer's warning signs; she advised listeners to see a physician if they noticed symptoms and to get an annual physical examination. Rogers closed the program by praising the late Marie Curie, who "gave her life to a cause just as much as any one of France's heroes upon the battlefields." She likened Curie to a "modern Joan of Arc, who has led the fight against the most insidious, dread disease our world has suffered."[78]

Don't be defenseless against cancer was their joint message to Americans in the year before World War II began. How many people heard the broadcast can't be known. Congress did heed Rogers's suggestion. It passed a bill designating April as "Cancer Control Month," a tradition that continues to this day.

The cancer society was more visible than ever. Yet in March 1938, the ASCC had just over a thousand members and was losing money. To celebrate its twenty-fifth anniversary, it held a "quiet" dinner in New York City. At the dinner Waldemar B. Kaempffert, the *New York Times* science editor and president of the National Association of Science Writers, spoke on behalf of the press, the Associated Press reported.[79]

Needing money, the ASCC pushed hard and successfully for WFA recruitment, dubbing April "Enlistment Month." In a celebratory coast-to-coast radio show, actor Spencer Tracy talked up the women's "army" with three expert men: Surgeon General Thomas Parran, C. C. Little, and Dr. Ellis Fischel of St. Louis. In preparation for Enlistment Month, the society distributed over a million pamphlets and hundreds of thousands of WFA enlistment pins and stickers.[72,73,80]

"Public interest in the cancer problem is now at the highest point in history," said Dr. James Ewing in April 1938. Ewing, a pathologist at New York's Memorial Hospital, was one of the world's most renown cancer experts. As a teenager, he'd suffered for much of two years with a deep leg bone infection. Contemporary physicians and John D. Rockefeller Jr., the hospital's benefactor, held the famously "crippled," kind, and brilliant physician in high esteem. Ewing was on the receiving end of John D. Rockefeller Jr.'s checks through his employment at Memorial Hospital. At this time, construction was underway for a new building on Manhattan's east side, at a cost of around $5 million, which would open the next year.

Speaking before the National Academy of Sciences in Washington, DC, Ewing credited the cancer society with a "radical change" in cancer publicity since 1913. While the organization had "failed to reach" those who are uneducated, the WFA entered new "territory" by discussing cancer in schools and canvassing "the lower classes," Ewing said. "The Women's Field Army is one of the most significant efforts yet made in the history of cancer control in this or any country."[81–83]

Ewing cautioned philanthropists about hype: naïve donors, whose approach to cancer is "highly emotional, which perhaps is not to be deprecated, but at the same time it is gravely lacking in intelligent comprehension of the nature of the problem" are vulnerable, he considered. Like patients, donors might get swindled by sensational reports of investigators promising rapid success. Cancer is not one disease, Ewing reminded his 1938 audience. Finding cures would take time.[84,85]

When Dr. Anna C. Palmer launched the Cured Cancer Club in 1938, she wasn't looking for camaraderie. Her goal was to persuade the public that cancer is curable. Palmer, a retired Massachusetts physician, felt fine eighteen years after breast cancer treatment—and she wanted everyone to know it! Palmer traveled to New York City for the ASCC's anniversary dinner, spoke at the opening of a "Cancer Can Be Cured" exhibit at Rockefeller Center, and met with national WFA commander Illig. As if on tour, she visited Buffalo, where she posed for photos with other Cured Cancer Club members at the State Institute for the Study of Malignant Disease (figure 4.6).[86,87]

That April, Florida's *Tampa Tribune* ran a story, "Cured Cancer Patients Will Organize Club." Mrs. Wayne Thomas, a Florida WFA captain, set up the chapter. Mrs. L. A. Dreyfus, of Staten Island and Daytona Beach, volunteered as its charter member. Palmer's group—the earliest known patient organization for people affected by cancer—did not welcome impostors: "Membership is limited to cases vouched for by recognized physicians." Eleven states besides Florida had established chapters, the *Tribune* reported.[88]

The club grew. "I have had cancer and I have been cured of it," said James P. Roe, a businessman, in April 1939 on CBS radio in an afternoon *Highways to Health* program sponsored by the New York Academy of Medicine. Until recent years, mentioning cancer was taboo, Roe said. He described several close friends who were stricken: "They were palsied with fear. They tried to conceal the affliction even from themselves. Delay was their fatal mistake." Roe told his story. After he noticed a lump at the back of his tongue, his doctor immediately

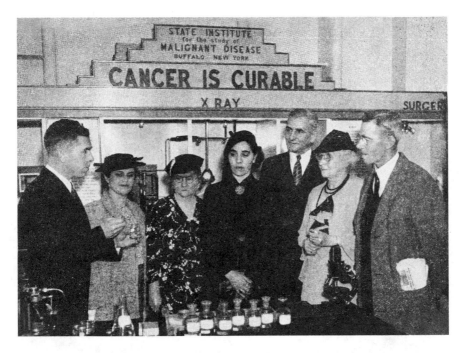

4.6 Cured Cancer Club members visiting a "Cancer Is Curable" exhibit at the State Institute for the Study of Malignant Disease in Buffalo, NY (*ASCC Bulletin*, May 1938)
Courtesy of the American Cancer Society and New York Academy of Medicine Library

referred him to a specialist who diagnosed a malignancy. The next morning, Roe began x-ray treatments. After the tumor shrank, doctors injected radium seeds. Roe acknowledged experiencing discomfort and losing his sense of taste. But it was worth getting treated: "Now I feel well," he said. "In common with the thousands of men and women who have been cured of cancer, I go about my daily work."

Deaths from cancer stem from "neglect," Roe told CBS radio listeners. Harm results from "delay in detecting, disclosing and treating" cancer and "dalliance with other than proper treatment," he said. "Other dread diseases have been conquered because fear of them had been dissipated. . . . The same applies to cancer. It is my hope that people generally—in all walks of life—will become cancer conscious." In retrospect, Roe's wish that everyone become "cancer conscious" sounds like a plea for awareness. And that is exactly what the first Cured Cancer Club was about: boosting perception that cancer could be successfully treated.

Dr. Palmer next took the microphone. Decades earlier, when she was in medical school, "even the best informed physicians were gloomy about the chances of recovering from cancer," she said. On the radio, Palmer didn't utter the word "breast" or detail her case: "I was operated upon. Two weeks later I was discharged from the hospital. Since that time I have been in the best of health, without pain or soreness or any sort or physical difficulty." Despite so much education, newspaper and radio programs, "many people still feel that cancer is incurable," she lamented. This is "one of the great tragedies of the present day."

"Men and women will talk about almost any disease except cancer," Palmer said. "Those of us in the Cured Cancer Club want to change all that." She would soon turn eighty-three and expressed delight: "I can imagine no better way of celebrating my birthday tomorrow than by receiving letters from people who are interested in the Cured Cancer Club, or in the work of the Women's Field Army against cancer."

The CBS broadcast was unprecedented. "Never before has there been a radio program in which the two principal participants were patients who had been cured of cancer," said Dr. Frank E. Adair, a cancer surgeon of Memorial Hospital, in the concluding segment. "A few years ago, it might have been considered difficult to find patients who had been cured of cancer. But not so today!"[89,90]

As war in central Europe became imminent, the WFA marched on. The ASCC commended women for their fieldwork. Little gave awards to Palmer and four WFA commanders at a dinner at New York's Roosevelt Hotel. Speaking at that March 1939 event, Dr. Bowman C. Crowell, a pathologist, justified an "army" against cancer:

> Surely an invader who killed 140,000 of our countrymen every year by force of arms . . . would be stoutly opposed by as great an aggregation of warriors and armament as the country could command. The million and a half cancer victims of the past ten years deserve the same kind of avengement . . . and the same chance for escape, that the defenders would give the civilians in a besieged city.

Women inject "drama, romance, [and] appeal to the public's fighting instinct against a destructive, cruel enemy," Crowell said. He flattered the WFA leaders, praising their knowledge of cancer and treatment. Women could deploy an innate quality, "a certain propensity for finesse and strategy" with which they are endowed, he indicated. "I adjure you, officers of the Women's Field Army, to look to the medical profession for your orders."[91]

In April 1939, George Gallup's American Institute of Public Opinion confirmed that cancer was the most unwanted disease: 76 percent of Americans said they'd "hate" to have it, as compared with tuberculosis (13 percent), heart trouble (9 percent), or pneumonia (2 percent). Four in ten Americans thought cancer is "catching" or might be so. "Fortunately, the majority of Americans have already realized that cancer can be halted or cured," Gallup noted. Attitudes varied by region, age, and income. In eastern states, people tended to view cancer as curable "if caught in time," while southerners and westerners held more pessimistic views. In general, younger and wealthier individuals were better informed. The ASCC touted the survey findings to support its educational mission.

"Almost every other person has some theory about what causes cancer," Gallup wrote in a syndicated newspaper article. Respondents named all sorts of culprits:

> Smoking, drinking, vaccinations, colds, infections, warts and moles, a bad diet, canned foods, certain kinds of cooking vessels, modern diet, too much milk, lack of vitamins, electric shocks and burns, using dirty dishes, adulterated food, the use of vinegar, the use of food preservatives, too much acid-forming foods and drinks, swallowing phlegm, swallowing uncooked foods, swallowing seeds, coal dust and sunburn.

Gallup's list continued. Some people thought that mental states including "jealousy," "resentment," and "bad thoughts" could be cancer-inducing, he reported. Neither he nor the ASCC clarified which of these putative causes were incorrect.[92–94]

The cancer society tried variously to convey statistical information (figures 4.7 and 4.8). At the Minnesota State Fair, the WFA exhibited two enlarged Telefact charts. One depicted the aging U.S. population; another compared cancer deaths with the number of men killed during the first World War. The Telefact charts came, with permission, by way of Pictorial Statistics, a New York firm directed by Mr. Rudolf Modley. In the late 1930s, demand for visual representations of scientific information was such that Modley employed a team of designers who prepared figures—infographics—for advertisers, newspapers, and other clients. As told in the *New Yorker*, Modley and his mentor, Otto Neurath of Vienna, ascribed to the view that people struggle to comprehend numeric facts expressed in words: to be sure the average man grasps an idea, "you'd better resort to pictures." Nearby the Telefact charts at the Minnesota fair, the women placed a six-foot-high woodcut of a "large flaming sword" above a removable base that read "WOMEN'S FIELD ARMY."[95,96]

In Colorado, Mrs. A. G. Fish manned a booth at the National Western Stock Show where, in January, a predictable influx of crowds provided opportunity to distribute cancer pamphlets and enlist members. Wherever people gathered—at fairs in rural regions, or urban hubs like department stores and train stations—the WFA set up shop. For Americans who had no other way of finding reliable information about cancer, ASCC materials may have been a lifeline.[97]

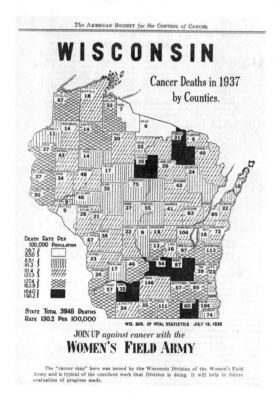

4.7 "Cancer map" issued by the WFA Wisconsin Division (*National Bulletin of the ASCC*, December 1939)

Courtesy of the American Cancer Society and New York Academy of Medicine Library

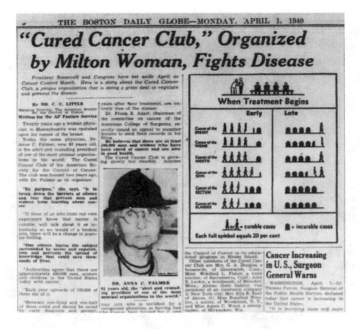

4.8 1940 Associated Press story on the Cured Cancer Club by C. C. Little with infographic on early and late cancer detection. Each walking figure ("curable") or tombstone ("incurable") represents 20 percent of cancer cases treated early or late.

(*Boston Daily Globe*, April 1, 1940)

Four months before World War II started, the World's Fair opened in Queens, New York. At an exhibit sponsored by the NYC Cancer Committee and curated by Frederick Hoffman's daughter, Ella Hoffman Rigney, "Cancer Woman" was a standout attraction (figure 4.9). Onto a life-size Bakelite woman's figure, a "spot of light" indicating breast cancer would appear and then momentarily enlarge, representing a tumor's local growth. Successive points of light marked cancer's spread to glands of the armpit and neck, then to lungs and bones. Cancer Woman demonstrated that "cancer invariably starts in one spot and can be eradicated more readily in its early stages," Rigney explained. The exhibit drew more than a million visitors, she reported in the NYC Cancer Committee's *Quarterly Review*.[98,99]

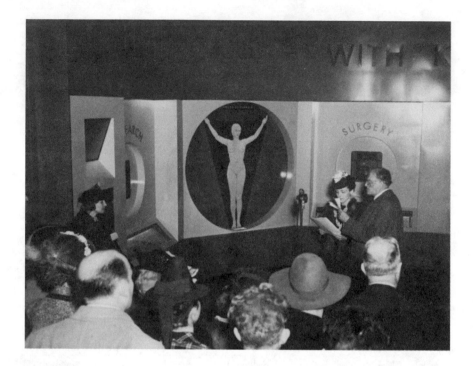

4.9 "Cancer Woman" in an exhibit on cancer by the NYC Cancer Committee of the ASCC
at the 1939–1940 World's Fair in Flushing Meadows, Queens, New York

New York Public Library Digital Collections, https://digitalcollections.nypl.org/
items/5e66b3e8-7aa1-d471-e040-e00a180654d7.

Not surprisingly, the women's army of lay cancer educators met resistance from
doctors. The ASCC publicist Clifton Read recounted these harsh words of a
"leading" physician: "They tell me that chronic irritation causes cancer. Well, if
you want my opinion, cancer publicity must cause a lot of cancer. It's the most
irritating stuff I've ever read." Read responded to "this rather sour comment" by
advising anticancer troops to avoid "an irritating approach." Instead, they should
encourage hope. "What they do need is courage gained from the knowledge that
the disease can be cured in its early stages," Read wrote. With these concerns in
mind, WFA slogans emphasized optimism—as in "Cancer Can Be Controlled"
and "Early Is the Watchword for Cancer Control" (figure 4.10).[100]

The ASCC insisted its educational programs were helping patients, and armed
women with information supporting that claim. At a northeastern regional WFA

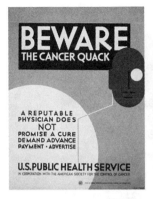 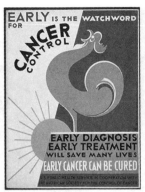 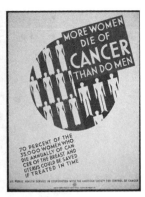

4.10 Cancer education posters produced by the U.S. Public Health Service in cooperation with the American Society for the Control of Cancer, 1936–1938
(Library of Congress)

assembly, Dr. Adair reported supportive studies. For instance, one institution found that in 1920 54 percent of breast cancer patients had "arrived too late" for surgery and by 1937, at the same hospital, only 13 percent were inoperable. "Education among women is catching hold rapidly and is of life-saving value," he stated. "From the medical profession in nearly every state come reports that there has been a definite increase . . . in early diagnosis and treatment, particularly among women," Illig wrote. "No news could be more heartening than this."[96,101]

Reports about cancer were amplified in Americans' minds by tragic stories in books and movies. In April 1939, Warner Bros. released *Dark Victory* starring Bette Davis as a vivacious young equestrian with brain cancer. This Hollywood movie has a straightforward central cancer plot: the protagonist receives a malignant diagnosis, and dies. The details are telling: Davis's character falls in love with her neurosurgeon, a Manhattan doctor who smokes and drinks. After he performs a neurological exam, orders x-rays, and advises surgery, she's plainly terrified: "I don't want to be a guinea pig," she says, expressing a common fear about cancer treatment. On screen, her doctors weigh telling her the truth—that the malignancy will recur—and decide against it. Telling her would be pointless, they say. Soon enough, however, the patient happens upon her open file. She

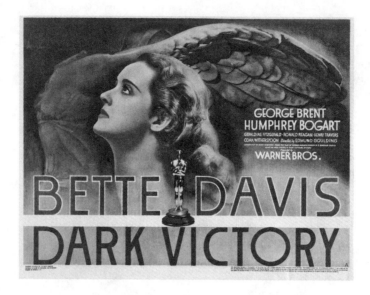

4.11 Poster for the 1939 movie *Dark Victory*, about a young woman who dies from brain cancer.

reads "prognosis negative" and realizes she will die. The film, based on the 1932 play *In Time's Course* by George E. Brewer Jr., earned admiring reviews and three Oscar nominations (figure 4.11).[102–105]

The ASCC sought to counter narratives it considered unduly negative. "An Appeal to Writers" stated, "Popular attitudes towards cancer have lagged behind medical progress. This is tragic since one's attitude toward the disease may determine the outcome of an encounter with it." The society singled out cancer in Daphne du Maurier's *Rebecca* as "the final shocking note in a study of terror." Alfred Hitchcock adapted the best-selling 1938 novel into a 1940 movie which won multiple Oscars including best picture.

Although malignancy enters late in *Rebecca*, it plays a pivotal role. The dark, romantic tale is narrated from the perspective of a young woman who marries an English landowner, Maxim de Winter. Their marriage is threatened by de Winter's haunting memories of his beautiful first wife, Rebecca. It turns out she'd been cruel and promiscuous. De Winter killed her. When Rebecca's body is found in a sunken boat, de Winter is suspected of murder. After an inquest deems the death a suicide, her cousin questions the verdict: Rebecca was strong-willed; she never would have taken her life, he insists. Only at the novel's end, upon an interview with a London doctor whom Rebecca had secretly consulted, does the reader learn that she was suffering from cancer:

"The pain was slight as yet, but the growth was deep-rooted," [the doctor] said, "and in three or four months' time she would have been under morphia. An operation would have been no earthly use at all. I told her that. The thing had got too firm a hold. There is nothing anyone can do in a case like that, except give morphia, and wait."

Once it's established that Rebecca knew she had cancer, her suicide becomes plausible. Her cousin no longer challenge the verdict and de Winter is cleared of murder charges. The story reflected common understanding of cancer as a death sentence.[106,107]

The ASCC took issue with several other works of fiction. In *Night Music*, Clifford Odets's short-lived Broadway play, "the detective, A. L. Rosenberger, suffers bitter agonies from incurable cancer." *Of Lena Geyer*, a 1936 novel about an opera singer, ends with "a vivid description of cruel death "And in *Idiot's Delight*, a Pulitzer–winning play and 1939 movie starring Clark Gable, a character suggests that cancer is incurable: "Dr. Waldersee in 'Idiot's Delight' remarks inaccurately that there is as yet no remedy for cancer," the ASCC complained in its bulletin.[108]

After Germany invaded Poland in September 1939, WFA activities continued. In Colorado, Boy Scouts delivered tens of thousands of WFA flyers to residents of Denver and Colorado Springs. "Each Boy Scout is to take six pieces of literature, ring the doorbell, and hand it to the lady of the house," detailed the state commander, Mrs. Emily G. Bogert. Personal delivery would ensure the ASCC's message would be received: "Boy Scouts are respected, and I do not believe many of these will be thrown in the waste paper basket without reading," she wrote. In 1941, a WFA booth at the Florida State Fair attracted so many thousands of visitors that counting became "impossible." Many who stopped by were "Latins" including "Spaniards and Italians," reported Mrs. A. Malcolm Smith. "Negroes seemed especially interested and were invited to pass literature on to their friends," she said. Supplies of a pamphlet on "Cancer Facts for Men" ran out.[109,110]

Military metaphors seem not to have troubled contemporary participants in the anticancer crusade. During World War II, the ASCC doubled down on military style and phrases. The society published a U.S. map-like illustration highlighting "cancer defense" forces (figure 4.12). "April is our battle month," Illig

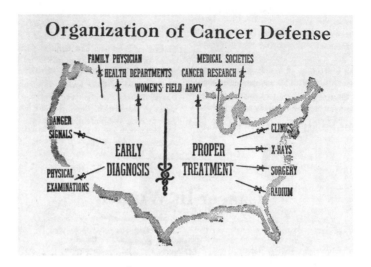

4.12 Wartime illustration of U.S. anticancer defenses (*ASCC Bulletin*, April 1941)
Courtesy of the American Cancer Society and New York Academy of Medicine Library

declared in a February 1941 speech. "Our foe is a stealthy one; it has rightly been called the fifth column disease".[111]

"War cancels national assembly," the society announced in January 1942. A month after the Pearl Harbor bombing, WFA leaders finally cut back. Regional activities continued in Montana and a handful of other states where the ASCC sponsored multiday cancer "training schools" to educate WFA officers about cancer biology and treatments. Little remained defiant, however, refusing to let the World War kill the war against cancer. In March 1943, he decried the "somewhat hysterical rush towards any obvious war activity." In 1944 a new group of cancer fighters, led by Mrs. Mary Lasker, took over the ASCC and renamed it the American Cancer Society.[112–115]

By the end of World War II Americans were more familiar with cancer even if they didn't talk about it much. Most doctors remained fatalistic, and public demand for standard treatments stayed low. What did advance in the 1930s was cancer activism by ordinary people. The WFA aroused hundreds of thousands of women. Their messages of optimism seeded post-war enthusiasm for research and care of cancer patients.

CHAPTER 5

A CELEBRITY CAUSE (1945–1960)

When Henrietta Lacks entered the Johns Hopkins gynecology clinic in January 1951 she was worried about a "knot" on her womb. For a while, she'd sensed something was wrong. She'd been bleeding irregularly and experiencing pain during intercourse. Lacks consulted a local practitioner, who initially thought she had syphilis. After a test for that venereal disease came back negative, he advised her to get checked by experts at the Baltimore hospital.

Lacks was thirty years old, Black, and suffering from cervical cancer. She, a mother of five, lived with her family in Turner Station, east of Baltimore. Henrietta and her husband, David, a Bethlehem Steel worker, came from Virginia. As children they'd harvested tobacco. At fourteen, Henrietta delivered her first baby and her education stopped. Segregation was legal in 1951 Maryland. Some hospitals wouldn't treat Black patients. At Johns Hopkins, Black people received care in separate clinics and wards provided by doctors and nurses who were, for the most part, white.

A doctor reached Lacks by phone the next week. A biopsy, taken at the clinic, showed cancer. She should return to Johns Hopkins for treatment, he said. During surgery, doctors stitched radium to her cervix and, without her knowing, sent a bit of her tumor to a research lab. After Lacks left the hospital, it seemed her tumor had disappeared. Back at home and feeling well, she didn't mention the cancer to relatives or neighbors.

Doctors were so pleased with Lacks's response to radium that they prescribed x-ray treatments, daily on weekdays, for a month. By giving extra, or *adjuvant*, external radiation therapy, physicians hoped to prolong her remission. Of course these terms would have sounded like gibberish to Lacks or most anyone. Like most patients then, she accepted whatever doctors prescribed. There was no pretense of understanding risks or probability of treatment's benefit.

Lacks realized she'd need help with transportation to her daily radiation treatments, and then told her cousins about the cancer. Radiation was grueling in 1951. It charred her torso and caused nausea and fatigue. She was too exhausted to take the bus to and from Baltimore. As we'll see, modern cancer patients disclose their conditions for all sorts of reasons. Lacks's motivation to share her diagnosis was pragmatic: had there been no treatment, she might have stayed mum.

The malignancy returned by that summer, unfortunately. Lacks had difficulty walking and developed anemia and kidney failure. She re-entered Johns Hopkins for palliative treatment. When word about her condition got around Turner Station, relatives and neighbors lined up to donate blood. Lacks died at thirty-one in October 1951.[1]

Today we know about Henrietta Lacks because researchers immortalized her malignant cells in a laboratory. "HeLa" cells, as they're called, proved useful to scientists around the world. Yet Lacks never gave permission for doctors to use her tumor in this way. Nearly sixty years later, journalist Rebecca Skloot illuminated her story in best-selling book *The Immortal Life of Henrietta Lacks*. While investigators purchased and used HeLa cells for experiments, her family remained impoverished and under-educated.

Lacks's story speaks volumes about the plight of an ordinary cancer patient. With a limited grade school education, she was vulnerable to doctors' recommendations—good or bad. And as a Black woman, she was susceptible to racist behavior of some practitioners. She sought care and followed advice of physicians at a leading medical institution, received support from her family and community, and died nonetheless. An observer might have deemed her treatments futile.

Confidence in American science surged after World War II. Yet clinical progress against cancer remained modest. In this era, scientists applied powerful electron microscopes to visualize cell compartments, acquiring knowledge of biology that would be crucial for elucidating how cancers grow. Chemists deciphered how proteins fold, enabling subsequent investigators to envision and probe how hormones bind receptors. The 1953 discovery of DNA's structure by

Watson and Crick, Franklin and Wilkins led to gene sequencing. But that took decades! These laboratory developments—now applicable to everyday cancer care—would have been imperceptible to most doctors and patients in the early postwar years.

Chemotherapy was the main advance. Before 1945, specialists disapproved of using medicines to treat cancer. Experts insisted that surgery, external x-ray (radiation) treatments, or radium applied internally, were the only valid remedies. After World War I, scientists knew that mustard gas, used as a chemical weapon, halted growth of white blood cells; some inferred that it might reduce malignancies of those cells (lymphomas and leukemias). In 1943, the bombing of an American ship holding a stash of chemical weapons in the Italian port of Bari exposed servicemen and civilians to toxic gas. Hundreds died, and autopsies showed depletion of blood cells—a clue to the chemical's power. Around this time, a Yale surgeon observed that nitrogen mustard shrank lymphoma patients' cancerous glands. As later reported by Dr. Vincent DeVita Jr. in *The Death of Cancer*, information about the potent chemical was restricted until the war's end. This knowledge boosted doctors' enthusiasm for trying chemical therapy— chemotherapy—against cancer. Antibiotics against bacteria were becoming available in the 1940s. The concept of deploying chemicals, like "penicillin for cancer," appealed to physicians and the public.[2–7]

Cancer specialists began experimenting with antimetabolite drugs—compounds that interfere with DNA replication and cell growth—and observed encouraging results in children with leukemia or lymphoma. Most remissions were transient, however, and few adults with "solid" tumors—like melanoma, breast or colon cancer—responded favorably to these agents tried singularly. Chemotherapy made patients feel and look sick. It caused nausea and vomiting, hair loss, permanent hearing loss; it damaged bone marrow, kidneys, and other organs. It weakened patients' immune systems, enabling killer infections. Because these medicines were so harsh, "chemotherapists"—the administering physicians—earned a bad reputation even among doctors. Chemotherapy's benefits were far from evident, while toxicity was obvious.

It would be a long time, around fifty years, before many cancers could be treated and a good fraction cured. To this day, many people believe chemotherapy treatment is worse than the disease.

～

In August 1948, baseball legend Babe Ruth died from cancer. The "Bambino" was said not to know of his diagnosis; he never spoke of it publicly. While he was hospitalized at New York's Memorial Hospital for the Treatment of Cancer and Allied Diseases, newspapers headlined the ups and downs of his medical condition with language of sports pages: "Babe Reported Rallying Today," "Keep Slugging, Babe," and "Ruth Loses Ground In Life Battle." They said he suffered from a cold or "throat ailment," and did not use the word "cancer."

George Herman Ruth was a physically strong, big-hearted and imperfect man, beloved by baseball fans everywhere. He had a rough childhood, rocky career, and volatile marriage. Before his eighth birthday, Ruth's parents had sent him to a Baltimore reform school. By age nineteen, he'd signed with the Boston Red Sox. During World War I, he became famous hitting home runs. In 1920, he joined the New York Yankees. His popularity was such that when the new Yankee Stadium opened in 1923, people called it the "House That Ruth Built." He shattered records. Ruth's personal life was tumultuous, however, and his behavior self-destructive. He drank and ate heavily. Before doctors labeled tobacco a carcinogen, he enjoyed smoking cigars and often chewed tobacco.

In 1946, Ruth's voice became hoarse. At fifty-one, he complained of left eye pain and headaches. His face became swollen, he had difficulty swallowing and lost eighty pounds. That fall, doctors found a mass at the base of his skull. He had surgery during a long hospitalization in New York City's French Hospital. Radiation treatments caused his hair to fall out. By the next spring, Ruth appeared well. In April 1947, he celebrated "Babe Ruth Day" at Yankee Stadium before a crowd. By June 1947, however, Ruth's cancer recurred. He received an experimental chemotherapy (teropterin, an antimetabolite) by injection over six weeks from Dr. Richard Lewisohn, a surgeon at New York's Mount Sinai Hospital. Ruth's doctors thought he had a laryngeal (voice box) tumor. But as reported fifty years later, review of his medical charts and autopsy indicate that he had nasopharyngeal cancer, a rare malignancy of the throat.[8–10]

It's hard to believe that Ruth didn't know he had cancer. Although it's been reported that he didn't provide written consent for his treatment, Ruth did understand its investigational nature: "I realized that if anything was learned about that type of treatment, whether good or bad, it would be of use in the future to the medical profession and maybe to a lot of people with my same trouble," he told a biographer. Initially, the drug appeared to help: doctors observed reduction in his swollen neck glands. Ruth felt better and ate comfortably.[11,12]

Without naming the celebrity patient, Lewisohn reported on Ruth's case at a medical conference. Word leaked. On September 11, 1947, the *Wall Street Journal* ran a front-page headline about a possible cancer cure. "Success on 'Famous Figure,'" the article proclaimed. It detailed the case of a male celebrity, age fifty-two, treated by Lewisohn in New York. An announcement by Lederle Laboratories, teropterin's manufacturer, prompted this news. Lederle had reported that two chemicals demonstrated promising anticancer activity in mice and some "hopeless" patients. The *Journal* referred to nearly a hundred patients in Boston trying Lederle's anticancer drugs.[13,14]

Ruth's second remission was short-lived. In June 1948, he was admitted to Memorial Hospital where his treatments included radiation and implanted gold seeds.[10] On July 26, he left the hospital for a few hours to see the premiere of *The Babe Ruth Story*. Outside of Broadway's Astor Theatre, a police cordon insulated Ruth from a pushing, cheering crowd. He was "a sick man," the *New York Times* observed: "Ruth walked slowly into the theatre, supported by both arms, perspiring heavily, and seemingly too ill to do anything but smile wanly." Ruth left halfway through, the *New York World-Telegram* reported. Producers arranged for a private viewing inside Memorial Hospital (figure 5.1).

It was Ruth's final outing. One can only imagine what it was like for a dying man to see his life and unstated medical condition enacted on the big screen, reviewed and discussed. At the movie's end, Ruth's character submits his body to science. A body on a stretcher is wheeled down a hospital corridor. Ruth said he thought the movie was "wonderful." Critics disagreed. Writing for the *New York Herald Tribune*, theater critic Otis Guernsey Jr. called it "the Babe's worst inning."[15–18]

Memorial Hospital employed a spokesperson to provide updates on Ruth's condition. Boys sat on a stoop outside waiting and, reportedly, praying. Photographers grabbed and published photos of his wife, sister, and daughter when they visited. He died at age fifty-three in August 1948.

Babe Ruth wasn't the only famous cancer patient of 1948. As told by Dr. Siddhartha Mukherjee in *The Emperor of All Maladies*, Einar Gustafson, a twelve-year-old boy with lymphoma, became the face of the Children's Cancer Research Foundation, a Boston charity. For fundraising purposes, organizers gave him an

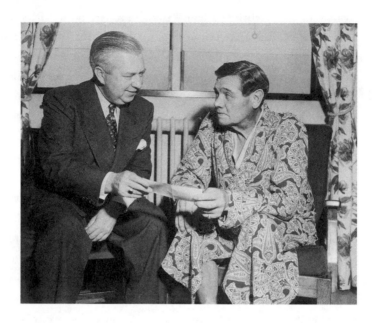

5.1 Babe Ruth, right, at Memorial Hospital, with Steve Broidy of Allied Artists movie studio, accepting a check for the Ruth Foundation, July 29, 1948
AP photo (with permission)

American-sounding name, "Jimmy." They may also have wanted to protect Gustafson's privacy.

"Jimmy is suffering from cancer. But he doesn't know he has it," said Ralph Edwards, host of the popular radio show, *Truth or Consequences*, to a nationwide audience. He's a "swell little guy" who loves baseball, Edwards said before reaching Gustafson by phone in a Boston hospital room. The boy greeted listeners and, responding to a question, said he hoped the Boston Braves would win that year's baseball pennant. Soon Braves team members filed into his hospital room bearing gifts. On radio, "Jimmy" led the team in singing "Take Me Out to the Ball Game." After the call, Edwards asked listeners to aid cancer research by donating to the Children's Cancer Research Foundation.

The show delivered over $200,000 and terrific publicity for the "Jimmy Fund," as it became known. In this new charity, the Variety Club of New England had joined with Dr. Sidney Farber, a Harvard pathologist who was treating hospitalized children with experimental chemotherapy. The fund would build a brighter facility for cancer patients and researchers, and it succeeded by crowdfunding.

Famous baseball players supported this cause and encouraged fans to give. Ordinary people chipped in: at sports stadiums, people dropped coins and bills into Jimmy Fund cans; at movie theaters, filmgoers did the same. Boys in Little League baseball uniforms went door-to-door asking for contributions. While cash amounts collected were generally small—financially trivial, compared to donations registered at gala dinners—the Jimmy Fund fostered an "everyman's" feeling of responsibility for the cancer hospital.[19–21]

In New England, the Jimmy Fund became a community cause. Celebrities added visibility. In 1949, the actor Burt Lancaster was photographed breaking ground for the Jimmy Fund building, with Dr. Farber at his side. The facility opened in 1952. Later, the philanthropist Charles Dana began directing large grants to this charity. The institution widened its scope of care, admitting children and adults. It became the Dana-Farber Cancer Institute, a leading cancer hospital. In 1980 Billy Starr, a young man who'd lost his mother to melanoma, decided to raise money for this cause by organizing a bike ride and soliciting contributions. By 1982, a 187-mile marathon from Sturbridge in south-central Massachusetts to Cape Cod's Provincetown benefited the fund. Today, the Pan-Mass Challenge bikeathon brings hundreds of researchers, patients, family members, students, and other cyclists together to raise money for the Jimmy Fund. Annual proceeds, in the tens of millions of dollars, support "the Farber," as oncologists call the institute.[22–28]

"Jimmy," it turns out, did well too. For fifty years the public remained unaware of his healthy survivorship; many presumed him dead. In 1998, a tip from Gustafson's sister led journalists to the gray-haired, sixty-two-year-old truck driver. Newspapers around the country noted his height, at six feet and five inches, and fertility: he had three daughters and six grandchildren. Gustafson was "a picture of stamina and good health" and "in fact, thriving," the *Washington Post* reported. He ran a small business and owned houses in Maine and Buzzards Bay, Massachusetts. The *Boston Globe* headlined "Jimmy Fund Gets 50th Anniversary Gift: 'Jimmy.'" Gustafson's excellent outcome offered vital testimony. His wellness affirmed long-term benefits of cancer care and research.[29–31]

"We were taught when we were kids you didn't talk about those things. You didn't talk about sickness," Gustafson told the *Boston Globe* in 1998. As a child, "Jimmy" helped break that taboo. He died in 2001, at sixty-five years.[32]

Meanwhile the nation's largest cancer charity was operating under new management in New York. Between 1943 and 1945, Mary and Albert Lasker had taken over the ASCC and renamed it the American Cancer Society (ACS). Previously the society had aimed to educate doctors and the public by dispelling myths and spreading knowledge. Research had never been its goal. The Laskers prioritized science and installed business-minded friends on its board: Emerson Foote, an adman; Elmer Bobst, a pharmaceutical executive; and Eric Johnston, head of the U.S. Chamber of Commerce and upcoming president of the Motion Picture Association, assumed leadership positions.[33,34]

Mary Woodward Lasker would have a lasting impact on cancer philanthropy and medical science. Her education was remarkable: A Radcliffe graduate from Watertown, Wisconsin, she'd traveled through Europe and, before landing in New York City in the 1920s, studied briefly at Oxford. During the Great Depression, she started a successful fabric business and became secretary of the Birth Control Federation, a Planned Parenthood predecessor. In 1940, she married Albert D. Lasker, the creative, brilliant, and rich owner of the Lord & Thomas advertising agency who'd famously promoted Lucky Strike cigarettes. Albert had children from a prior marriage; Mary had none. After Albert's death in 1952 from colon cancer, Mary's dedication to the research cause became all-consuming.

A story about her motivation, shared by Lasker, is that as a child she'd accompanied her mother to visit a laundress who lived in poverty with seven children after having both breasts removed for cancer. After suffering "mutilation," the laundress continued working for many years, Lasker told an interviewer. "I recall noticing that cancer didn't have to be fatal even though it was very cruel." Decades later, after a household cook in New York City succumbed to cancer, Lasker was appalled by the lack of progress.

In 1943, she chatted up the subject with her friend Lois Mattox Miller, a *Reader's Digest* editor, and persuaded the journalist to write about cancer. Miller, for her part, persuaded the *Digest* publisher, DeWitt Wallace, to print a request for donations. Miller's three articles, starting in October 1944, led to an inundation of the ASCC's office with mail and contributions totaling over $120,000. Lasker soon gained a spot on the cancer society's board. She disagreed with the agency's director, C. C. Little, on matters of style and substance. By 1945, he was out. From then on, through Nixon's 1971 declaration of "war on cancer," a glitzier ACS raised millions to support cancer research.[35-41]

Mary Lasker's privileged volunteerism resembled that of Ellin Speyer, years earlier, and Elsie Mead. These well-connected, intelligent, and persistent women shared a passion for fighting illness and a willingness to ask acquaintances for donations. Doctors still talk about Lasker. That's in part because the Lasker Awards are among the most prestigious medical honors. And because she advocated for research, persuading politicians and donors to support their work. Dr. Jonas Salk, inventor of the polio vaccine, called her "a matchmaker between science and society."[36]

At the war's end, money poured into Memorial Hospital. On August 7, 1945—between the bombings of Hiroshima and Nagasaki—Alfred P. Sloan Jr., chair of General Motors, and Charles Kettering, GM's research director, held a press conference. The two friends announced a $4 million gift to establish the Sloan-Kettering Institute for Cancer Research affiliated with Memorial Hospital.[42]

The hospital's publicity department shifted into high gear, steering donations to the Memorial Cancer Center Fund and cranking out radio announcements with messages like these:

Cancer may not be the hopeless disease everyone thinks it is. At Memorial Cancer Center in New York City, extensive research and treatment has reduced the rate of deaths from those suffering with cancer of the breast by 30 percent.

Cancer kills more children than infantile paralysis.

Never say die! Leading doctors and scientists are working to find the control and cure for cancer.

"Hope" is replacing "Despair" in the treatment of cancer—for progress is being made toward control of this dread disease.

Business leaders set up Memorial Fund committees by industry: aviation, book publishing, chemical, liquor, retail banking, theater, etc., and by occupation: doctors (and, separately, doctors' wives), furriers, lawyers, shoemen, stockbrokers, and so forth. Memorial's fundraising plan differed from the geographically arranged ACS appeals, which followed lines of former ASCC "territories."

In December 1945, Mrs. Edward (Clelia) Delafield, chair of the Women's Division, spoke before a capacity crowd of a thousand over dinner at New York's Biltmore Hotel. She said, "The financial means to make a cancer crusade possible must come from every walk of life, from every race, color and creed. Cancer does not discriminate when it strikes one person out of every nine."[43]

New York City Mayor William O'Dwyer dedicated a week for this cause in February 1946. In department stores, hotels, restaurants, and theaters, volunteers solicited donations. That week, the Federation of Jewish Women's Organizations asked members to give. Local unions signed onto the campaign with the American Federation of Labor's approval. As did Memorial Hospital's night-time volunteers and nurses' aides. The season's debutantes, led by Miss Jean Coffin of Park Avenue, contributed. In 1948, fashion models employed by the elite Powers and Thornton agencies spent evenings canvassing: the attractive "Night Raiders" entered clubs at dinnertime, requested donations from each patron, and then returned at 11:30 p.m. for another round.

Speaking at a Lawyers' Club luncheon, Edward Delafield said that the fight against cancer had been handicapped by a "hush hush" attitude toward the disease. One purpose of Memorial's campaign was to overcome this attitude so that cancer would be treated early, while a cure is feasible, Delafield said. "People used to say that cancer was something to be ashamed of," he said. "Surely there is nothing disgraceful about such a disease."[44-45]

As Memorial Hospital enlarged so did the ACS. At annual galas co-orchestrated by the NYC Cancer Committee and ACS, scientists and philanthropists mingled. The local and national cancer campaigns were interrelated and, in general, synergistic. Well-heeled donors to the NYC Cancer Committee, nominally an ACS chapter, sought to improve care close to home. Elsewhere in the country, hospitals needed trained cancer surgeons. For this reason, the ACS supported fellowships at a handful of institutions including Memorial Hospital, expecting that trained specialists would settle in other U.S. regions—spreading expertise.[46-49]

It needs be said that Dr. Cornelius P. ("Dusty") Rhoads, who directed Memorial Hospital and research at the Sloan-Kettering Institute in the postwar era, was a racist with a profoundly disturbing history. In 1931, while in Puerto Rico working on a Rockefeller-funded anemia project, he'd drafted a letter to a colleague. Puerto Ricans were "beyond doubt the dirtiest, laziest, most degenerate and thievish race of men," he'd written. "What the island needs is not public health work but a tidal wave or something to totally exterminate the population. I have done my best to further the process of extermination by killing off eight" and by "transplanting cancer into several more." Rhoads said he was drunk when he penned this letter, which went unmailed and was found near his desk. It was "a joke," he claimed.[50-53]

Although the incident sparked outrage in Puerto Rico, mainland newspapers barely covered it. Rhoads's work—piloting clinical trials of chemicals against cancer—was celebrated by colleagues, by philanthropists, and by *Time* magazine on its cover. The Sloan-Kettering Institute, which he led, states on its website: "Rhoads's ties to the military and charges of unethical human experimentation would later sully his reputation as a pioneer of chemotherapy." Unfortunately, Rhoads was not singular in his racism; he was exceptional in his fame, in part because he worked at New York's prestigious Memorial Hospital. Modern scholars of racism in medicine, including oncology, are only beginning to uncover the prevalence of this issue.

An energized ACS, restructured under the Laskers' leadership, aimed for corporate efficiency. The Women's Field Army was deemed unsophisticated and dismantled. Old-fashioned education and fundraising continued (figures 5.2 and 5.3). Many business owners didn't want to simply write a check "for cancer"; they sought visibility in supporting the ACS. Gulf Oil, for instance, offered sixty days of its Louisiana billboard space to the society. F. W. Woolworth—a retail giant with thousands of stores, in large and small cities—approved use of Woolworth store windows for ACS displays. The U.S. postal service, for its part, shipped ACS posters to offices in every state, enough to place on both sides of nine thousand mail trucks. "This means 18,000 posters roving through the streets of the nation to help the cause," an ACS bulletin stated: "Watch for them in your community!".[54]

As the ACS grew, new cancer charities formed. An early spin-off, the Damon Runyon Cancer Research Foundation, exists to this day. Runyon was a popular journalist. After Runyon's 1946 death from throat cancer, his pal Walter Winchell, a gossip columnist and radio show host, set up a memorial fund. In 1949, comedian Milton Berle hosted the first charity telethon; the sixteen-hour

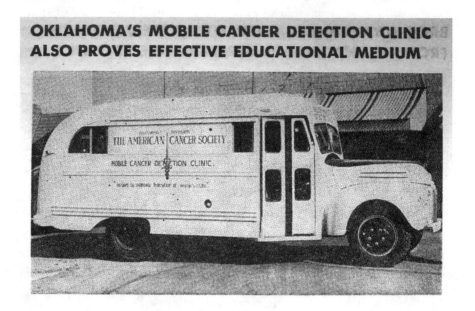

OKLAHOMA'S MOBILE CANCER DETECTION CLINIC ALSO PROVES EFFECTIVE EDUCATIONAL MEDIUM

5.2 ACS mobile cancer detection unit sponsored by the Oklahoma Federation of Women's Clubs (*Field Army News* 5, No. 9, September 1946)
Courtesy of the American Cancer Society, scan courtesy of Ebling Library, UW-Madison

NBC broadcast raised over $1 million for this cause. Also in New York, Rudolph and Antoinette de Villiers founded the Robert Roesler de Villiers Foundation after their son, Robbie, died from leukemia at age sixteen; their organization became the Leukemia Society and, eventually, the Leukemia & Lymphoma Society. Another agency, the Cancer Research Institute, focused on nonsurgical cancer treatments. Around this time, Cancer Care in New York began providing practical support for patients. While none of these charities approached the ACS in size or scope, they reflected a widening set of priorities among donors.[55–62]

In April 1946, more than a hundred women gathered at Toronto's Royal York Hotel to establish a Cured Cancer Club and "by their very presence [dispel] the bogey that the dread disease is incurable," the *Globe and Mail* reported. Each was alive at least five years after cancer treatment. "By no means invalids, the group last night was as keen and lively as school girls and talk of jobs, travel and future

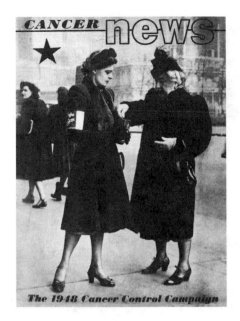

5.3 March 1948 cover of *Cancer News*, an ACS magazine

plans floated from table to table." The Toronto group had no apparent ties to the original Cured Cancer Club founded in 1938 by Dr. Anna Palmer, who had died during the war at age eighty-seven.[63,64]

By 1960, Cured Cancer Clubs had popped up in Baltimore; Boston; Lansing, Michigan; Cedar Rapids, Iowa; and elsewhere. In Washington, DC, a tireless Mrs. Oliver S. Kern—alive long after surgery for "intestinal cancer"— led a most active chapter involving dozens of men and women. In May 1950, the Washington club staged a fashion show at the Willard Hotel to benefit its "gift and loan closet" which provided cancer patients with suitable clothing after surgery. Models wore American-themed costumes such as a gown handed down from Dolly Madison and a plaid dress from "the wife of an officer in Lee's army." The *Washington Post* occasionally reported on the group's events such as dinners at the Fairfax Hotel or Capital Club, and tea at the Egyptian embassy.

The DC club wasn't only about patients being visible to demonstrate cancer's curability, as Palmer had intended. The Washington group took on new functions: camaraderie, peer support for survivors, and fundraising. "The important thing, which the Cured Cancer Club is doing, is to keep hope alive while avoiding false hope," the *Post* observed. (figure 5.4)[65–69]

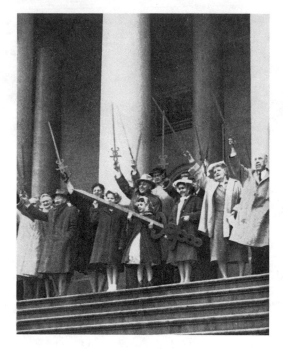

5.4 "Swords-up Salute to Cancer Crusade," Delegates to the first "Cured Cancer Congress" on steps of the U.S. Capitol (ACS *Bulletin* 7, no 5, April 28, 1958)

Courtesy of the American Cancer Society; scan courtesy of the Countway Library, Harvard Medical School

Unaffiliated individuals spread the "cured" message, too. In these years, Edward F. Reid—an Alabama lawyer who lived after colon cancer surgery—wrote, spoke, and toured the country as "Mr. Cured Cancer." Reid's national reputation was such that the Los Angeles ACS chapter flew him to California to give a keynote lecture at a luncheon kicking off its 1955 campaign. Reid was one of the first patients to speak, essentially as an advocate, before an audience of doctors and potential donors.[70–72]

The Washington, DC Cured Cancer Club impressed U.S. Senator Prescott Bush of Connecticut. At a 1956 ACS dinner in Hartford, he mentioned the group and, with hundreds of volunteers listening, urged formation of a local chapter. At the dinner, Dr. Matthew H. Griswold, head of Connecticut's cancer control group, received an award for compiling ninety thousand Connecticut case records. The comic pianist Victor Borge was glad to be seated next to Dr. Griswold, the *Hartford Courant* reported. "'He's supposed to know all about cancer,' Borge observed, 'and he's been smoking all night long. That's good for me because a close friend of mine just wrote a book about the evils of smoking, and it was so horrible that I decided to give up—reading.'"[73]

Deaths from lung cancer were rising and people wondered why. Many considered cigarettes culprits. In England, health officials acknowledged the smoking link ten years before their U.S. counterparts. In February 1954, a British medical committee found a complex but "established" relationship between smoking and lung cancer.[74,75] After the health minister told the House of Commons that young people should be cautioned about smoking's ill effects, American newspapers reported it variably. The *Baltimore Sun* placed "Sure Smoking–Lung Cancer Link" near the bottom of page 1; that story, printed in an inverted "L," framed another: "Smoker-Grandma Dies At Age Of 101." The *Los Angeles Times* squeezed "British Medics Link Smoking With Cancer" into the middle of a page 7 column. The *New York Times* gave little attention to the matter except in the stock pages: "Tobacco Issues Decline In London."[76–79]

Public debate over tobacco's role in causing cancer surfaced. *U.S. News & World Report* published a story titled, "Is There Proof That Smoking Causes Cancer?" featuring Q&A "with Dr. E. Cuyler Hammond," a Yale epidemiologist and ACS director of statistical research. In a gigantic nationwide ACS study led by Hammond and psychologist Daniel Horn, nurses and volunteers interviewed over 185,000 American men about their smoking habits and then monitored who developed cancer. Hammond and Horn spoke at the 1954 AMA meeting and published their findings and conclusion—that cigarette smoking almost certainly causes lung cancer in men—in the American Medical Association's journal. But doctors ignored the ACS report. Scientists such as Dr. Wilhelm Hueper of the NCI insisted that other factors, like auto fumes and air pollution, were greater causes.[80–82]

Newspapers highlighted doubts. Skeptics insisted that correlation does not mean causation; it could be that smokers are more cancer-prone than nonsmokers, they suggested. A *New York Times* piece, "Doctor Lauds Smoking," quoted a Harvard radiologist about a purported upside of cigarette smoking—that it "gives more pleasure to man than anything else."[83]

By this time, leaders of America's largest tobacco companies had decided to jointly counter emerging evidence of smoking's harms. They hired an aggressive PR firm, Hill and Knowlton, and formed the Tobacco Industry Research Committee. In the summer of 1954, tobacco industry representatives met with *New York Times* publisher Arthur Hays Sulzberger, *New York Herald Tribune* chair Helen Rogers

Reid, and *Time* and *Life* owner Roy Larsen, among others. The committee began funding scientists, many credible, who would either question the smoking-cancer link or dilute findings with information on other potential causes. As later told in *Merchants of Doubt*, they would "fight science with science" so that the public would keep on wondering about the validity of the ACS's and others' findings.[84]

The evidence against tobacco was "overwhelming," Hammond told reporters at the October 1954 ACS meeting in New York. Even a half-pack of cigarettes per day could be harmful, Hammond said. Former ASCC director C. C. Little led the industry-funded Tobacco Industry Research Committee. Little disagreed with Hammond, citing many "unknowns" about tobacco. Industry would support more definitive research, Little said. As reported in the *Times*, Little, "for many years a leader in cancer research," said, "All the chips aren't down yet."[85]

Fear of cancer led patients to fraudulent practitioners. Journalists could out but a few. *Collier's* magazine ran a 1951 exposé, "Cancer Quacks," by Bill Fay, outlining a range of deception—from a "secret serum" sold by Dr. Hett of Ontario, Canada, to Glyoxylide, a homeopathic tincture sold by Dr. William Koch through Detroit's Christian Medical Research League, to "bizarre cultists . . . advocating the 'Orgone Theory' propounded in the pseudo-Freudian writings of Dr. Wilhelm Reich" in New York. Meanwhile, Hoxsey's Dallas enterprise remained open for business and lucrative, Fay reported.[86]

Countering cancer misinformation wasn't easy. The Spears Chiropractic Sanitarium and Hospital in Denver, said to be worth $8 million, advertised unconventional medical services in a confusing brochure "Cold Cancer Facts" (figure 5.5). Inside, disturbing photographs revealed patients' bodies after surgery or radiation.[87] In Pittsburgh, Lillian Lazenby, previously a cafeteria worker, and Philip Drosnes, formerly a tire salesman, sold Mucorhicin as a "cure" despite journalists' reporting on their fraud and complaints by University of Pittsburgh faculty and local health authorities.[88,89]

"The difficulties of prosecuting cancer quacks cannot be blamed entirely on loopholes in federal and state drug laws," Fay wrote. "There also are serious human factors involved. . . . For example, the reluctance of victims to admit they have been deceived frequently hampers investigators," he considered. "Many credulous victims are firmly convinced that they have been helped by the quacks," he

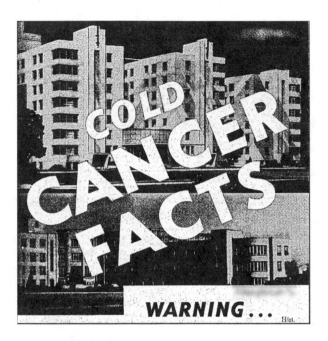

5.5 Cover of counterfactual brochure for the Spears Chiropractic Sanitarium and Hospital
Courtesy of the Ebling Library Rare Books & Special Collections, UW-Madison

added. "The sad truth of the matter is that the quacks seem destined to survive and prosper until science provides a complete cure for all types of cancer."

The ACS got people talking about cancer, but only to a point. Manners kept many from chatting about health problems. Outside of doctors' offices, detailing one's illness was often considered impolite. And if an ordinary person did choose to reveal a malignant diagnosis, their words didn't go far. Unlike today, when most anyone can post to the internet, few people had access to printing or broadcasting equipment. As we'll see, journalists led the way in public cancer disclosures. They did so, in part, because they could: they were professional storytellers with audiences at their disposal.

One of the first patients to chronicle her experiences for an audience was Lorna Doone Burks, a literary agent who died in 1945. With entries titled "The

Importance of Jelly Doughnuts" and "Ambulance At My Door," her book, *I Die Daily*, reads like the grandmother of all cancer blogs. She, a self-described devout Christian, aspired to educate: "My experience might teach someone else. That's why I'm recording it." she stated. While her condition declined, her husband, Arthur J. Burks, a Marine officer and professional writer, was stationed abroad. After Lorna's death and war's end, Arthur edited and published her words.[90]

I Die Daily contains unpleasant details and traces of anger. Unlike upbeat stories popularized by the "cured" clubs, Burks's account lacks a happy ending. Or start. Her uterine cancer progressed after surgery and radiation, before the book's beginning. She has an incurable disease and then she declines. Her text is studded with descriptions of excruciating pain. She details palliative care received at home and finally at Saint Joseph's Hospital in Burbank, California.

Burks's attitude differed from the ACS party line: she didn't quite trust doctors. She questioned conventional medical wisdom. After writing that "cancer can be cured in many cases if taken [out] in time, she recounts the discomfiting story of a relative whose cancerous breast was removed in 1906: "She had been operated on in San Francisco and went home . . . just in time to escape the Great Fire. It might have been better for her if she had not escaped," Burks wrote. "A specter went with her" for thirty years until "she died of the cancer which had presumably been destroyed."

She blames herself for having advanced cancer. After failing to get checked promptly, she held an "account" with "the Father" needing payment. She writes of being punished through the cancer ordeal, for self-neglect. Her skepticism delayed care, Burks admits: "I knew very well that pride was the cause of my being where I am now. I had refused to be examined by doctors many times when reason told me I should have been examined." She describes shame: "I felt that it was a shameful thing and to say one had it was like coming out in public and saying: 'I am a syphilitic!'" Her feelings were tinged with guilt: "It *is* unclean, this cancer. But it is not disgraceful—unless you deliberately refuse to do something about it. Then it is a disgrace of the most flagrant kind. I know. If I had accepted knowledge sooner, I might not be where I am now."

Costs of treatment weighed on Burks. "At this moment monthly expenses run to a little more than twice my husband's entire salary," she wrote. After she'd depleted their savings, her family resorted to selling their car. When Burks realizes that her caregiver, an empathetic Dominican woman, has quietly used an uncle's money to cover Burks's mounting medical bills, she contemplates, "It would be better for all concerned if I died quickly."

Cancer rendered Burks dependent on others, and she resented it. She harps, understandably, on the indignity of using a bedpan. She perceived her condition as unworthy of a physician's time, writing, "None wanted me, when told that I was dying of cancer—not even for experimental purposes. Doctors simply didn't want a losing case!" During the war, scarcity of manpower aggravated her sense of worthlessness, of being a burden: "No busy doctor in wartime wished to be chained to a hopeless case."

In a compelling episode, Burks describes being admitted to an unnamed hospital with unsympathetic staff:

> I became aware of something: the nurses who had me in charge disapproved of me! Was it because I had the effrontery to develop cancer? I hadn't done it purposely, just to cause them inconvenience. I might have made a mistake in my life, might have been careless, or in some fashion neglectful—I've heard doctors and nurses say that cancer is caused by some sort of neglect, which is perhaps true—but I hadn't deliberately acquired cancer!

The nurses call her a "hophead"—a drug addict. They think she's feigning cancer to get narcotics: "You ought to be ashamed of yourself!" one says. "You'll get no hourly morphia *here*, I can promise you *that*!" When another asks "what is the trouble?" Burks's nurse responds, "Oh, an old hophead! She just came in. Gave me the old cancer story to get morphia."

Denied morphine, Burks becomes agitated. "The pain began to mount, mount. I confess I kept stabbing the bell for the nurse, and she did not come. I bit my lips until they bled, and the blood was salty on my tongue," she wrote. "I was not afraid to die, but *this* wasn't dying, this was living—and torture beyond anything a concentration camp commander could think of." During a nightmarish period, while feeling as if every "atom" in her body were on fire, Burks loses and regains consciousness. When the nurses finally learn that she really has cancer and give morphine, it comes as a relief to the reader.

I Die Daily was not a best seller. In April 1947 the *New York Times* mentioned it alongside a longer review of a more upbeat book, *Cancer Can Be Cured* by Dr. Alfred J. Cantor. The *Times* called *I Die Daily* "courageous, pathetic, terrifying . . . and morbid."[91]

~

The story of Robin Bush, told by former first lady Barbara Bush in a memoir, illustrates how constrained were conversations about cancer. In early 1953, Barbara and future president George H. W. Bush were living in Midland, Texas, when their daughter was diagnosed with leukemia at age three. George, a Navy veteran and Yale grad, worked for Dresser Industries, an oil company supplier. Barbara, who'd left Smith College to marry George, cared for their children: George W., Pauline Robinson (Robin), and Jeb, an infant.

One day Robin appeared listless. A trusted pediatrician, Dr. Dorothy Wyvell, suspected something serious, drew a blood sample, and later summoned the young parents to her office. There is no cure for leukemia, Wyvell told them. "Her advice was to tell no one, go home, forget that Robin was sick, make her as comfortable as we could, love her—and let her gently slip away." George asked if Wyvell might contact his uncle, Dr. John Walker at New York's Memorial Hospital, and she did. "Uncle John also thought Robin had little chance to live, but he thought we should by all means treat her and try to extend her life, just in case of a breakthrough," Barbara recalled.[92]

It's noteworthy, but not surprising, that the Bushes didn't seek leukemia care at MD Anderson Hospital in Houston. That University of Texas–affiliated institution first opened to patients in 1944. Monroe Dunaway Anderson, its namesake, was a Tennessee-born cotton trader and banker who had cofounded the world's largest cotton-trading firm. He died in 1939. Eventually, MD Anderson would become a leading cancer center, but in 1953 it was a relatively primitive facility with some units converted from army barracks. While researchers elsewhere were developing antileukemia drugs, MD Anderson Hospital primarily offered cancer surgery and radiation treatments. It moved to its current location in 1954.[93,94]

Robin received leukemia treatments at New York's Memorial Hospital. She went in and out of remission until October 1953, when she died. During those months, Barbara stayed in a Walker family apartment near the Manhattan hospital. The experience affected her deeply. Other patients' families suffered financial problems, "which made the ordeal even tougher." Memorial didn't charge those who couldn't pay. Barbara wrote,

> But there were so many other expenses involved. I remember one precious little boy named Joey, whose mother had a big family in upstate New York.

Her husband was a laborer. . . . She worried all the time. She had no Ganny Walker to put her up nine blocks from the hospital, and no Mom Bush to help with the children. . . . Joey's mom had a cheap room out in the Bronx and commuted every day on the bus and subway in her bedroom slippers.

Years later, Barbara volunteered with Ronald McDonald House Charities, an organization that provides housing and support for families of children receiving cancer treatment.

Against the pediatrician's advice, the Bushes did open up about Robin's condition. Their family and church proved to be a source of support, Barbara wrote. Misunderstandings arose, however. After taking her ailing daughter to Connecticut and, briefly, home to Texas, she recalled, "Many people thought it was catching and did not let their children get near Robin. In those days, cancer in general was only whispered about, and some people just couldn't cope with a dying child."

Few public figures admitted having cancer. One woman who courageously did so was Olympic track and field champion and golfer Mildred ("Babe") Didrikson Zaharias. She was the world's most famous female athlete in 1953 when she underwent surgery for cancer involving the rectum with permanent colostomy (an artificial conduit from the large intestine to the abdominal wall, with a stool-catching pouch). "This cancer was the toughest competition I'd faced yet. I made up my mind that I was going to lick it all the way," she wrote in her autobiography.[95,96]

After cancer, Zaharias stunned observers by winning the 1954 U.S. Women's Open. Doctors told her to take it easy, but she was determined to set an example for cancer patients. Zaharias traveled frequently for ACS benefits, radio and TV appearances, and to play golf. "Every time I get out and play well in a golf tournament, it seems to buck up people with the same cancer trouble I had," she wrote.[96]

"The cancer problem should be out in the open. The more the public knows about it the better," Zaharias stated. She took awareness to a new, perhaps uncomfortable, level. She described when the doctor found her cancer. She was matter-of-fact about the colostomy. When her cancer recurred, she was open about that, too. She died in 1956, at age forty-five. The *New York Times* printed on page 1, "Babe Zaharias Dies; Athlete Had Cancer."[97]

～

As the ACS annual budget ballooned—from less than $1 million in 1944 to over $20 million a decade later—cancer publicity turned from nagging to spectacular. On April 1, 1954, President Dwight D. Eisenhower played golf with Zaharias before lighting a seventy-foot high ACS "Sword of Hope" in Times Square. He did so remotely from Washington, somehow by waving a wand tipped with radioactive cobalt, setting off clicks on a Geiger counter; the sounds were amplified by a microphone and transmitted by telephone to an ACS booth in Times Square, completing an electric circuit and turning the sword's lights on. This technological gimmick reflected optimism and excitement about the possibility of using isotopes, developed as weapons in the Cold War, against cancer.[98–100]

Entertainers provided free publicity. While few admitted having cancer themselves, many tied their names with this cause. Lena Horne, Nat King Cole, Louis Armstrong, Count Basie, and other "sepia" musicians asked fans to give, the *Chicago Defender* reported. In 1954, actor Audrey Hepburn and her *Ondine* costar Mel Ferrer appealed to theatergoers in a backstage public service announcement. Ferrer appeared in costume, dressed as a knight, which, Hepburn noted, matched the ACS crusade's theme (figure 5.6).[101,102]

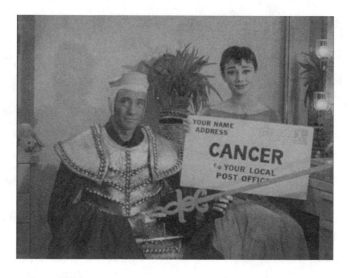

5.6 Actors Audrey Hepburn and Mel Ferrer in a "public service announcement" appeal for the ACS from backstage in a 1954 Broadway production of *Ondine*.
Sherman Grinberg Film Library (reproduced with permission)

Churches contributed. On April 1, 1955, church bells rang in the ACS crusade: "As parishioners pause from their daily activity for 10 seconds of meditation, the city's church bells will toll the beginning of 'Cancer Control Month' at 12 noon Friday," the *Shreveport Journal* reported. Notices for this event appeared nationwide. "The purpose of the meditation and sounding of bells throughout" America is "to remind us that cancer can be controlled and ultimately defeated if we all work together toward that end," said the ACS crusade leader of Silver Bow County. After hearing the bells toll, "armed with lifesaving cancer literature, workers will call upon homes and businesses throughout the country to dispense knowledge," a Los Angeles paper reported.[103–106]

Merchants participated with cause marketing. A famous episode involved the tiny town of Funkley, Minnesota. In 1953, the Pacific Mills company flew nearly its entire population of twenty-five, including a baby, on an all-expenses-paid trip to New York City to reward their anticancer volunteerism. *Life* magazine captured photos of the citizens' send-off and travel. For two years, the ladies of Funkley and nearby acquaintances had met monthly, turning old bedsheets into surgical dressings for cancer patients. To support this effort nationwide, Pacific Mills offered a credit of fifty cents for old sheets toward new purchases. The "Funkleyites" toured Manhattan in a decorated bus, took in a baseball game, and appeared on television. They met with President Eisenhower, who lauded their efforts (figure 5.7).[107–111]

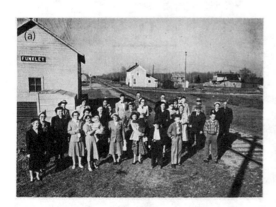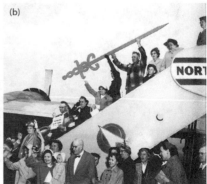

5.7 People of Funkley, Minn. were recognized for their anticancer efforts with an all-expenses-paid trip to New York City sponsored by Pacific Mills Co. (a) The "Funkleyites" in *Life* Magazine, May 1953 (*LIFE* Picture Collection); (b) arrival at LaGuardia Airport, *courtesy of the American Cancer Society*

~

Under new management, the ACS produced short educational films like *The Traitor Within* (1946) and *Man Alive* (1952). Together with the NCI and U.S. Public Health Service, the ACS produced *Breast Self-Examination*. This fifteen-minute documentary instructed women how to check their breasts for lumps. It debuted at the May 1950 biennial convention of the American Nurses Association in San Francisco and played before a "standing room only" crowd at the AMA's 1950 annual meeting. Upon release, it was shown at women's clubs, factories, state health departments, and film festivals in Venice, Italy, and Montevideo, Uruguay. *Breast Self Examination* circulated widely in the United States with daytime showings in public movie theaters. By 1955, it had been seen by over seven million people (figure 5.8).[49,112–114]

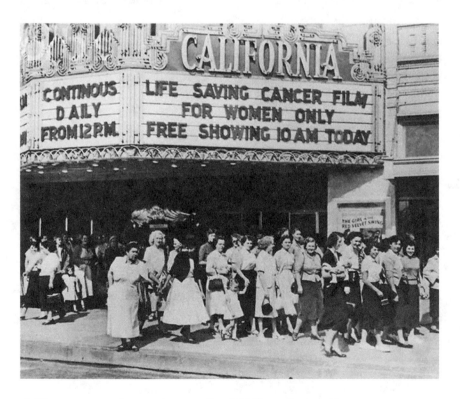

5.8 Women exiting a daytime showing of an ACS film on breast self-examination, 1955. *Photo by Otto Bettmann (Getty, with permission)*

Most Hollywood films avoided cancer. *No Sad Songs for Me* was an exception. This tearjerker, based on Ruth Southard's 1944 novel, opened at Radio City Music Hall in April 1950. Margaret Sullavan portrayed Mary Scott, a middle-aged woman stricken with advanced cancer affecting her womb. As in the 1921 film *The Reward of Courage*, at this story's center is a prosperous white family. Mary lives in a well-appointed house and employs a housekeeper. Her circumstances echo old ASCC messages that wealth does not protect against malignancy. But this commercial film differs from *The Reward* in two key respects: the woman with cancer is not easily fooled, and she dies. In retrospect, *No Sad Songs* is revealing—about how doctors spoke with female patients and how women's sacrifices, for family, were prized.

In an early scene, Mary visits the doctor. He knows she's got cancer; already he's reviewed her x-rays and biopsy with experts. The doctor planned to tell Mary's husband first, but she insists on hearing of her condition: "I want you to go into the exact medical details," she asserts. "I realize that there are some people who shouldn't be told bad news, but I should." When the doctor begins to explain her diagnosis, Mary is stunned: "This isn't . . . I can't even say it. It isn't," she pauses, "cancer?" Once she realizes what's wrong, Mary interrogates the doctor about the possibility of surgery or radium treatments. "But there are things you can do," she implores.

"It's too late," the doctor tells her. Consistent with the state of cancer care in 1950, he has no medicines to offer other than painkillers, which he prescribes. When Mary asks about how long she's got, he answers directly: ten months.

"Thank you for telling me the truth," Mary responds.

The portrait is one of a woman's emotional strength. Facing death, Mary encourages and embraces an attractive, smart, young woman as a future wife for her husband and substitute mother for her daughter. Mary is admirable—a hero!—for not succumbing to despair.

Writing for the *New York Times*, Bosley Crowther gushed over the film's "high ideals" and star's performance: "Miss Sullavan plays with such sincerity, such dignity and restraint that the morbid and tearful situation of this poor woman is cloaked in gallantry. . . . Not since Bette Davis played 'Dark Victory' several years ago has a subject of such peculiar anguish been handled so delicately."[115,116]

∼

Cancer stories appeared in literature. William Saroyan's postwar play, *Don't Go Away Mad*, depicted men's conversations in a San Francisco cancer ward. Performed off Broadway at Indiana University and later in Oakland, California, this drama received critics' praise and small audiences. "Its mere subject is almost certainly taboo in the commercial theatre," noted one critic. Saroyan, a prolific and Pulitzer-winning author, placed a Black man, "Greedy Reed," at this cancer story's heart. The uneducated Greedy craves knowledge before dying. He requests that the entire dictionary be read aloud by other cancer ward denizens, starting with the word "a." A young Chinese man on the ward begins this undertaking and dies promptly. Another patient is limited by his language, Greek, and another by blindness. Ultimately, Saroyan's story is about men leveled by cancer. The play's title reflects the idea of accepting death. Originally it was called *The Incurables*.[117-121]

Reviewers praised *Death Be Not Proud*, a memoir by John Gunther, upon its 1949 publication. This moving account, in which the writer stoically reports his son's decline before dying at seventeen from brain cancer, was later adapted as a television movie.[122] A few years later, Mark Harris's novel *Bang the Drum Slowly* broke new ground with its exploration of relationships among men on a team when one gets cancer. Bruce Pearson, a baseball catcher of limited intellect, is "doomeded" from Hodgkin's disease. The team's pitcher and story's narrator, "Author" Henry Wiggen, reports his teammate's suffering with sensitivity. Long before this story reached the big screen in 1973, it was adapted for television on *United States Steel Hour* with Paul Newman as Author and Albert Salmi as the dying catcher.[123,124]

Tennessee Williams depicted a memorable cancer-stricken patriarchal figure, Big Daddy, in his Pulitzer-winning play *Cat on a Hot Tin Roof*. Big Daddy suffers from cancer, but no one will speak of it. The 1958 film starring Burl Ives, Elizabeth Taylor, and Paul Newman was widely seen, reinforcing popular views of cancer as a death sentence.[125-127]

The AMA attempted to dent pervasive cancer fatalism by producing *Medicine U.S.A.—The Living Proof*. Notes for this 1956 television program, hosted by veteran CBS journalist H. V. Kaltenborn, appear in publicity records of Memorial Hospital, which was involved in production. The script calls for Kaltenborn to sit on a leather seat in a library or study with a "strongly masculine" tone and remark on "hundreds of thousands enjoying life in good health five, ten, or more years" after cancer treatment.

The program's spin was one hundred percent positive. Before filming, eight cancer patients received physician-vetted scripts. One was Mrs. Joan Hargrett, a forty-two-year old woman with Hodgkin's disease. Dr. David Karnofsky, her physician, referred Hargrett to the show's producers, noting, "Despite the continuous presence of the disease, she has responded well to treatment, and has been able to lead a normal life and care for her family."

Details, such as mastectomy, were skirted on TV. When Kaltenborn questions Mrs. Edith P. Carl, a sixty-eight-year old "homemaker" of a Boston suburb, "Was the necessary surgery extensive?" she responds, "It was." But there was no need for her family to worry. She adds, "I'm fine!" TV listings indicate that the AMA's cancer program aired occasionally on local channels such as Chapel Hill, North Carolina's WUNC-TV; Wilmington, Delaware's WPFH-TV; and Reno, Nevada's KZTV.[128]

One April 1958 evening, a force of thirty-five thousand men and women engaged in house-to-house canvassing for the Los Angeles ACS. The "crusaders" gave donors receipts on which were printed seven "danger signals" about which health-minded citizens should be vigilant, the *Los Angeles Times* reported. Cancer campaigning had become extreme, involving tens of thousands of Americans distributing information of uncertain benefit. Yet few had the audacity to question the society's tactics, priorities, or finances.[129]

Richard Carter wrote *The Gentle Legions*, a biting critique of health-related charities, around this time. He depicted a volunteer with cynicism: "Tentatively, and with no sense of commitment, she tried cancer as one might try window-box gardening or canasta. She might have looked into polio or muscular dystrophy, but the Cancer Society was conveniently located, and a friend of hers had died from cancer not long before." She finds preparing surgical dressings "drudgery" but enjoys transporting patients and chatting with their families. She attends funerals. These efforts challenge the volunteer: "She sometimes caught herself pitying those who were to die soon, and she prayed that the emotion would not show." She is promoted and "serves on local and state committees concerned with educating the public." She attends conferences, "associating happily with others who share her dedication," Carter wrote. "She finds that her life is in focus." Through cancer charity work, the woman finds purpose—not unlike Ellin Lowery and friends many years earlier.

The cancer volunteer had become demanding, he wrote: "Every April she raises more money than she did during the previous April." And fierce: "She descends on friend and neighbor with her cancer literature and her impressive determination. . . . It is difficult to fend her off." And annoying: "She hectors you about seeing your doctor." Worse yet, her aims were questionable.

Were the millions of dollars collected by the ACS put to good use? Carter was unconvinced, observing, "The Cancer Society is forever educating itself to educate others."[130]

PART II

CANCER COMES OUT

This section reveals how cancer became an everyday subject of conversation. We'll see how journalists, celebrities, and other public figures opened up about their personal cancer experiences. After the AIDS epidemic began, people with cancer became increasingly vocal and visible. The internet revolutionized patients' ability to communicate and share their stories.

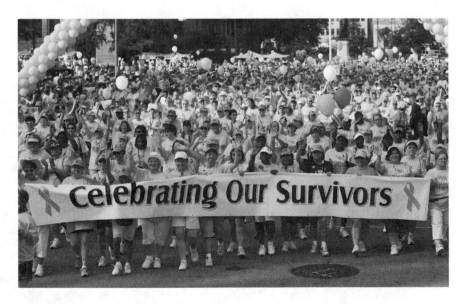

St. Louis Race for the Cure, June 16, 2007.
Photo by Bill Greenblatt, UPI (with permission).

CHAPTER 6

OUR BODIES, OUR DECISIONS (1960–1980)

Wearing a dark wig and horn-rimmed glasses, Rachel Carson testified before a U.S. Senate subcommittee in June 1963. The biologist and author spoke of pollution and health hazards of pesticides. At fifty-six, she was debilitated from metastatic breast cancer, arthritis, healing ulcers, and a heart condition. Carson was exhausted. Her wig hid thinning hair. Yet her forceful words and best-selling book rocked the chemical industry (figure 6.1).

In *Silent Spring*, Carson reported on widespread use of synthetic chemicals in agriculture and in homes as a threat to nature, including humans, and tied that to cancer. Excerpts appeared in a June 1962 *New Yorker* series and immediately caused a stir. That September, Houghton Mifflin published the book. A review captured the gist with this headline: "There's Poison All Around Us Now." The language is potent. Chapter 3, for instance, is titled "Elixirs of Death." Carson named DDT, a common insecticide, and aminotriazole, a weed killer, as carcinogenic. Citing American Cancer Society (ACS) statistics, she expressed alarm over high cancer rates. Childhood cancers might be caused by fetal exposure to chemicals in the womb, she suggested. *Silent Spring* ignited the environmentalist movement. Carson's legacy includes the Clean Air Act of 1963, federal legislation protecting wildlife, creation of the Environmental Protection Agency (EPA) in 1970, and the Clean Water Act of 1972.[1-6]

Carson's critics, many affiliated with industry, insinuated she was a communist, questioned her objectivity, and likened her to a witch. Velsicol, the manufacturer of chlordane and heptachlor pesticides, threatened lawsuits. That fall, Monsanto produced "The Desolate Year"—a *Silent Spring* parody describing a world plagued by insects. But it wasn't only industrial chemists who disputed

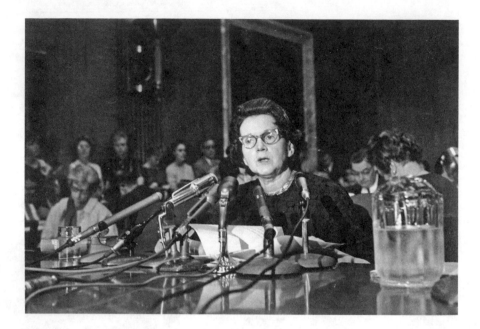

6.1 Rachel Carson testifying before a U.S. Senate subcommittee on pesticides, June 1963. AP photo (with permission)

her work. *Time* magazine called her words "unfair, one-sided, and hysterically overemphatic." Nutritionists said the United States couldn't feed its population without using chemicals in agriculture.[7–9]

Serious allegations came posthumously. Academics criticized her conclusions. Bruce N. Ames, the University of California, Berkeley, biochemist who invented the eponymous "Ames test" for carcinogens and his colleague Lois S. Gold wrote of the "Rachel Carson fallacy" in a 1997 review: "Neither toxicology nor epidemiology supports the idea that synthetic industrial chemicals are causing an epidemic of human cancer." Long after the EPA's 1972 ban of DDT, Carson was accused of causing hundreds of millions of deaths from mosquito-borne diseases like malaria. A 2014 Breitbart news headline called Carson "the 20th Century's Greatest Female Mass Murderer."[10–14]

Carson was an unlikely firebrand. Contemporary journalists described the aging biologist as a frail spinster. Born in 1907, her passion for nature—and pen—took her from poverty in western Pennsylvania to Pittsburgh's Pennsylvania College for Women, to Johns Hopkins University where she studied zoology, to the U.S. Department of the Interior, to fame as a writer. She first glimpsed the sea's edge as a student in Woods Hole, Massachusetts, and was smitten. After *The Sea Around Us* won a 1952 National Book Award, Carson, who by then lived in Silver Springs, Maryland, bought property in coastal Maine. In her last decade, she cared for her mother, adopted a young grandnephew, and had an intimate relationship with Dorothy Freeman, a married woman and Maine neighbor.

Hers was a household name. President John F. Kennedy was a fan; he kept two of her books in his Cape Cod home. During an August 1962 press conference, he responded to a journalist's question about DDT by mentioning "Miss Carson's book." On CBS television, an hour-long April 1963 feature was titled "The Silent Spring of Rachel Carson."[15–19]

Carson didn't admit much about her health. In April 1960, she underwent mastectomy after a biopsy showed breast cancer. Months later, the cancer recurred near her breastbone. She received radiation and consulted Dr. George ("Barney") Crile Jr., a forward-thinking surgeon at the Cleveland Clinic. Getting a second opinion was not unheard of in Carson's time, but it was unusual. Doing so reflected both her income and disposition to taking initiative. As a patient, Carson was neither passive nor unquestioning. But having money and access to experts could not alter the course of her disease.

Effective drugs against breast cancer were lacking in the 1960s. Some doctors prescribed radiation to body parts, *whac-a-mole*, when and where a tumor spread. In 1963, cancer invaded her left pelvis; Carson had difficulty walking. Already it had infiltrated her spine, causing pain. She tried Krebiozen, a bogus treatment not recommended by her doctors. Under Crile's advisement, she took testosterone injections. Although there was no evidence to support its use, that hormone was sometimes given as treatment for breast cancer. These were to no avail.[20]

She tried to conceal her illness. In public appearances—on Capitol Hill and on TV—Carson wore a wig because she didn't want people to perceive her as a cancer victim lashing out at the chemical industry. But that was not the only reason. In May 1962, Carson attended a dinner where she overheard gossip of another prominent woman with cancer, Senator Maurine Neuberger. Months earlier, the Oregon senator had undergone surgery for an intestinal tumor. "She can't last," someone said of Neuberger. This remark upset the writer. Carson didn't want people talking about her health, or pity. (Senator Neuberger, then in her fifties, lived to age ninety-three.)

Carson's condition deteriorated. In October 1963, while traveling to San Francisco to give a lecture, she needed a wheelchair. In early 1964, with cancer infiltrating her liver, she flew to Cleveland for experimental neurosurgery at Crile's directive. After doctors injected yttrium-90, a radioactive isotope, to ablate the pituitary gland at the base of her brain, Carson became gravely ill. She was hospitalized in intensive care before traveling home with assistance. She died in April 1964.[21,22]

Carson's story illustrates two points about personal attitudes toward cancer. Like most patients of the 1960s—and many today—she preferred not to reveal her diagnosis. And until her last days, she hoped that scientists would find an effective treatment. Carson didn't give up until the very end.

The 1960s and 1970s were a socially turbulent time. Many Americans demonstrated against racial discrimination and against the Vietnam War. People marched for women's liberation and for nuclear disarmament, while a blossoming counterculture tugged at conventions. In 1970, the Boston Women's Health Book Collective published the first edition of *Our Bodies, Ourselves*, a powerful pre-internet example of peer-to-peer health information.[23,24] In 1973, the Supreme Court's *Roe v. Wade* decision reflected increasing respect for women's personal and reproductive choices. Greater openness about sexuality became the norm, along with talk of gay rights.

Amid these cultural shifts it's not surprising that people became more comfortable saying *cancer*. Americans were living longer than ever. Because age is a risk factor for malignancy, cancers became more frequent. Statistics were hazy, however. A few states maintained registries and the American College of Surgeons tracked patients after surgery, but it wasn't until 1973 that the National Cancer Institute (NCI) established the Surveillance, Epidemiology, and End Results (SEER) Program to gather nationwide cancer information. Without an inclusive registry, statisticians could only estimate its incidence.

As people became more aware of cancer, many wondered about its causes. Radiation, an established mutagen, was on people's minds. During the Cold War schoolchildren ducked and covered in drills. People worried about fallout from atomic weapons and, as nuclear power expanded, power plant accidents.[25,26] Smog blanketed Los Angeles and other cities. People couldn't help but notice the poor air quality. Images of a massive 1969 fire on the Cuyahoga River in Cleveland, Ohio, fueled by industrial waste, woke Americans to the extremity of chemical pollution in waterways.[27] Many considered environmental and household toxins likely culprits.

Genetic causes were not yet appreciated. Dr. Henry Lynch, working in Nebraska, deduced that a cancer disposition could be inherited. But east coast experts resisted his conclusions, which countered ACS dogma and the long-standing message that cancer is not hereditary.[28]

Surgery and radiation remained the mainstays of cancer treatment. Most patients died within five years. Although physicians today consider five-year survival a poor measure of treatment outcomes, then it was an unfortunately telling statistic. In the 1960s, fewer than half of men with colon cancer lived five years after diagnosis. With acute leukemia, five-year survival stayed below four percent.

After a half century of educational campaigns, three decades of NCI effort, and countless testimonials that cancer is curable, for most cancer patients the odds of long-term survival remained low.[29]

In January 1964, U.S. Surgeon General Luther Terry reported that smoking tobacco causes lung cancer. A ten-man advisory committee found that men who smoked cigarettes were at least nine times more likely to develop lung cancer than nonsmokers; among heavy smokers, risk exceeded twenty-fold. The panel also determined that smoking cigarettes contributes to heart disease, laryngeal cancer, and breathing ailments. To minimize rattling of stock markets, Terry released the report on a Saturday.[30,31]

The findings—while controversial—were hardly surprising. Doctors already knew that smoking tobacco disposes to lung cancer. Ordinary people knew it too. The connection was so apparent that by 1952, *Reader's Digest* had run a story titled "Cancer by the Carton." In his 1962 novel, *A Clockwork Orange*, Anthony Burgess plainly called cigarettes cancers.[32,33]

"Cigarette smoking far outweighs all other causes of lung cancer in men—and the findings as to women point in the same direction," stated a front-page *St. Louis Post-Dispatch* summary. The surgeon general's "bold and devastating" findings cannot be ignored by smokers or "blown away by the tobacco industry's spokesmen," said a *New York Times* editorial. While smoking shouldn't be prohibited, the government should discourage young people from this habit, it stated. America's leadership was at stake: "Surely this country ought not lag behind

Great Britain, the Soviet Union and Denmark, whose public health ministries already use posters and other means to warn against smoking."[34-36]

Yet people didn't stop lighting up. Americans' avidity for tobacco was nearly unbreakable. Historians trace the U.S. smoking epidemic to World War I, when soldiers stationed in France received cigarettes in ration kits. By that time, the Duke family's American Tobacco Company and its rivals had implemented automated rolling machines in cigarette factories—speeding production, lowering manufacturers' costs, and accelerating distribution of their addictive, carcinogenic product. Before the 1920s, only a small fraction of adults, predominantly men, regularly smoked cigarettes. Tobacco companies invested heavily in advertising and began targeting women, who took up cigarettes in unprecedented numbers. Albert Lasker's slogan for Lucky Strike, "Reach for a Lucky instead," appealed to those seeking to lose weight; it drew on the view that smoking makes it easy to stay slim (figure 6.2).[31,37,38]

Cigarette consumption dipped during the Great Depression and then resumed rising. Smoking's allure involved sex and attractiveness. Movie stars—Clark Gable, ASCC friend Spencer Tracy, Joan Crawford, Bette Davis, Rita Hayworth,

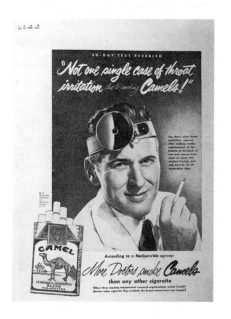 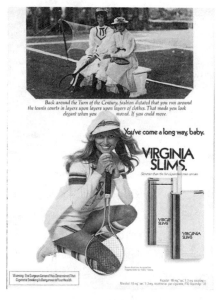

6.2 1949 ad for Camels (left); 1972 ad for Virginia Slims (right).

(Stanford Research Into the Impact of Tobacco Advertising, https://tobacco.stanford.edu/)

Fred MacMurray, Ronald Reagan, and John Wayne, to name a few—endorsed brands. The biggest Hollywood studios arranged for cigarette commercials featuring actors with whom they held contracts. While its leaders were aiding the cancer society, the motion picture industry was selling tobacco products.[37,39]

Physicians, for their part, were in denial. Many enjoyed smoking and were hooked. Until the early 1950s, manufacturers advertised to doctors in medical journals including the American Medical Association's journal, *JAMA*. At a 1947 AMA conference, Philip Morris sponsored a lounge where doctors might "Drop in. Rest . . . read . . . smoke . . . or just chat." As reported by Bernard DeVoto in *Harper's Magazine*, companies gave away free cigarettes at medical conferences and doctors "lined up by the hundred" to receive them. To counter perception of cigarettes' untoward health effects, tobacco firms promoted images of doctors smoking. An R. J. Reynolds advertisement boasted a nationwide survey finding, "more doctors smoke Camels than any other cigarette!" In the 1950s, campaigns featuring actors Fredric March and Barbara Stanwyck proclaimed, "L&M filters are just what the doctor ordered."[40–42]

A postulated link between tobacco and cancer goes back far.[43] Evidence was limited by its observational nature, that it's hard to prove cause and effect from exposures—especially if past cigarette use is estimated from surveys based on smokers' recollections. Aggravating the issue were poor statistics; lung cancer was "invisible" and underdiagnosed. Operating on lungs was so risky that, before the 1950s, it was rarely performed. X-rays couldn't reliably distinguish between infection and cancer. For these reasons, doctors connected smoking with lip, mouth, tongue, throat, and larynx (voice box) cancers—in patients like the former president Ulysses Grant, President Grover Cleveland, and Babe Ruth—decades before the relationship with lung cancer became apparent.

Skeptics maintained that there was no proof of causation.[44–46] Some suggested there might be something about smokers, an attribute, that disposes them to getting cancer. In one remarkable line of industry-funded research, investigators explored a putative relationship between smoking and "weakness of the masculine component." Harvard men deemed physically unsuited for muscular work, emotionally "sensitive," and who tended to major in "art, letters, and philosophy," were identified as more nervous and inclined to smoke. A 1959 *Science* paper concluded that research was warranted to see if those traits—rather than smoking—caused lung cancer and heart disease in men.[47,48]

Tobacco was a huge industry in 1964. Over over half of American men and a third of women smoked regularly. People lit cigarettes in workplaces including

schools and hospitals, on trains and airplanes, in restaurants and theaters—
everywhere. After the surgeon general's report, tobacco firms resisted advertising regulations. Other groups did too. Because cigarette taxes delivered billions
of dollars to state and federal governments, many politicians opposed limits.
The U.S. Department of Agriculture took the position of tobacco farmers, that
evidence of smoking's ill health effects was not yet definitive.

In 1965, Congress passed a law requiring that cigarette packages carry a warning that "cigarette smoking may be hazardous to health." This soft language did
not contain the word "cancer." Starting in 1971, federal law banned cigarette
advertising on radio and television. Still, tobacco ads were permitted in print—on
billboards, in newspapers and magazines. "Cigarettes were the most advertised
product in America and far and away the most important source of advertising revenue for many publications," Patterson wrote in *The Dread Disease*. This
income dependency led some magazines to self-censor tobacco-related content.
The industry's clout was amplified by corporate relationships. R. J. Reynolds, for
instance, owned Canada Dry soda and Del Monte Foods; Philip Morris, another
giant tobacco firm, owned Maxwell House coffee, Kool-Aid, and Birds Eye foods.[49]

Americans' cigarette use peaked in the 1960s. But it would take three decades
for lung cancer rates to fall.[50] This lag resulted from cancer's long latency and,
also, that many individuals kept on smoking—or first began. The problem wasn't
only that people enjoyed cigarettes and became addicted, but that many people
didn't want the government telling them how to behave. Some adults continued
smoking "because they did not respond readily to the experts—epidemiologists,
researchers, government bureaucrats, middle-class health professionals, do-good-
ers," Patterson wrote in 1987. "To smoke was to assert the right to be free, to be
an American." The issue involved a clash of values and differing attitudes toward
health, illness, and the medical profession.[49]

Several famous men had lung cancer, elevating public concern. Before his 1964
lung cancer surgery, John Wayne advertised Camels and reportedly smoked five
packs a day; after his diagnosis, the tough-guy actor appeared in television spots
for the ACS. "I licked the big C," he told *Playboy* in 1971.[51,52]

The popular singer Nat King Cole died just weeks after lung cancer surgery at
age forty-five. In 1965, he was one of the first Black celebrities to publicly admit

having cancer. "When the serious nature of Cole's illness was disclosed, he was deluged with mail, telegrams and calls—more than had been received by anyone else in the hospital, which often has celebrity patients," the *Los Angeles Times* reported in Cole's obituary.[53]

Some doctors mistakenly thought that cancer primarily affects white people. This falsehood arose in part because cancer is more frequently detected in people with access to physicians. Before 1965, when the government established Medicare and Medicaid, cases arising in poor Americans were undercounted. As historian Keith Wailoo details in *How Cancer Crossed the Color Line*, only as Black Americans entered "the insurance experience" did their health conditions become diagnosed and statistically known. Besides, early awareness campaigns had overlooked communities of color. This double fault—of not collecting data, and not educating—led to fewer Black patients getting timely care, underreporting of disease, and higher cancer death rates.[54]

The myth of cancer as a "white" disease was perpetuated by a paucity of Black characters with cancer in popular books and movies. One story that helped break this color barrier was John A. Williams's 1967 novel, *The Man Who Cried I Am*. The story details the experiences of an "American negro" who is dying from cancer. The protagonist constantly feels the need to urinate and senses his body's foul odor, "the cancer smell of rot and death." Wailoo writes that this Black man's cancer story reflected the era: it was as "an angry, intimate, personalized, and politically charged health identity that made a sharp break with earlier sanitized portraits."[55,56]

Carson McCullers's novel *The Heart Is a Lonely Hunter* includes a central "negro" character, Doctor Copeland. In the 1968 movie version, Percy Rodriguez portrayed a proud Black physician who suffers silently and reveals his cancer only to a man who literally cannot speak. This film, with its broad audience, bolstered perception that cancer is an equal-opportunity killer.[57]

While we in the twenty-first century consider breast cancer treatable and possibly curable, back then it was terrifying. Although few people think in statistical terms, the preponderance of deaths from breast cancer, even after treatment, must have influenced perception of the disease and discouraged patients from seeking proper care. In the 1940s, nearly half—47 percent—of breast cancer patients succumbed within five years of the diagnosis. In the 1960s and 1970s, adults would have recalled relatives or neighbors who'd died after mutilating surgery. And those memories would have been reinforced: five-year survival hovered around 65 percent; one in three breast cancer patients still died within five years.[58,59] And treatment was awful. Radical mastectomy, the usual operation, meant losing a breast, chest muscles beneath, and a few dozen glands from the armpit. Chronic arm swelling was a frequent complication.

In this context, it's credible that a central character in Jaqueline Susann's 1966 sensational novel, *Valley of the Dolls*, commits suicide rather than having a mastectomy. Sharon Tate portrayed Jennifer, the affected beautiful young woman, in the 1967 movie. The story draws on old ideas of cancer as divine punishment: Jennifer receives her cancer diagnosis after living in a way some would consider immoral; needing money to support her disabled husband, she'd appeared nude in films. In reality, Susann underwent mastectomy in 1962 and took numerous treatments including chemotherapy before she died from metastatic disease in 1974. Like Carson, the author kept her diagnosis out of the spotlight. She feared loss of lucrative book contracts and her glamorous image.[60–63]

Women worried about breast cancer, with reason. It was the most common cancer affecting American women, with nearly seventy thousand diagnoses and thirty thousand deaths annually, and those numbers were climbing.[64] Connecticut cancer registry data, though geographically limited, indicated a rising incidence: up by 1 percent per year, on average, from 1940 to 1980.[65] Magazines published updates. A 1962 *Ladies' Home Journal* article on "weapons against breast cancer" detailed chemotherapy drugs, like thiotepa, and hormonal agents. A 1963 *Good Housekeeping* story on "A New Test for Early Detection of Breast Cancer" explained how mammography works.[66,67]

As more patients accepted cancer treatments, some began chatting directly, peer to peer. Conversations started in doctors' offices, in waiting rooms before daily radiation, and inside hospitals where some spent weeks recovering after surgery. Those impromptu discussions among patients and caregivers formed the roots of modern patient advocacy. At this time, doctors were beginning to lose control of conversations about cancer. Yet organized cancer support groups were rare and physicians generally frowned on lay advice.

One peer support network did exist. Reach to Recovery, founded by Terese Lasser, involved women who'd "been there" greeting and offering practical tips to postmastectomy patients. In 1952, Lasser was devastated when after surgery in New York's Memorial Hospital she'd woken up to find her breast gone. As was standard then, she'd signed consent for the surgeon to remove her breast if a pathologist's quick review of the biopsy, a "frozen section," revealed cancer. While recovering, Lasser's mind surged with questions—about exercising her arm, where to get a prosthesis, if she could have sex, and what to tell her sons. No one offered answers. In Lasser's time, most surgeons expected patients to feel relieved that the cancer was out and shrugged off patients' concerns.

"How I ached to talk to another woman who had had the same experience and come through it, and so could counsel, and reassure, and understand!" she wrote in her 1972 book. Lasser made it her mission to assist other women after breast cancer surgery. She began by visiting postmastectomy patients in Memorial Hospital. She delivered gift boxes, each with a temporary breast prosthesis, so women might feel less self-conscious receiving visitors, and a squeezable ball for exercises to reduce post-surgical arm stiffness and swelling. The Reach to Recovery program, as she called it, expanded as affected women whom Lasser visited reached out to other mastectomy patients in other hospitals.

The message was strictly upbeat: Lasser advised Reach to Recovery volunteers to dress smartly and brightly and to speak positively about life after breast cancer. As told by medical historian Dr. Barron Lerner in *The Breast Cancer Wars*, while some doctors appreciated Lasser's visiting their patients, others considered her a bother; she threatened their authority. One surgeon likened the volunteer network, disparagingly, to Alcoholics Anonymous. After years of controversy—because many doctors disapproved of patients giving advice one to another—in 1969 the ACS embraced Reach to Recovery as an official program. For some affected patients and doctors, this leant legitimacy to the organization.[68-71]

Reach to Recovery had only limited influence, however. Its volunteers contacted patients only with surgeons' permission. The program engaged relatively few women of color and few in rural hospitals. It succeeded because so many women were diagnosed with breast cancer, and a good percentage lived years after mastectomy. For people with rare malignancies or cancers with lesser survival rates, peer support did not take off until much later.

Around this time, doctors were debating breast cancer surgery and, in particular, the appropriateness of the "Halsted" radical mastectomy. A few surgeons—notably Dr. Oliver Cope at Harvard and Dr. Crile at the Cleveland Clinic, whose wife had died from breast cancer—developed less drastic procedures: modified radical mastectomy, in which the breast is amputated but chest muscles are retained; and lumpectomy, in which only the affected breast part is removed. When those innovative surgeons reported survival results comparable to results after radical mastectomy, their colleagues rebuked them for performing smaller operations. At medical conferences, men argued about the rationale and ethics of randomized trials of breast cancer surgery. The debate spilled into the public realm. After the *Radcliffe Quarterly* published Cope's "Breast Cancer: Has the Time Come for a Less Mutilating Treatment?" in 1970, stories on breast cancer surgery appeared in *Vogue, Woman's Day, Ebony,* and other magazines.[72–75]

Women's preferences began to matter. Yet when Babette Rosmond, an editor at *Seventeen* magazine, insisted on separating her 1971 breast biopsy from definitive surgery so that she could weigh options, a surgeon called her "a very silly and stubborn woman." Nor was the issue deemed fit for proper conversations. Macmillan published Rosmond's book *The Invisible Worm* under a pseudonym. In 1972, the *New York Times* reported that after being told that she'd be "dead in three weeks," the author, "Mrs. Campion," "flew to the Cleveland Clinic, where only the visible tumor was removed in a highly controversial operation called a 'lumpectomy.'"[69,76,77]

Popular movies ratcheted up sympathy for cancer patients. *Love Story,* a 1970 blockbuster, starred Ali MacGraw as Jennifer, a Radcliffe student who falls in love, marries, and dies, and Ryan O'Neal as Oliver, the couple's preppy, wealthier half. No one says "leukemia" or "cancer" in this film. As was common practice, a doctor informs Oliver of his wife's diagnosis before telling Jennifer. After an off-camera discussion, she states that the hematologist (blood specialist) spoke frankly; she understands she has little time. In the hospital, she accepts blood transfusions but declines "antimetabolites"—what we'd call chemotherapy. After Jennifer dies, Oliver may be reconciled with his estranged father.[78,79,80]

Audiences wept. This sad tale appealed to millions. The book by Erich Segal dominated best-seller lists for over a year and was read widely in translation. Some critics gave *Love Story* glowing reviews. Writing for the *New York Times,* Vincent Canby called the film "beautiful," "romantic," and "possibly as sophisticated as any commercial American movie ever made." Pauline Kael, for the *New Yorker,* was less impressed by the "shlock classic." It was a cheap cry that inspired self-righteousness: "Those who sob away can flatter themselves that the picture must have been beautifully done—or they wouldn't have been so affected." Kael predicted a "return of the weepies."[81-83]

Indeed. On a Tuesday evening after Thanksgiving, 1971, one in three American television sets tuned to *Brian's Song*. ABC's "Movie of the Week" focused on the interracial friendship between Brian Piccolo, a twenty-something Chicago Bears football player who died from testicular cancer,* and his Black teammate Gale Sayers. The film was adapted from Sayers's 1970 memoir, *I Am Third*.[84,85] The account was so moving, it was said, technicians cried during production. "The film left no possible manipulation of the emotions unmanipulated," wrote John J. O'Connor in the *Times*. The tremendous success of *Brian's Song* on TV led to its distribution in theaters.[86-90]

Next came *Bang the Drum Slowly*. In the 1973 movie, Robert De Niro portrayed Bruce Pearson, a baseball catcher with Hodgkin's disease, and Michael Moriarty played Henry Wiggen, the team's pitcher and story's narrator. The movie opens with Pearson exiting the Mayo Clinic in Rochester, Minnesota, a place that codes for cancer treatment. Secrecy surrounding cancer is central to the plot. Wiggen knows of Pearson's diagnosis but won't tell anyone. The team's coach and managers are so determined to find out what Pearson was doing in Rochester, they hire a private investigator. Ultimately, when Pearson suffers recurrent symptoms and the men learn of his condition, they rally in support of their dying teammate.[91]

What's striking about these three films—*Love Story*, *Brian's Song*, and *Bang the Drum Slowly*—isn't just that each cancer-stricken character dies, but that there's no dramatic possibility that they might be cured. Even in fiction, their deaths are inevitable. And in each case, cancer brings people together. It mends rifts, as if the condition has "healing" powers for those other than the patient.

A year after *Love Story* opened in theaters, President Richard Nixon declared "War on Cancer." This culminated years of lobbying by the "cancer alliance" led by Mary Lasker, Dr. Sidney Farber, the ACS, and NCI officials. In April 1971, Lasker's friend Esther ("Eppie") Lederer—whose pen name was Ann Landers, the widely read syndicated advice columnist[92]—had appealed to the public, writing, "How

---

* Piccolo had embryonal cell carcinoma, a rare form of testicular cancer.

many of us have asked the question, 'If this great country of ours can put a man on the moon why can't we find a cure for cancer?'" Lederer urged readers to contact their senators.[93-95] Many did. A "blizzard" of letters reached the Capitol.[96-98]

Nixon signed the National Cancer Act on December 23, 1971. He hoped the Christmastime announcement would distract attention from the Vietnam War. "I hope that in the years ahead that we may look back on this day, and this action, as being the most significant action taken during this Administration," he said. "We find that more people each year die of cancer in the United States than all the Americans who lost their lives in World War II." Nixon affirmed a "total national commitment" to the cancer cause. He concluded with this caveat: "We would not want to raise false hopes by simply the signing of an act." But "for those who have cancer . . . they at least can have the assurance that everything that can be done by government . . . now will be done."

Support for expanding the federal cancer research program was bipartisan and seemingly universal. At the White House ceremony, Senator Edward (Ted) Kennedy, a Democrat and political opponent, crossed the stage to shake Nixon's hand and stood behind him in photographs.[99] If politicians had reservations about the measure, they would not vote against it. The Senate vote, earlier in December 1971, was 85–0.[100,101]

Newspapers covered the declaration, but not as lead story. On page 6, the *Wall Street Journal* emphasized the boon for scientists: "Cancer Bill, Signed by Nixon, Seen Having Major Impact on Future Medical Research." The $1.6 billion "federal crusade against cancer," as the *Washington Post* called it, would nearly triple research into causes and treatment. The *Times* relegated the National Cancer Act to page 16.[102-105]

A few journalists questioned the mission. In her November 1971 "The Politics of Cancer," Lucy Eisenberg considered Capitol Hill debate over the Conquest of Cancer Act, an earlier version of this legislation. "Proponents, who are mostly laymen, claim that breakthroughs in cancer are imminent, and that given enough money and the proper management techniques, man can conquer cancer just as he split the atom and landed on the moon," she wrote in *Harper's Magazine*. Critics complained that the NCI already had plenty of money, that it was run too much like a business, and that funding was misspent on its notorious chemotherapy program. "The prime mover behind the Conquest of Cancer Act is Mrs. Mary Lasker, a woman of wealth, charm, and social position who has extensive contacts in the scientific world," Eisenberg wrote. "Mrs. Lasker's opinions on research policy do not always coincide with those of many research scientists or even top

NIH officials, but when they don't, it is often Mrs. Lasker's that prevail," she continued. "Virtually the entire scientific community" opposes the legislation.

"At the heart of the matter, I think, there is a real difference in scientific opinion," Eisenberg offered. While some experts think "cancer is ready" for rapid implementation of research, enabled by money and effective administrators, others say, "What holds up research isn't management but ideas." Politicians were so "bewitched by words" that at one point, "Congressman John Rooney declared that cancer should be cured by 1976 as 'an appropriate commemoration of the 200th anniversary of the independence of our country,'" Eisenberg noted. "It is a pretty thought: announcing a cure for cancer on July 4, 1976. But wishful thinking won't make it happen and neither will Congressional resolutions."[106]

This was the ACS's heyday. Few charities specialized in particular cancer types. If people gave money "for cancer," usually they gave to the ACS. Celebrities such as comedian Bob Hope helped shape the society's image while the ACS's enormous budget expanded. Between 1970 and 1975, public donations rose from around $50 to $79 million yearly—a 58 percent spike; total revenue soared to $122 million annually.[107]

Before 1970, marathon fundraisers—walkathons, bikeathons, swimathons, etc.—were almost unheard of. The idea of holding large-scale participatory events for health charities may have evolved as an outgrowth of social demonstrations. In LaGrange, Georgia, for instance, thousands of junior and high school students marched in an anticancer "protest." The ACS's *Cancer News* published images of marching bands, football teams, and local businesses participating.[108]

In October 1972, the cast of ABC's *The Partridge Family*, a TV show about a musical family, pedaled two-wheelers in a "Ride for Life." Shirley Jones, the actor and Partridge "mom," invited viewers to ride for the ACS. Promotions featured teen idol David Cassidy and other Partridge stars. Dr. A. H. Letton, the ACS president, emphasized that leukemia often strikes young people; he hoped the *Partridge Family* cast's involvement would inspire real families to support the cause. That fall, ACS bikeathons dotted the country—in Florida, Pennsylvania, Illinois, South Dakota, California and elsewhere (figure 6.3).

Americans were not yet familiar with marathon fundraisers, so newspapers explained: volunteer bike riders asked acquaintances—friends and family,

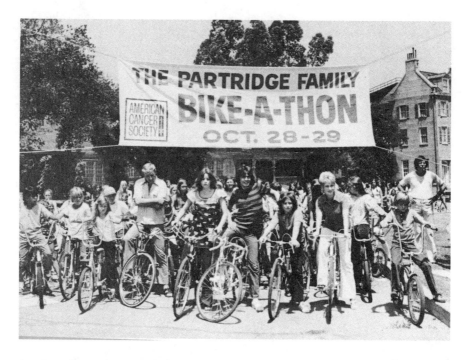

6.3 *Partridge Family* stars including David Cassidy and Shirley Jones set off on an ACS bikeathon, October 1972.

ACS Cancer News image courtesy of the American Cancer Society; scan by Countway Library, Harvard Medical School

coworkers and neighbors, local business owners—to pledge an amount for the ACS per mile traveled. Cyclists could travel short or long distances based on their ability and time. In Florida, where some rode as far as two hundred miles over two days, the minimum donation was ten cents per mile, the *Orlando Sentinel* detailed. The 1972 bikeathon reportedly netted around $250,000 for the society—and inspired future marathons long after the Partridges went off-air in 1974.[109–113]

The marathon fundraising strategy caught on, morphed, and grew. On college campuses, dance marathons took hold.[114,115] The idea likely jumped from the 1969 movie *They Shoot Horses, Don't They?* This film, based on a 1935 novel, depicts desperation of participants in a Depression-era dance marathon.[116] That endurance craze started in the 1920s and had nothing to do with charity: couples danced for days and even weeks, exhausting themselves for prize money. For paying onlookers, marathon dances provided entertainment and opportunity for betting. In

California in 1927, after marathoners collapsed during a grueling dance from the pier in Venice Beach to a Los Angeles dance hall, the Humane Society, which then dealt with cruel treatment of people, halted it. In the 1930s, contestants entered for food and shelter. In some states, extreme endurance events became illegal. The fad petered out.[117–119]

At Penn State today, the monumental event held each winter called "THON"—involving hundreds of dancers and over fifteen thousand spectators filling a sports arena, plus virtual onlookers—began in February 1973 when seventy-eight paired students danced for thirty hours at the campus Hub in State College, Pennsylvania, raising $2,000 for the "Butler County Association for Retarded Children." Leaders of the interfraternity and pan-Hellenic (sorority) council planned this activity, which, besides fundraising, provided indoor entertainment for students during wintertime. The dance marathon proved so successful that the council expanded it, delivering thousands of dollars to the American Heart Association in 1974, Easter Seals in 1975, and Muscular Dystrophy Association in 1976. When the council selected Four Diamonds, a local charity established by the family of Christopher Millard, a boy who'd died from cancer, as its 1977 cause, Penn State's football team got involved, and the relationship stuck. Since then, THON has raised over $160 million to support pediatric cancer research and care at nearby Hershey Medical Center.[120–122]

Newspapers and magazines promulgated the notion that psychology plays a role in cancer's growth. This was not a new idea. *Cosmopolitan* magazine, for instance, had run a 1960 article titled "Cancer and Your Emotions, in which the ACS president Dr. Eugene Pendergrass, a radiologist, said cancer can flare during emotional stress. He suggested "the distinct possibility that within one's mind is a power capable of exerting forces which can either enhance or inhibit the progress of this disease," *Cosmopolitan* reported.[123] The idea didn't fade. Doctors didn't dismiss the role of emotions in disease, especially as those affect women.

In 1972, a *Ladies' Home Journal* feature, "Personality Traits That May Lead to Cancer," by Howard R. and Martha E. Lewis, authors of *Psychosomatics: How Your Emotions Can Damage Your Health*, covered this subject with apparent depth. The Lewises described work of the popular psychologist Lawrence LeShan. With all the vagaries of a fortune-teller, LeShan had outlined a "life pattern" common among cancer patients: a lonely childhood, possibly with traumatic loss, development of meaningful relationships and "full life" experience in young adulthood, followed by a devastating event and feelings of hopelessness. Six months to eight years later, cancer patients developed symptoms, he claimed. The Lewises invoked pseudoscience, stating "psychological attitudes can affect the production of hormones," to support LeShan's theory.[124,125]

The Lewises also detailed the work of Dr. David Kissen, a Scottish pulmonologist who'd written on lung cancer's psychological causes.[126,127] Kissen's interest had been piqued upon meeting a woman who "had never smoked [but] she had lung cancer," the Lewises reported. After observing her "inability to acknowledge emotional conflict and deal adequately with it," Kissen interviewed "almost 1,000" patients and became convinced that many with cancer suffered from "poor outlets for emotional discharge." It's not mentioned in the *Ladies' Home Journal*, but Kissen had died unexpectedly in 1968. He'd been expected to travel to the second Conference on Psychophysiological Aspects of Cancer sponsored by the New York Academy of Sciences (NYAS).[128,129] Kissen had organized the first such NYAS conference at which papers presented included "An Emotional Life-History Pattern Associated with Neoplastic Disease" (by LeShan) and "The Significance of Personality in Lung Cancer in Men" (by Kissen).[126,130] An academic tribute to Kissen appears in the 1969 NYAS proceedings, authored by Claus Bahnson, a professor of psychiatry at Philadelphia's Jefferson Medical College who later accepted funds from the Council for Tobacco Research (previously the Tobacco Industry Research Committee).[131,132]

Kissen, it turns out, received tobacco money.[132,133] The idea that cancer stems from repressed emotions was useful to cigarette manufacturers. The tobacco industry was, most everybody realized, downplaying smoking's harms. But it was doing so in unobvious ways. The Council for Tobacco Research paid for research into causes of cancer unrelated to smoking. Besides supporting bogus psychology, it sponsored investigations into cancer's environmental triggers and, in an era when oncologists doubted heritable causes of malignancy, cancer genetics. And to discredit the ACS—which at this time was mounting nationwide anti-smoking campaigns—the tobacco council promoted unfavorable reports about the cancer society.

Enter "Cancer, Inc.," a 1978 *New Times* magazine article by Ruth Rosenbaum.[134] This puzzling piece—reproduced and distributed by the Council for Tobacco Research—appears to be a left-leaning attack on the "cancer establishment."

Rosenbaum likened the NCI to a "dollar pump," highlighted cancer-causing radiation from "X-rated mammography," and called out ACS statistics as dishonest. "Rosenbaum was fêted as a lefty maverick, but a search of the tobacco industry's archives reveals a more sinister story," Robert Proctor, a historian of science, later noted. Hill & Knowlton, the tobacco industry's PR firm, assisted Rosenbaum in writing the article, Proctor reported.[135]

Rosenbaum's piece followed a critical 1975 *Columbia Journalism Review* article by Daniel S. Greenberg, a science journalist. In Greenberg's view, the ACS and NCI officials were providing too rosy a picture of progress. "With the acceleration of the so-called federal War on Cancer, now in its third year, it is useful to contemplate certain curious and gruesome parallels that are beginning to appear between the reporting of this 'war' and the early bulletins from Vietnam," he led. The *Washington Post* republished this commentary in which Greenberg questioned the merit of using medicines (chemotherapy) to treat cancer. "One does find speculation among experts that some newly devised 'treatments' may actually be adding to the toll," he wrote.[136,137]

Greenberg's piece was one of the earliest to challenge the "war on cancer." Over time, more journalists piled on. "The 'cancer establishment' came under attack from both the Right and the Left," Proctor wrote in *Cancer Wars*. On the right, conservatives argued that the cancer society, NIH-funded research programs, and organized medicine (the AMA) conspired to suppress unconventional practitioners and alternative treatments. G. Edward Griffin of the John Birch Society suggested in his 1974 book, *World Without Cancer*, that the FDA be disbanded; in Griffin's libertarian view, patients should be free to try whatever drugs they want. On the left, critics suggested that cancer scientists aligned with industry avoided implicating chemicals as carcinogens and gave inadequate attention to cancer prevention.[138,139]

Americans built new cancer hospitals and expanded old ones. In Memphis, Tennessee, St. Jude Children's Research Hospital became a pediatric cancer mecca. The hospital's namesake is Jude Thaddeus. For Catholics, St. Jude is the patron saint of desperate and hopeless causes. Danny Thomas, the comedian and actor, led appeals for this hospital.[140,141] In Seattle, Dr. William B. (Bill) Hutchinson established a research center after his brother Fred, a baseball player and

Cincinnati Reds manager, died at forty-five from lung cancer. When "the Hutch" opened in 1975, Senator Warren G. Magnuson of Washington took to the podium, along with Ted Kennedy and Joe DiMaggio.[142–145]

Advances in radiology were instrumental to improving cancer care. The earliest CT (or CAT, computerized axial tomography) scanners rolled out in the 1970s, followed by NMR (nuclear magnetic resonance) machines, which soon became known as MRI (magnetic resonance imaging).[146] The capacity to measure tumors in three dimensions enabled doctors to gauge cancer patients' treatment responses. By mapping tumors internally, radiation oncologists could take narrower and more precise aim at cancer, reducing toxicity from x-rays hitting nearby organs.

As more people sought cancer care, oncologists specialized: surgical oncologists performed surgery; radiation oncologists gave radiation; medical oncologists, "chemotherapists," administered anticancer medications. Still, many doctors hesitated to refer their patients for chemotherapy and many patients preferred not to receive it.

While many people with breast cancer stayed quiet, public patient voices gained attention. Days after her 1972 mastectomy, the former child movie star Shirley Temple Black took the unusual step of speaking to reporters from her Stanford Hospital room in California. She deliberately publicized her operation so that women who noticed breast lumps wouldn't "sit home and be afraid." At forty-four, she wore a coral negligee and a white gardenia over one ear, the *New York Times* reported. "Don't let vanity get in your way," Black advised. The *Times* used the occasion to detail surgical options: a biopsy before definitive surgery, simple mastectomy, and lumpectomy. "There is a controversy in medical circles over which procedure is safest and best," it noted. Black wrote of her experience for *McCall's* magazine, offering this progressive stance: "The doctor can make the incision; I'll make the decision."[147–149]

A series of famous women revealed they had breast cancer. Weeks after First Lady Betty Ford underwent mastectomy in September 1974,[150–152] Happy Rockefeller, the vice president's wife, noticed a lump and underwent the same.[153–155] Doctors credited news surrounding their diagnoses for a subsequent uptick in mammography.[156,157] Meanwhile Marvella Bayh, the Indiana senator's wife, had been diagnosed in 1971 and—until her death from the disease in 1979 at age forty-six—spoke for the ACS, advocating breast self-examination and mammography.[158,159] Betty Rollin, an NBC News television correspondent, wrote about her cancer experience in *Family Circle* magazine and tell-all book titled *First, You Cry*. Notably, there was cross talk among these prominent patients. In *First, You Cry*, for instance, Rollin describes thinking of what Bayh had gone through. Before social media, many patients relied on published narratives for information and inspiration.[160,161]

In 1976, the singer Minnie Riperton was one of the first Black celebrities to open up about having breast cancer—and one of the youngest. She became an ACS spokesperson. Tragically, Riperton, a mother of two, died from breast cancer at age thirty-one in 1979. Although her treatments failed, Riperton's case raised discussion of cancer in communities of color where, in general, the subject was taboo.[162–166]

After her 1974 diagnosis, the Maryland journalist Rose Kushner applied her reporting skills to breast cancer. She visited the National Library of Medicine in Bethesda, one of few places where medical journals were available to the public. She read up on breast cancer and decided against having a radical mastectomy. But Kushner's research didn't inform only her personal choice; she laid out options about which she thought all patients should be aware in the *Washington Post*.[167] She set up the Breast Cancer Advisory Center and hotline where lay volunteers responded to queries about breast lumps and surgery. About her 1975 book, *Breast Cancer: A Personal History and an Investigative Report*, another journalist told Kushner of her embarrassment reading in public: "I put another jacket on it so I could read it on the subway." Subsequent editions were published with the title *Why Me?* and, later, *Alternatives*.[168–170]

While many Americans were not yet comfortable talking about breast cancer and even less ready to hear a patient discuss how it should be treated, Kushner attended medical conferences, uninvited. She was famously booed for questioning surgeons about radical mastectomy.[170] Eventually her pushiness paid off, though. Kushner later served alongside doctors on national cancer policy committees and published perspectives in medical journals. As considered by Ellen Leopold in *A Darker Ribbon*, Kushner reconstructed "her own ordeal to expose, at every turn, the entrenched medical practices that had remained unchallenged and unproven."[169]

Kushner died from breast cancer in 1990, after making a lasting impact on patient advocacy.[171] Like her colleague Babette Rosmond, who'd written anonymously in 1972, Kushner formed her own opinions about cancer treatment. For these "difficult" women Lasser's program, which had been so controversial in the 1950s and 1960s, wasn't cutting it. Rosmond called Reach to Recovery "a supportive parade of so-called well-adjusted fellow sufferers." Over just twenty years, patient activism had changed!

Cancer support groups formed, facilitating patient-to-patient chatter and questioning. Hotlines proliferated. If you had a question about cancer, dialing was the easiest way to get information. In 1975 the NCI, cooperatively with the ACS, established regional call centers (figure 6.4). Charities like Y-ME, based in Chicago, offered toll-free numbers.[172]

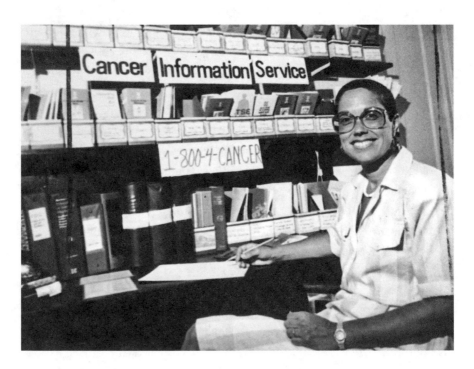

6.4 Launch of the NCI's Cancer Information Service at Yale Cancer Center, 1976

Courtesy of Yale Cancer Center

Dr. Eugene Thiessen, a Manhattan surgeon, started one of the earliest cancer support groups in 1976 after realizing that his breast cancer patients were eager to talk among themselves. A dozen women showed up to the first meeting at the Strang Clinic.[173] The Post Mastectomy Support Group, later known as SHARE, met regularly from then on. SHARE expanded to include people with gynecological cancers and caregivers. It meets to this day.

In March 1977, support group members banded with the National Organization for Women in one of the first acts of patient activism: a demonstration supporting cancer patients' right to fair employment. "Twenty women cut their Saks Fifth Avenue charge cards into pieces in front of the Fifth Avenue store yesterday to protest the store's recent refusal to hire a woman who had had a cancerous breast removed," the *New York Times* reported. Jacqueline Bleiberg of Bayside, Queens, "recently divorced," said she'd been offered a $140-a- week job selling handbags, but the offer was rescinded after Bleiberg told Saks's nurse that she'd had a mastectomy. Protesters, some in fur coats, "marched in a circle in front of the store during the lunch hour, chanting: 'Don't shop at Saks.'" Before the protest, the Saks CEO apologized for how the episode had been handled, and Bleiberg was again offered the job.[173]

In her landmark 1978 essay, "Illness as Metaphor," Susan Sontag dissected words and images surrounding malignancy.[174] She, a writer, rejected metaphorical thinking—the representation of cancer as anything other than it is—as hurtful. Because cancer is demonized and stigmatized in stories, and its reality clouded by paternalistic physicians, patients could not know their interests, she reasoned. The solution she offered is truth-telling, "to rectify the conception of the disease, to de-mythicize it."[175]

Her ideas were grounded in her experiences as a patient, which she hardly mentions. While Sontag argued against applying military terms to cancer or its treatment, she battled the disease hard and repeatedly. Sontag's breast cancer, with numerous involved lymph nodes, came at age forty-two in 1975. As later detailed by her son David Rieff, she had stage 4, metastatic disease. After consulting doctors at the Cleveland Clinic who advised a less drastic approach, she opted for radical mastectomy, a "Halstead," followed by chemotherapy and an experimental immune treatment. According to Rieff, Sontag believed her exceptional response—a complete and durable remission—was a consequence of her choosing the most aggressive course, her grit. Later, while in her sixties, Sontag was treated for a uterine cancer. Then she developed a preleukemic condition called myelodysplastic syndrome (MDS) that was likely a complication of prior cancer treatments. Most doctors considered MDS incurable. Against advice of some physicians, in her last year of life Sontag traveled to Seattle for a risky bone marrow transplant. She died in 2004 after the transplant failed, at age seventy-one.[176,177]

As a patient, Sontag wrestled with psychological theories of cancer.[178] As a writer, she dispatched these as absurd. "According to the mythology of cancer, there is generally some steady expression of feeling that causes the disease," she wrote, charging an Austrian-born psychiatrist, Dr. Wilhelm Reich, with disseminating that notion. "The source for much of the current fancy that associates cancer with repression of passion is Wilhelm Reich, who defined cancer as 'a disease following emotional resignation—a bio-energetic shrinking, a giving up of hope.'" Blame-the-victim conjecture seeps into all kinds of writing about disease, she noted, citing W. H. Auden's "Miss Gee," which refers to the mystery of cancer's causes and "foiled creative fire"; and preposterous statements by her contemporary, Norman Mailer, "who recently explained that had he not stabbed his wife (and acted out 'a murderous nest of feeling') he would have gotten cancer and 'been dead in a few years himself.'" Sontag stated, "As far as I know, no oncologist convinced of the efficacy of polychemotherapy and immunotherapy in treating patients has contributed to the fictions about a specific cancer personality." She added, "Widely believed psychological theories of disease assign to the luckless ill the ultimate responsibility both for falling ill and for getting well."

Like Rachel Carson's, Sontag's writing and medical decisions demonstrate confidence in medical science. Without naming Greenberg, Sontag called out his downplaying of progress: "Reporters covering the 'war on cancer' frequently caution the public to distinguish between official fictions and harsh facts; a few years ago, one science writer found American Cancer Society proclamations that cancer is curable and progress has been made 'reminiscent of Vietnam optimism prior to the deluge.'"

In Sontag's view, journalists' doubtfulness can be harmful when it borders on denialism. "It is one thing to be skeptical about the rhetoric that surrounds cancer, another to give support to many uniformed doctors who insist that no significant progress in treatment has been made," she wrote. Truth about cancer lies between "twin distortions" of military rhetoric—the American cancer establishment's tireless hailing of "imminent victory over cancer"—and pessimistic specialists who talk "like battle-weary officers."

As we'll see, balancing hype, skepticism, and legitimate optimism would challenge physicians, journalists, and patients for years to come.

CHAPTER 7

CANCER IN THE TIME OF AIDS (1980–1990)

I was twenty-three years old, a first-year medical student, when *Terms of Endearment* opened in movie theaters. Debra Winger vibrantly portrayed Emma, a young mother with terminal cancer. You may recall, as I did over many years, the scene when she's in a hospital room saying goodbye to her sons. My eyes dampened watching, as did pretty much everyone's. The 1983 drama featured Shirley MacLaine as Emma's widowed mother Aurora, a youthful Jeff Daniels as Emma's deadbeat husband, and Jack Nicholson as hesitant companion to Aurora who, after her daughter's death, takes charge of raising her grandchildren. *Terms of Endearment* won several Oscars, including Best Picture. It avoided cliché. Emma's diagnosis arrives amid other problems in her life; her home is broken before cancer strikes. Yet in some ways it is the same old story: Emma dies.

It's a deeply American tale, adapted from Larry McMurtry's novel of the same name. While McMurtry's text focuses on Aurora's life and relationships, the film centers on Emma's unhappy marriage and death. Evidently in 1983, producers felt confident that moviegoers would flock to a picture in which cancer kills and is said aloud.[1–3]

Midway through the film, Emma pleads for openness: "Tell them it's OK to talk about the cancer!" she shouts to her best friend after an awkward lunch with acquaintances. In a sense, the film accomplishes Emma's wish: *Terms of Endearment* "talks" about cancer. And it's likely to have precipitated real-life discussions: "I don't want to die in a hospital"; "Who will take care of my kids?"; "I don't want chemo if I'm going to die anyway"; and "I don't want my kids to see me looking pale and sick," etc.

Viewed now, Emma's plea marks how conversational norms have changed since 1983. Talking about cancer has migrated from private to public spaces.

The 1980s represent a turning point in cancer's story. In this decade, patients' prospects shifted from bleak to iffy: overall, around half lived five years after diagnosis. Gradually people began to perceive cancer differently, as treatable in some cases and not necessarily a death sentence.

The *survivor* term was new in oncology. After World War II, its use generally had been reserved for people who'd survived the Holocaust. As the number of Americans living after a malignant diagnosis expanded from five to seven million between 1987 and 1987, it gained traction. Progress became apparent as an emerging cohort of cancer survivors became visible.[4,5]

As some patients and families opened up in their communities and workplaces, others followed. Still many people didn't mention it. Before social media, public arguments about cancer were rare. There was little debate over prices of cancer drugs, and there weren't many to try. Cancer conversations were dominated by expressions of hope, encouragement, or comfort, as in *Terms of Endearment*. For cancer's "victims," sympathy abounded.

Cancer's station as the "emperor" of maladies had been secure in the postwar era. Tuberculosis had long since waned. Many Americans believed that infections would be conquered through a mix of sanitation, antibiotics, and vaccines. After doctors took aim at vascular diseases, death rates from heart attacks and strokes were declining. No illness inspired so much fear as cancer. Until AIDS.

On July 3, 1981, the *New York Times* ran this page 20 headline: "Rare Cancer Seen in 41 Homosexuals." After doctors in New York and California had diagnosed an "often rapidly fatal" malignancy in dozens of gay men, Dr. Alvin Friedman-Kien, a New York University dermatologist, alerted physicians to the "rather devastating" outbreak of Kaposi's sarcoma. The *Times* story revealed brewing anxiety—before the panic—about a disease that was not yet called AIDS. It hinted that victims would be blamed, and how: "Doctors said that most cases had involved homosexual men who have had multiple and frequent sexual encounters with different partners, as many as 10 sexual encounters each night up to four times a week." Doctors didn't know what caused this mysterious disorder. "Cancer is not believed to be contagious," and, according to a spokesperson from the Centers for Disease Control (CDC), "there was no apparent danger to nonhomosexuals," the *Times* assured readers.[6]

Upon reading this article, the gay activist and playwright Larry Kramer was compelled to action. "This is our disease and we must take care of each other and ourselves," he wrote in the *New York Native*.[7] In August 1981, some eighty people, mainly gay men, crammed into Kramer's Manhattan apartment to hear from experts what was known about the emerging disease, and to raise money for research. Friedman-Kien spoke at this meeting, which recalls the cancer society's 1913 origin, when concerned citizens gathered in Dr. Cleveland's Park Avenue home. Within a few months, Kramer and others founded the Gay Men's Health Crisis (GMHC). From its start, GMHC borrowed strategies from cancer organizations but aimed to help those affected faster—as in the "crisis" designated by its name.[8,9]

Gay men soon realized that they couldn't rely on doctors for advice or facts about the emerging disease. Most physicians in North America had never seen a case of Kaposi's sarcoma. Before the web, information tended to spread locally—on bulletin boards and flyers, by lecture and word-of-mouth. Only if a story reached an editor's desk and was deemed of broad interest, might it be covered in major news outlets. Newsletters enabled subscribers to keep abreast of developments, but those could take weeks to arrive by snail mail. There was no mechanism for real-time, nationwide discussion of medical updates.

In San Francisco, Bobbi Campbell printed a "Gay Cancer" flyer with photographs of his purplish Kaposi's skin lesions. He posted this in the window of the Star Pharmacy on Castro Street so that at-risk individuals might recognize this rare malignancy—even if doctors missed it—much as, decades earlier, the ASCC had used shop windows to raise awareness of cancer's "danger signals." To provide information directly to his community, San Francisco dermatologist Dr. Marcus Conant cofounded the Kaposi's Sarcoma Research and Education Foundation. In Los Angeles, a group later known as AIDS Project Los Angeles emerged.[10–12]

Some doctors called the disease "Gay-Related Immune Disorder," or GRID. *New York Magazine* called it the "Gay Plague." The situation in New York City, where many early cases were diagnosed, was dire. In neighborhoods like Chelsea and the West Village, dying men visited and cared for one another inside hospitals and homes. While physicians knew that AIDS affected people with hemophilia, people who inject drugs, people who'd received blood transfusions, and others, the homosexual link captured the public's attention. In September 1982, the CDC called it the "acquired immune deficiency syndrome," or AIDS.[13,14]

Fear of catching AIDS was so rampant that gay men were shunned by dentists and doctors, fired from jobs, evicted from housing, and denied funeral parlor services. Inside hospitals, workers avoided touching patients who needed assistance with showers, food, and bedpans. In San Francisco, nurses and physicians set up the first ward for AIDS patients: General Hospital's Ward 5B. In some ways, that early AIDS unit resembled cancer pavilions of the early twentieth century where, at least in principle, specialists provided treatment in a compassionate and expert manner to people with a dreaded condition.[9,15–17]

These avoidance behaviors—reflecting ignorance and stigma—were reminiscent of how cancer patients had been treated many years earlier but more extreme. Cancer could happen to anyone, most people understood, while AIDS seemed an illness affecting others. Or that's how many Americans chose to see it.

In gay communities, a sense of urgency bred a more assertive brand of patient advocacy than cancer organizations had previously demonstrated. Some people with AIDS chose to counter stigma by rendering their illness visible. In June 1983, at a Denver conference on lesbian and gay health, activists unfurled a parade-style banner reading "Fighting for Our Lives." That month, some 1,500 people attended a memorial service in Central Park for Ken Ramsauer who died from AIDS at age twenty-eight (figure 7.1). When many patients hid their condition even from their families, Ramsauer had been open about having AIDS in a televised documentary. Images of memorial-goers appeared in news. That October, vigils took place in over a dozen U.S. cities, raising AIDS awareness. In Washington, DC, more than a thousand people walked by the White House in a candlelight procession.[11,18–21]

While in medical school, I read constantly: newspapers, textbooks, and medical journals during the day; novels at bedtime. Until my fourth year, I had no TV. Like most people then, I had no personal computer. The internet was inaccessible. Inside hospitals we used clunky computers to access patients' lab results and

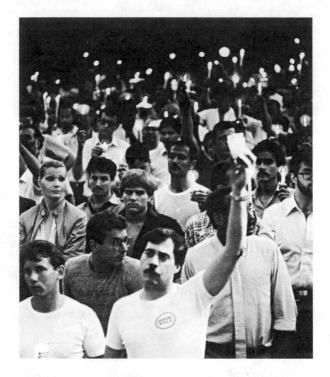

7.1 June 1983 vigil in Central Park for Ken Ramsauer who died from AIDS.
Photo by Lee Snider (with permission).

that was about it. What I learned about cancer, I learned from my professors, resident physicians at the hospital, books, and my patients. Patients most of all.

Yet I was shamefully oblivious to patients' ideas about illness. Unlike today—when many physicians take pride in "listening" to patients, and some openly exchange information and banter on social media—there was little crosstalk. Among those whose insights I overlooked was Audre Lorde, a self-described Black feminist lesbian poet whose *Cancer Journals* were published in 1980, two years after her mastectomy.[22]

Openness about breast cancer is essential because it is therapeutic, Lorde asserted. Women shouldn't "move on" after breast cancer surgery by hiding their grief or disfigurement. "Other one-breasted women hide behind the mask of prosthesis or the dangerous fantasy of reconstruction," she observed. "But I believe that socially sanctioned prosthesis is merely another way of keeping women with breast cancer silent and separate from each other."

In her community, breast cancer was hidden. Only after her mastectomy, for instance, did Lorde learn of an affected relative.[23] Rendering wounds invisible doesn't just isolate cancer patients; it delays healing and, ultimately, disempowers: "The emphasis upon wearing a prosthesis is a way of avoiding having women come to terms with their own pain and loss, and thereby, with their own strength."[24]

Lorde rejected pressure to be upbeat about cancer. After recounting a visit from a well-intentioned Reach to Recovery volunteer, she wrote, "Every attempt I made to examine or question the possibility of a real integration of this experience into the totality of my life . . . was ignored by this woman, or uneasily glossed over by her as not looking on 'the bright side of things.'"[25] Medical providers reinforced the importance of appearances, she observed. After mastectomy, Lorde felt confident of her looks and style. But when she entered a surgeon's office without a breast prosthesis under her clothing, a nurse ushered her into an exam room and chastised her: "You will feel so much better with it on," the nurse said. "Besides, we really like you to wear something, at least when you come in. Otherwise it's bad for the morale of the office.'" Indignant, Lorde compared her postmastectomy figure to Moshe Dayan, the Israeli leader who wore an eyepatch over his empty eye socket, a war wound. "Nobody tells him to go get a glass eye, or that he is bad for the morale of the office," she wrote. "The world sees him as a warrior with an honorable wound, and a loss of a piece of himself which he has marked, and mourned."[26]

Lorde wanted to be considered a combatant against cancer, not its victim. "Women with breast cancer are warriors," she wrote. "I refuse to have my scars hidden or trivialized behind lambswool or silicone gel. I refuse to be reduced in my own eyes or in the eyes of others from warrior to mere victim, simply because it might render me a fraction more acceptable or less dangerous to the still complacent."[26]

In the four decades since *Cancer Journals* was published, pugilistic cancer language has fallen out of vogue.[27-29] But in Lorde's time, when many people followed doctors' orders unquestioningly, "battling" cancer suggested a daringly active role for patients—that they didn't have to suffer passively, that their knowledge and choices could make a difference.

Lorde's words on breast cancer foreshadowed the "Silence = Death" message popularized by AIDS activists a few years later. "If we are to translate the silence surrounding breast cancer into language and action against this scourge, then the first step is that women with mastectomies become visible to each other," she wrote. "For silence and invisibility go hand in hand with powerlessness." By accepting breast prosthetics or reconstruction, mastectomy patients reinforced their isolation.* "Surrounded by other women day by day, all of whom appear to have two breasts, it is very difficult sometimes to remember that I AM NOT ALONE."[30]

Meanwhile, cancer's visibility had been notching up. One person who contributed immeasurably to this trend was Terry Fox, a Winnipeg-born athlete who aspired to run across Canada to raise money for cancer research. Fox was no ordinary runner. At age eighteen, his right leg had been amputated for osteosarcoma, a bone cancer. In April 1980, at age twenty-one and with a prosthetic leg, he set out from Newfoundland, on Canada's Atlantic coast, toward the Pacific. He ran for over four months, averaging twenty-six miles daily and traversing more than 3,300 miles. Along his route, crowds greeted Fox as media attention—and donations—grew. In September, when Fox reached Ontario's Thunder Bay, he stopped because he'd become short of breath. The cancer had spread to his lungs. He could run no farther.

Fox called his tour a "Marathon of Hope" (figure 7.2). Canadians were moved by the young man's effort. Isadore Sharp, the Toronto-born CEO of Four Seasons Hotels, sent a telegram to Fox's family, stating, "You started it. We will not rest until your dream to find a cure for cancer is realized." Days later, the Canadian television network CTV ran a telethon that raised $10 million (Canadian) in pledges for the Canadian Cancer Society.

Fox died in 1981. Since the 1980s, the Terry Fox Foundation has raised hundreds of millions of dollars for cancer research. Marathons of Hope have taken place throughout Canada—and in Brazil, Hong Kong, India, and Vietnam. Forty years later, his legacy continues to expand: in 2019, his family announced that the foundation will fund "Marathon of Hope Cancer Networks." With the Canadian government's support, this initiative will advance precision oncology—an approach to cancer care that was inconceivable during his lifetime.[31-33]

* In a footnote, Lorde attributed this idea to Maureen Brady, a contemporary feminist writer.

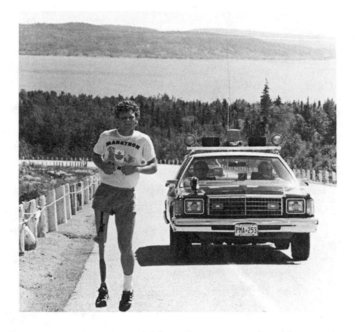

7.2 Canadian Terry Fox ran over 3,300 miles in his 1981 "Marathon of Hope." Photo by Ed Linkewich (with permission)

The deaths of two celebrities around this time demonstrate the continued appeal of alternative cancer treatments. Actor Steve McQueen had mesothelioma, an incurable malignancy of the lung lining. When doctors diagnosed his tumor in 1979, the "King of Cool" had already quit smoking. McQueen took chemotherapy and radiation, but when those didn't work he traveled to Rosarito Beach, Mexico, near Tijuana, where. Dr. William D. Kelley, a dentist with a suspended Texas license, gave vitamins and minerals, coffee enemas, cells prepared from animal fetuses, and laetrile—a controversial "treatment" derived from apricot pits.

McQueen tried to keep his cancer a secret but the *National Enquirer* got wind of his condition and published "Steve McQueen's Heroic Battle Against Terminal Cancer." At first McQueen said the story was just a rumor. Then he acknowledged his illness. The reason for denying his cancer, he said, "was to save my family and friends from personal hurt and to retain my sense of dignity." He McQueen died at age fifty after surgery in a Mexican hospital, less than a year after his diagnosis.[34–36]

Bob Marley, the world-famous Jamaican reggae musician, died from skin cancer. In 1977, after injuring his right big toe playing soccer, he'd developed a painful nonhealing wound. After a biopsy revealed malignant melanoma, a doctor advised toe amputation. Marley, then thirty-two, declined surgery. Later he sought "integrative" and unproven immune cancer treatments at the West German clinic of Dr. Josef Issels. Marley died in 1981, at thirty-six, with tumors involving his lung, liver, and brain.[37]

Since Marley's death, dermatologists have used his story to teach medical students that people of African heritage can develop melanoma, a tumor of melanocytes (skin cells containing melanin pigment). Some doctors mistakenly believe that Black people are not at risk for skin cancers, which tend to occur after sunburns. Acral melanoma, what Marley had, tends to arise on palms, soles of feet, and nailbeds.[38,39]

I didn't know of Marley's diagnosis until 2018, when I read Tara Westover's book, *Educated*. "From the Internet I learned about the cancer that had been discovered on Bob Marley's foot," she wrote. Rastafarian beliefs had led him to refuse surgery, Westover noted, "while an operable melanoma was, at that moment, metastasizing." Westover had been homeschooled and previously had avoided immunizations. Her mother was an herbalist. After considering what happened to Marley, Westover became open to receiving modern medical care. She decided to get vaccinated.[40]

In 1983, the evangelist Oral Roberts sent a letter to his followers, said to number a million, asking each to contribute $240 for the City of Faith Medical and Research Center in Tulsa, Oklahoma. The complex, with three high-rise buildings including a sixty-story clinical tower on Tulsa's Oral Roberts University campus, opened in 1981 but stayed unfinished.[41–43] "God said to me . . . 'I am going to bring mighty and greater breakthroughs for the cure of cancer,'" Roberts wrote to his "prayer partners," the *Washington Post* reported.[44]

Cancer couldn't save the City of Faith, however. The facility remained somewhat empty and was losing money.[45–47] In 1989, Roberts decided to shutter the hospital and an affiliated medical school.[48–50] The next year, Cancer Care Centers of America (CCCA), which later became Cancer Treatment Centers of America, took a thirty-year lease on space in the thirty-floor hospital building, sparing Roberts's enterprise some debt.[51,52]

Tulsa's cancer center became second in an expanding CCCA network. Unbeknownst to many patients, the original CCCA facility in Zion, Illinois, had run into trouble under another guise: American International Hospital. In 1980 the

Chicago Tribune had exposed that institution for peddling harmful "cures": hyperthermic treatments, a chemical called DMSO, coffee enemas, and laetrile. The newspaper revealed how desperate families were drawn to alternative therapies offered at the seemingly legitimate cancer center in Illinois.[53,54]

The *Tribune* detailed the story of Floyd Lewis, an Indiana trucker and father of six whose ten-year-old son had leukemia and died after receiving "metabolic" treatments at the Zion hospital. Initially, Lewis was appreciative of having options for his son, other than bone marrow transplant as had been advised by University of Minnesota doctors. At the Illinois facility, his son was put on a meatless diet. He was given intravenous vitamin C and coffee enemas. "They just kept brainwashing us that it would work," Lewis told the *Tribune*. "They just kept saying that he was getting better right up to the time he died."[55,56]

Perhaps no activity had a greater effect on cancer awareness than what started on a drizzly 1983 day at the Galleria Mall in Dallas, Texas. Hundreds turned out to cheer runners, clad in pink tee-shirts, at the Susan G. Komen Breast Cancer Foundation's first "Race for the Cure," as these events became known. Nancy Goodman Brinker, a wealthy and well-connected Dallas resident, founded the organization soon after her older sister, Susan Goodman Komen, died from metastatic breast cancer at age thirty-six in 1980. The inaugural Komen function—a planned polo tournament and luncheon—drew Betty Ford, the former first lady who'd had breast cancer. Other prominent women affiliated with the Republican Party got involved: Kay Bailey Hutchison, a lawyer and newscaster who'd served in the Texas state legislature and later became a U.S. senator, and Laura Bush, a young mother of twins and future first lady.

People in Dallas weren't keen on talking about breast cancer, Brinker considered. A run would get people involved, to donate—even if they wouldn't speak of it. By hosting races, gala parties, and other pleasant affairs, the organization raised several hundred thousand dollars annually. Although the charity later acquired a reputation for funding awareness *per se*, Komen's early grants supported clinical care and research at Texas institutions. In 1984, Brinker herself was diagnosed with breast cancer; she underwent surgery and received chemotherapy. Brinker "believes in being 'public' about her breast cancer—she even talks about her illness on public-service television announcements in Dallas,"

Judy Klemesrud reported in a syndicated 1985 *New York Times* story. Yet some news outlets couldn't—or wouldn't—use the word "breast" in covering the annual Dallas run. They could call it a race for "'female cancer' or 'woman's cancer,'" Brinker recalled.[57–62]

While numerous local breast cancer organizations existed, few had national reach. In 1986, Brinker teamed up with Rose Kushner and others in founding the National Alliance of Breast Cancer Organizations (NABCO). Amy Langer, who'd left her job as a Lehman Brothers investment banker after a diagnosis at age thirty, got involved. Using her personal Macintosh computer, a novelty then, working in a closet-like space within the New York office of Cancer Care, an established agency, Langer set up a database of NABCO members and a breast cancer information network. By 1990, she was NABCO's executive director.[63–65]

To educate women and promote screening, NABCO promoted October as "Breast Cancer Awareness Month." In doing so, it accepted support from Imperial Chemical Industries (ICI), a British-based company that manufactured tamoxifen, one of the earliest FDA-approved breast cancer treatments. Chicago's Y-ME—with its then-expanding network of support groups—also collaborated with ICI and accepted industry funds. Doctors' organizations including the American Academy of Family Physicians participated.[66,67]

The calendar event remained under most Americans' radar until after 1990, however. That's when Congress passed legislation and President George H. W. Bush signed a proclamation designating October as Breast Cancer Awareness Month.[68]

Having fun—planning a party, essentially—for cancer charities had been a successful fundraising strategy since the Ladies' Auxiliary of the New-York Skin and Cancer Hospital held its *kirmesses* in the 1880s. To draw crowds and donations, organizers developed elaborate and wacky event themes. The tradition continues today, as numerous cancer charities compete for the public's attention and dollars. Some indulge "guilty pleasures"—behaviors that would otherwise be forbidden—like gambling or pie-throwing, for the cause.

"Jail-a-thons" are a disturbing example. Rules varied by location. "Do you have someone you would like to land in the slammer? You can do it . . . And the bad deed can be a good deed," the 1985 *Pensacola News* told Florida readers. "The Jail-a-Thon means you donate $25 to ACS and they will have a real off-duty lawman haul your choice to the mall jail," it explained.[69] This was not an isolated event: cities hosting jail-a-thons to benefit the ACS included Hartford, Connecticut; Asheville, Chapel Hill and Rocky Mount, North Carolina; Indiana and Bethlehem, Pennsylvania; Flagstaff, Arizona; and Casper, Wyoming.[70–78]

In Lawrenceville, Georgia, an Atlanta suburb, organizers in 1984 erected a temporary jail on the county courthouse lawn. For a $25 donation, an ACS volunteer would mock-arrest most "anyone—a boss, friend or spouse." At the courthouse Lawrenceville's mayor, other local politicians, and the Gwinnett County police chief judged and set "bail" for "prisoners." The event grew bigger. In 1986, KISS 104 FM radio sponsored a "Jail and Bail" for the ACS at Atlanta's Greenbriar Mall. Proceeds would support cancer research, patient services, and educational programs. "Participation is strictly voluntary," the *Atlanta Daily World* assured.[79,80]

The jail-a-thon fad spread to the West Coast where, in Southern California, LA Rams cheerleaders assisted Orange County Sherriff's Department officers in "incarcerating" individuals to be released upon "bail" payment to the cancer society. "Arrestees were allowed as many phone calls as they needed to raise their bail, which was set by a 'judge' and 'jury,'" the *Los Angeles Times* reported.[81]

By the 1980s, public concerns about chemical carcinogens were fading. Warning after warning about cancer-causing substances—artificial sweeteners, red dye no. 2, flame retardants, hair dyes, and chemicals like polychlorinated biphenyls (PCBs)—had resulted in alarm fatigue. (figure 7.3).

"The parade of chemicals that cause cancer seems endless," science journalist Philip M. Boffey wrote in a 1984 *New York Times* article.[82] There had been a "striking shift of opinion" among many researchers, he reported. Then U.S. Secretary of Health and Human Services, Margaret M. Heckler—a Reagan appointee and former Republican congresswoman—emphasized smoking and low-fiber diets as causes. Boffey referred extensively to the findings of British epidemiologists Richard Peto and Dr. Richard Doll.[83] In their landmark report commissioned by the U.S. Congress, Peto and Doll attributed most cancer deaths to tobacco and diet. "By diet, they did not mean chemical additives or chemical pollutants that invade the food supply." Boffey clarified. "Rather, they meant such dietary factors as carcinogens that appear naturally in food," excess fats which raise the body's internal production of carcinogens, lack of fibers to "flush" toxins from the bowels, and other nutritional causes. Workplace exposures accounted for only four percent of cancer deaths and consumer products, like hair dyes and plastics, less than one percent, Peto and Doll had estimated, with this caveat: "There is too much ignorance for complacency." ACS and NCI officials agreed with Peto and Doll's estimates, Boffey reported. So did Berkeley biochemist Bruce Ames: "I think we got off on the wrong track. We're concentrating almost exclusively on little bits of pollution and manmade things and completely ignoring enormous amounts of natural mutagens and carcinogens," Ames said.

As attention to cancer's possible environmental causes diminished, genetics gained traction. Investigators developed ways to clone and sequence DNA

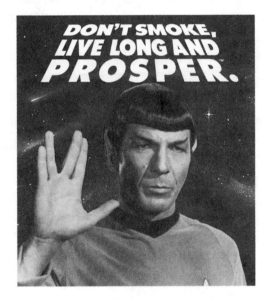

7.3 "Great American Smokeout" poster, c.1989

Courtesy of the American Cancer Society

more efficiently, and oncogenes—bits of genetic material implicated in malignant growths—were identified. In 1985 the polymerase chain reaction, PCR, was invented; now it's an essential tool for analyzing genes. Monoclonal antibodies were another advance. Although doctors already appreciated the structure of antibodies—natural substances that bind germs—pharmaceutical companies had not yet manufactured these for treating disease in humans. In the 1980s, they began developing uniform (monoclonal) antibodies to target malignant cells.

Yet there was little application of basic science in cancer care. In these years, medical oncologists tried to shrink patients' tumors by combining and upping doses of chemotherapy. Treatments were hard to take; patients became quite sick. When I was a student and resident, we lacked effective drugs for nausea. Patients getting chemotherapy retched horribly, sometimes tearing the esophagus. Growth factors to stimulate healthy white blood cells weren't available. Without those injectable agents—now in everyday use—many cancer patients died from infection. While chemotherapy is no "walk in the park" today, it's much less onerous than before 1990.

In July 1985, I entered my third and clinical year of medical school at New York University. AIDS patients were crowding Bellevue, NYU's main teaching hospital, and other New York City hospitals. My friends and I watched the epidemic unfold close-up on wards where we worked and in neighborhoods around the dorms where we lived. A good fraction of my patients had AIDS, and many of the cancer patients I recall from those years had Kaposi's sarcoma or AIDS-related lymphomas. There were no antiretroviral treatments. The disease appeared uniformly fatal.

That same month, Rock Hudson announced that he had AIDS. The movie star was credited with "putting a face" on the disease and he died less than three months later.[84,85] As with cancer charities, celebrities got involved. Judith Peabody, a prominent socialite, volunteered with GMHC. Elizabeth Taylor, Hudson's friend and *Giant* costar, led appeals for amfAR, the Foundation for AIDS Research.[86–88] But those organizations—while helpful in providing services and funding research—failed to channel the despair and anger of those affected.

When doctors removed a malignant polyp, glands, and two feet of President Ronald Reagan's gut in 1985, the operation was publicized. Reagan's surgery took place at the U.S. Naval hospital in Bethesda, Maryland. Before going under anesthesia, Reagan signed a letter assigning presidential powers to Vice President George H. W. Bush. The *Washington Post* headlined updates on page 1: "Reagan to Undergo Intestinal Surgery Today" (July 13); "Reagan Tumor Removed; No Cancer Evident" (July 14); "President, Recovering . . ." (July 15); and "Reagan Tumor Found to Be Cancerous" (July 16).[89–92]

"The President has cancer," the NCI's Dr. Steven Rosenberg stated at a press conference, prompting speculation about Reagan's status, if he was cured.[93] "Doctors Have a Tense Debate: Reagan 'Has' or 'Had' Cancer?" the *Los Angeles Times* recapped. Rosenberg used the verb "has," it reported. "A subsequent statement that, as far as doctors can tell, Reagan's cancer had not spread—has raised questions about why he used the present tense." The White House subsequently asked Rosenberg not to discuss the case with reporters, "so it is not possible to learn what prompted his choice of words," the *Los Angeles Times* added. Some experts disagreed with Rosenberg's tense. Dr. Kenneth Ramming, a professor of surgery at UCLA's medical school, stated, "My style is to say that he or she had a cancer and, thank goodness, we were there in time."[94]

When asked if the president, then seventy-four, could hold down a job as stressful and difficult as the presidency after colon cancer surgery, Rosenberg responded obliquely: Most patients can and should resume complete activity. "That will be my advice to the President as well," he told journalists. This discussion revealed how perception was changing, that a malignant diagnosis was not a death sentence. People were beginning to consider cancer like other medical conditions—a finite illness after which life's activities, including work, might resume.

Reagan's cancer story was said to ease discussion of the unmentionable: "The taboo against talking about colon and rectal cancer, about the elimination of wastes from the body, and about the bowels in general has been broken," Irving Rimer, an ACS communications specialist, told the *Los Angeles Times*. After newspapers published explainers on colon cancer screening and staging, calls to the NCI's information hotline spiked. SmithKline Diagnostics, a manufacturer of screening kits for blood in stool, a sign of possible cancer, reported increased demand; in some stores, supplies ran out. Although the president's case raised interest in screening, there was no measured public health effect such as reduced deaths from colon or rectal tumors.[95,96]

Being a cancer survivor was unchartered territory when Dr. Fitzhugh Mullan published his 1985 essay "Seasons of Survival: Reflections of a Physician with Cancer." Cancer memoirs were not yet common when he'd written *Vital Signs*—a doctor's firsthand account of what it's like to be on the receiving end of chemotherapy and radiation. Mullan, a pediatrician and father, decided to open up because he thought that doing so would help other patients, much as Dr. Anna Palmer had used her position, in 1938, to persuade a skeptical public that cancer could be cured. While many doctors didn't pay attention to patients' concerns, and comments about survivors' "unmet needs" would have registered as complaints, Mullan's voice hit home because he was a physician.[97,98]

Writing for an audience of doctors reading the *New England Journal of Medicine*, Mullan used medical terms to explain the need for survivorship care. If cancer patients were fortunate to be saved during the acute phase of diagnosis and treatment, as he'd been, they didn't receive adequate counseling about late complications: disfigurement, infertility, depression, and social problems including insurance and employment discrimination, all of which he mentioned. Cancer patients need long-term guidance, he emphasized. "Survival, in fact, begins at the point of diagnosis," he clarified. Although many people mistakenly apply the "survivor" term exclusively to patients in long-term remission, Mullan's definition of survivorship—from cancer diagnosis until death—remains in use by the NCI and other agencies; a person living with metastatic cancer is a cancer survivor.[99–102]

In 1986, Mullan spearheaded the National Coalition for Cancer Survivorship. For the inaugural conference, twenty-five participants representing the extant hodgepodge of support groups scattered around the country—Asheville North Carolina's Life After Cancer-Pathways, Cincinnati Ohio's Cancer Share, Seattle's Cancer Lifeline, and others—traveled to Albuquerque, New Mexico. National organizations including the ACS, Cancer Care (based in New York), Candlelighters Childhood Cancer Foundation (based in DC), and the Oncology Nursing Society, got involved. This was a much-needed advocacy organization. Before the web, many cancer survivors felt isolated and were eager to meet others.[103–105]

One enthusiastic member of the survivorship coalition was Kansas City, Missouri, business leader Richard (Dick) Bloch. Two decades after he and his brother founded H&R Block, the tax preparation firm, Bloch was diagnosed with lung cancer. After local specialists said there was no hope, Bloch thought he didn't have long to live. Days later at Houston's MD Anderson Hospital, doctors said otherwise. Two years after Bloch's 1978 surgery, doctors pronounced him cancer free.

Delighted and feeling appreciative, Bloch and his wife, Annette, established a foundation to help Kansas City residents affected by cancer.[106] He sponsored a hotline and the foundation supported a center where patients and families could meet. At the "R. A. Bloch Cancer Management Center," patients could obtain expert second opinions at no charge. Getting another opinion wasn't trivial. It necessitated time and means for medical appointments and travel, and nerve. Some cancer patients didn't want to hear anything beyond what local physicians advised. Many died without hearing of possible treatments and clinical trials available elsewhere.

In his book *Fighting Cancer*, Bloch cautioned against uninformed doctors and undue fatalism: "Often the physician who makes the initial diagnosis is a contributor to the problem. If he graduated medical school only 10 years ago, over half the cancers he was told were untreatable when he was in school are today curable to some degree," he wrote. Physicians who've seen their patients suffer through "primitive treatments" are unlikely to recommend oncology care; instead, they recommend that cancer patients "go home and make themselves as comfortable as possible." Physicians' knowledge and attitudes are crucial, Bloch considered. "Be positive!" he advised.[107]

At a June 1986 "Celebration of Life" rally in downtown Kansas City, Bloch spoke before a crowd of eight hundred.[108,109] "I'm not saying that everyone can beat cancer. Certainly, some people are going to die from it, no matter what they do," he acknowledged. "But . . . if a person doesn't try, there is no way they can beat it." A year later, Bloch coordinated a rally with the first "survivor's day." In 1988, with involvement of the ACS and the survivorship coalition, in cities like Pittsburgh and Rapid City, South Dakota, surviving cancer patients and families observed National Cancer Survivors' Day with picnics, rallies, and balloon launchings. Festivities took place near the old Pondville Hospital site in Norfolk, Massachusetts. The National Cancer Survivors Day tradition continues, managed by a foundation, with events held on the first Sunday of June.[110–115]

To counter pessimism about cancer, Bloch decided to build inspirational parks. "I asked myself what could Dick Bloch do for cancer sufferers. It was not a question of money," he told a journalist. "The Government devotes billions to cancer research, and there was not much I could do that would make a difference in that." As reported by the *New York Times* in 1990, Bloch "believed that 'the second greatest correctable cause of cancer mortality—smoking is No. 1—is relating death and cancer.'"

The Cancer Survivors Park in Kansas City—one of around twenty nationwide—opened on 2.5 acres of donated land in the business district. Planted with shrubs and flowers, it featured symbolism to inspire those affected. Sculptures depicted the "trauma of entering and enduring treatment for cancer" but also celebrated "hope of victory and the joy of realization," the *Times* noted. At its center, pedestals held plaques carrying messages of support and led to an arch. "This arch denotes passage," Bloch said. "You go out to that area and it's a celebration of life. People now think death and cancer are synonymous. The whole purpose is to explode that myth."[116]

I was in my final year of medical school when the FDA approved AZT, the first drug for treating HIV, in March 1987. Six months earlier, investigators had cut short a randomized clinical trial because patients in the control arm, taking a placebo, were dying faster than those receiving AZT. The FDA issued a narrow decision, however, recommending prescriptions only for people with AIDS or other specified conditions. Researchers said they didn't yet know if this medicine would benefit people with HIV who weren't yet ill. While studies were ongoing, many gay men and other people living with HIV, but not yet with AIDS and without AZT-qualifying symptoms, wanted this medicine ASAP. The drug's manufacturer, Burroughs Wellcome, set a price of around $10,000 for a year's supply.[117–120]

That month, the AIDS Coalition to Unleash Power (ACT UP) began. Larry Kramer, who'd left GMHC and penned *The Normal Heart*—a play of rage against the disease[121,122]—spoke before 250 people at New York's Lesbian and Gay Community Center, saying, "A new drug can easily take ten years to satisfy FDA approval. Ten years! Two-thirds of us could be dead in less than five years." Kramer mentioned the Lavender Hill Mob, a brash group of AIDS activists who'd gained attention at a CDC meeting in Atlanta: "They yelled and screamed and demanded and were blissfully rude to all those arrogant epidemiologists who are ruining our lives." He told the audience, "We have to go after the FDA—fast. That means coordinated protests, pickets, arrests."[86,123]

Days later, the FDA approved AZT. Rather than hailing the agency's move, Kramer published a critical op-ed. The FDA's decision was a "sop to the gay community—so they'll shut up," a doctor told him. With no other HIV medicines nearing approval and AZT, in Kramer's opinion, not being the best drug in the pipeline, he was furious. "AIDS patients do not have that long to live," Kramer wrote. "AIDS sufferers, who have nothing to lose, are more than willing to be guinea pigs," he said. "Double-blind studies were not created with terminal illnesses in mind. It is, again, inhumane to withhold drugs from terminally ill patients willing to take them."[124]

Images proved powerful in the fight against AIDS. When six hundred activists participated in the first ACT UP demonstration†—a March 1987 sit-in on Wall Street—television crews were on hand filming. Police officers and others called to the scene feared catching AIDS; they hesitated to touch protestors who lay down on the sidewalk. Meanwhile AIDS activists had plastered the city with posters that declared, beneath a pink triangle, "Silence = Death." Between 1987 and 1990, ACT UP organized protests at the New York Stock Exchange and St. Patrick's Cathedral, at the FDA campus in Bethesda, Maryland, and elsewhere. ACT UP chapters formed in other cities.[86,125,126] In October 1987, volunteers displayed another evocative image, the AIDS Quilt, on the National Mall in Washington, DC. The quilt joined more than 1,900 panels, each marking someone who died from AIDS. The quilt originated in San Francisco and grew larger each year as grieving patients' partners, family, and friends added to it.[127–129]

As AIDS activists gained visibility, controversy continued over patients' access to medicines. In December 1987 the *New York Times* headlined "Doctors Stretch Rules on AIDS Drug" on page one. Nine months after AZT's approval, off-label prescribing was widespread and splitting the medical community, Gina Kolata reported. "No useful scientific information" will result from dispensing AZT without gathering data; sound studies take time, experts emphasized. "The best thing to do now is to let the scientific community work this out," the NCI's

† The organization was not yet called ACT UP.

Dr. Samuel Broder told her. "In addition to AZT's dangerous side effects, another drawback of the drug is its expense . . . as much as $10,000 a year," she noted. But most insurance companies weren't "balking" at covering off-label prescriptions, she noted.[130]

While this might seem a digression in a book about cancer patient activism, these same arguments—over dying patients access to medicines, the pace of FDA approvals, off-label prescriptions, and drug prices—enter current oncology debates. While some patients, advocates, and doctors favor a measured approach with FDA decisions resting strictly on survival benefits demonstrated in randomized trials, others support speedier access; that is, allowing people with incurable cancer to try compounds that have been safety-checked in early-phase studies and evaluated using novel methods in clinical research, such as umbrella or basket trials, for their impact on survival and for side effects.

Many doctors and historians credit AIDS activists with accelerating the FDA's approval of early HIV drugs; those medicines enabled survival of people who otherwise would have died. While AZT helped thousands with HIV to live longer, it was not a curative drug. Gradually, other antiviral medicines became available. Combined retroviral therapy turned out to be effective, suppressing HIV to undetectable levels and lowering risk of transmission to almost nil. With medication, today someone with HIV is expected to live a full life span.

In 1990, Congress passed the Ryan White Act, named for a boy who'd received a blood transfusion and died from AIDS. This legislation elevated federal funds for AIDS care and research. U.S. deaths from AIDS peaked in 1995.[131,132] The profound hopelessness surrounding AIDS persisted through the late 1990s; it took a long time for perception to change.

Unlike many people living with AIDS in cities in the 1980s, advanced cancer patients had little opportunity to organize. Lung cancer was the leading malignant killer; it claimed over one hundred thousand U.S. lives each year. Because there were no effective treatments for advanced lung cancer and it was rarely caught in time for surgery, long-term survival was unusual. With exception, people with lung cancer rarely met, lacked newsletters, and died quickly. Breast cancer was also common but less lethal. For the year 1988, the ACS estimated there would be 136,000 new diagnoses and 42,000 breast cancer deaths, a terrible statistic. But within most regions of the United States, what doctors and the public "witnessed" were stage 4 patients outnumbered by those with early-stage breast cancer, so it didn't appear so often fatal.[133]

Cancer charities were often staffed by survivors of treatable tumors. Many volunteers were women who preferred cooperative tactics: behaving professionally and even demurely, nodding to doctors' expertise, not being confrontational. Survivors who were sufficiently well—to work, travel, and speak up about patients' needs and priorities—were generally less desperate than their AIDS-affected counterparts. The "incurables" with advanced cancer lacked representation.

Near the decade's close, Gilda Radner died at age forty-two from ovarian cancer. Humor made it easier for the original *Saturday Night Live* cast member to talk about the disease. "Cancer is probably the most unfunny thing in the world, but I'm a comedienne, and even cancer couldn't stop me from seeing the humor in what I went through," she said. Her memoir, *It's Always Something*, was published within weeks of her May 1989 obits.[134–136]

Radner's cancer account, a best seller, is not a prettified read. For instance, she doesn't gloss over the experience of getting a barium enema; she calls it a "photo session" with "a tube up your ass" while spinning in "the Rotor." She admits feelings of humiliation, being weakened by chemotherapy and radiation treatments which kept her vomiting for days, pale, thin, without hair, stumbling, and unable to drive. And shame: "with baldness like the mark on a house that was quarantined."[134]

Radner discovered camaraderie and hopefulness at the Los Angeles Wellness Community, a place where cancer patients met and encouraged one another, shared feelings, and traded information. There she learned that "the most magic thing we have [is] our ability to open our mouths and communicate with each other." Language mattered to Radner. Like other patient-authors of this time, she preferred "fighting" words: "I didn't want a 'coping with cancer' cover because that's not the way I was dealing with cancer," she said of her interactions with *Life* editors who put her on the magazine's cover. "I was fighting," she insisted.

Her story reflects the era. While Radner thought chemotherapy might be curative, a doctor told her husband, actor Gene Wilder, the truth: that cancer had spread to her gut and liver. She was in the dark: "The internist told Gene that I had only a twenty-percent chance of survival. . . . Gene, of course, never told me, but he was carrying that information all the time behind his smiling face." She refers to her medical oncologist as the "Alchemist"—a term reminiscent of "chemotherapist" still used by older physicians then, but with an optimistic twist—adding a sense of wonder or, perhaps childishly, magic to his powers.

It's Always Something is essential to Radner's legacy. As a celebrity, through humor and openness, she broke barriers. The comfort she experienced at the Los Angeles center—among peer patients—led to Wilder's co-founding Gilda's Club a few years after her death. By telling her story, she made a difference in other—and future patients'—lives.

CHAPTER 8

ENTHUSIASM (1990–2000)

Days after his fifty-first birthday in February 1992, Paul Tsongas won the New Hampshire primary for the U.S. Democratic presidential ticket. The former senator from Massachusetts vied for the top slot with Arkansas's Bill Clinton, California's Jerry Brown, and Iowa's Tom Harkin. Tsongas's candidacy was short-lived, however; he withdrew a month later. Nonetheless, Tsongas took first place in several primaries and received more than a quarter of votes in delegate-rich states like Florida and New York. For a brief time, Tsongas—a cancer survivor—was a serious contender for the nation's highest office.

Tsongas came from Lowell, Massachusetts. His Greek parents operated a dry-cleaning business where he'd worked during high school. Smart and ambitious, he swam competitively in college at Dartmouth, joined the Peace Corps, and spent time in Ethiopia before attending Yale Law School. In 1974, he was elected to the U.S. Congress. His career moved forward steadily; four years later, he was elected to the Senate. Tsongas didn't drink or smoke; in Washington circles, he became known as a moralizing teetotaler. He was married, a father to three girls, in 1983 when a lymphoma diagnosis upended his life and career. Instead of seeking reelection, he sought oncology care at Boston's Dana-Farber Cancer Institute. In 1984, Tsongas published a memoir, *Heading Home*. His cancer came back, however. In 1986, he received a bone marrow transplant, then experimental, for recurrent lymphoma.[1-6]

In March 1991, doctors proclaimed Tsongas cancer-free and fit for presidential office. Dr. George Canellos, Dana-Farber's chief of oncology, said a successful transplant had left Tsongas "as healthy as any 50-year-old I've ever seen." Tsongas appeared at the National Press Club in Washington alongside his physician,

Dr. Tak Takvorian, a transplant specialist. The candidate did his best to assuage concerns about his health, inviting journalists to watch him swim. C-SPAN aired footage of Tsongas wearing a Speedo, stretching on a pool deck, diving into the pool, and doing laps of the butterfly.[7–11]

The *Boston Globe* ran a piece on health concerns surrounding the politician: "A 'survivor' boldly confronts Americans' fear of the 'Big C,'" it headlined.[12] "Tsongas is less at risk of developing a debilitating medical condition than a presidential candidate with, say, high blood pressure," Renée Loth reported. "With a survival rate of 50 percent for all cancers (and approaching 90 percent for lymphoma), living with the disease could almost be seen as an acceptable risk," she noted. "But for a whole generation of living, voting Americans, to be stricken with cancer is to be marked for death."

People in other U.S. regions might not be comfortable with the candidate's medical history, Dana-Farber's director of social work, Naomi Stearns, told the *Globe*. "We live in a medical mecca in Boston," she said. "If you go into the small towns, there are people who, if they heard you once had cancer, would still give you a paper cup." The AIDS epidemic had changed the standing of cancer as the nation's most dreaded disease, the story suggested. "Now that's the disease with the stigma, and cancer has become respectable," Stearns said. "People find out they have cancer and say, 'Thank God it's not AIDS.'"

Looking back, it's unclear if cancer is what sank Tsongas's candidacy. In April 1992, the *New York Times* reported that Tsongas hadn't been forthcoming about his medical history: that he'd undergone radiation treatment to an affected lymph node in 1987, after the transplant. Dr. Lawrence K. Altman, a physician and journalist, obtained comments on Tsongas's condition from a lymphoma expert unaffiliated with Dana-Farber, where Tsongas was both a patient and trustee. "The significance of a relapse after a bone marrow transplant is huge because it means that the bone marrow transplant did not cure him," said Dr. James O. Armitage of the University of Nebraska. "His doctors and the Dana-Farber Cancer Institute in Boston, a Harvard teaching hospital, now acknowledge that they have not told the complete story," Altman reported.[13]

Although Tsongas entered remission, it didn't last. Later in 1992, Tsongas disclosed that the lymphoma had grown again.[14–16] Then he developed myelodysplastic syndrome, a malignant blood condition, sometimes called "preleukemia," that can arise as a complication of bone marrow transplantation. In 1996 he received another kind of transplant from his twin sister. His condition declined irreversibly and he died at age fifty-five in January 1997.[17-19]

Tsongas's run for president reveals a changing perception of cancer—that a survivor who'd received intensive chemotherapy might be elected to lead the United States. His story elevated public understanding of lymphoma, bone marrow transplantation, and survivorship. He raised debate over politicians' responsibility to reveal personal health information. "Cancer" was no longer monolithic in the public's eye. Americans understood that some malignancies could be effectively treated and possibly cured.

The 1990s were heady times for oncologists. In clinics, my colleagues and I were prescribing medicines to effectively treat some types of lymphoma and leukemia. New kinds of therapy, like monoclonal antibodies, were in the pipeline. The first of those approved by the FDA—Rituxan (rituximab) for lymphoma, in 1997—turned out to be a terrific drug; it's now in everyday use.[20,21] Herceptin (trastuzumab) was in clinical trials in the 1990s; we had no inkling how amazingly helpful this antibody would prove against HER2-positive breast cancer, an aggressive form.[22-24] Experiments by Harvard physician Dr. Judah Folkman using anti-angiogenic agents, substances that block cancer's blood supply, received attention in news.[25-28] Although that strategy later disappointed, oncologists looked forward to implementing the innovative approach. Optimism prevailed.

Research was humming along. At the NIH and elsewhere, scientists were sequencing the human genome. We anticipated that project would deliver clues for better treatments. Still there was a long gap between research and patient care. For people with advanced solid tumors, the prognosis hardly budged. With rare exception, unless those cancers were caught early and could be removed by surgery or zapped by radiation, there was little hope. We medical oncologists, "chemotherapists," had little to offer patients with lung cancer, for instance, even in clinical trials. In general, our expectations of targeting drugs precisely to tumors were low for the foreseeable future.[29]

The World Wide Web became public in 1993. Most Americans didn't have internet access at home, but a growing number used computers at workplaces. Starting around 1995, web pages displayed photographs and other visuals, literally changing how we see the world. Email, previously used by academics, became commonplace by this decade's end. Although we may not have realized it then, these advances in communications and informatics would be crucial for cancer science and clinical care.

While online journals (weblogs, later "blogs") were rare, internet chat rooms and bulletin boards enabled patients to post questions and personal musings. A few cancer organizations developed listservs to distribute information by email. In 1995, after his wife's breast cancer diagnosis, Gilles Frydman sought information about options beyond what her doctor offered. He founded ACOR, the Association of Cancer Online Resources.[30,31] By 1998, ACOR's website published updates like blog posts from individual patients: "GrannyBarb" with chronic lymphocytic leukemia, "June Brazil" with multiple myeloma, and others. Some ACOR pages functioned as online newsletters with links to resources about colon cancer, metastatic breast cancer, melanoma, and other conditions.[32]

For the first time, patients living most anywhere, with rare cancers or undergoing particular treatments like bone marrow transplant could communicate directly, peer to peer. Before social media, this was revolutionary. Yet few envisioned the connectedness—and torrent of information—the web would deliver.

When I finished my fellowship in 1993, hospitals around the country were building specialized units to provide high-dose chemotherapy and bone marrow transplantation (BMT), a lucrative procedure. Broadly speaking, there are two methods. In *autologous* BMT, cells from the patient's marrow—the body's main source of blood cells—are removed, frozen, and stored. After the patient receives high doses of chemotherapy and radiation to eradicate cancer, their cells are thawed and infused to "rescue" the wiped-out marrow. In *allogeneic* BMT, blood-forming cells from another person—a "match"—are infused after the high-dose treatments.* Either way, until the graft takes, patients are vulnerable to

---

* More recent articles refer to hematopoietic stem cell transplantation (HSCT), a variant of BMT in which blood-forming stem cells are obtained and purified from the patient's or donor's circulating blood rather than directly from bone marrow.

infections and other life-threatening complications. Allogeneic transplants such as Susan Sontag and Paul Tsongas received near the ends of their lives are riskier than autologous BMT but more likely curative.[33]

Autologous transplants were being given, amid controversy, to women with breast cancer deemed likely to relapse ("high risk") or metastatic cases. This was a blunt treatment without known survival benefit. In early-phase trials some patients had terrific responses—their tumors shrank—but other patients' deaths were accelerated by toxicity from the high doses of chemotherapy and radiation; overall, lives were not prolonged.[34,35] In the early 1990s, a slew of premature and hyped news reports led thousands of desperate people to request the procedure.[36,37] Insurers initially balked at covering transplantation for breast cancer, which cost around $100,000, calling it "experimental." But after some high-profile lawsuits—featuring sympathetic, dying plaintiffs—federal and some state insurers were required to pay.[36,38,39]

Yet many oncologists harbored doubts about providing BMT to breast cancer patients. In her 1996 book, *Waking Up, Fighting Back: The Politics of Breast Cancer*, Roberta reported that doctors were split on the issue. Dr. Susan Love, a breast surgeon, had reservations, suggesting that "the intuitive feeling" of many physicians that BMT "is the best treatment [was] based on the notion that more must be better," Altman wrote. "That was certainly the notion we used with radical mastectomy, but it turned out not to be true," Love told her.[40] The issue divided patient advocacy organizations.[41,42] Meanwhile doctors struggled to recruit participants for randomized trials because many people with advanced breast cancer, who were likely to die soon with standard treatments, didn't want to risk assignment to a control (non-transplant) arm in a study.[43-45] Only at this decade's end did it become clear that uniquely favorable results, reported by Dr. Werner Bezwoda of South Africa, had been fabricated, and this way of treating breast cancer was abandoned.[46,47]

A generation of patient advocates and many physicians draw a lesson from the 1990s experience of BMT for breast cancer. Citing this episode, some say the FDA approves cancer drugs too readily, that randomized clinical trials must demonstrate a survival benefit before a new medicine is made available by prescription and covered by insurance.[48-50] On the other hand, as Larry Kramer wrote about AIDS and investigational drug access in 1987, people with terminal conditions don't have years to wait for completion of randomized studies.[51] It's unlikely such an episode could happen today. That's because data on a novel treatment's side effects and toxicity, including deaths, would be collected and reported much faster than was feasible then, and with greater transparency.

No symbol captured this era's hopeful sentiment about oncology—that suffering could be reduced by earlier detection and research into better treatments—so fabulously as the pink ribbon for breast cancer awareness. The fad traces to an old American tradition that a strand of yellow fabric worn, or tied around a tree, signifies a state of waiting—for return of a prisoner from war, for instance or, during the Iran hostage crisis, a captive's release. Yellow ribbons conveyed a message that a loved one's absence was never out of mind.[52,53]

The trend of wearing ribbons to connote illness took off in June 1991, when Jeremy Irons and other actors donned red ribbons—silently representing concern for AIDS—at the televised Tony Awards.[54,55] Pink ribbons probably debuted in October 1991 at the first Susan G. Komen Breast Cancer Foundation "Race for the Cure" in Central Park. That low-key event with some 2,500 runners received little media attention.[56–60] Otherwise there was little East Coast chatter about pink ribbons before September 1992 when a *New York Times* "Surfacing" column alerted readers: "The pink ribbon: to wear on your lapel in October in recognition of Breast Cancer Awareness Month."[61]

There is debate over the pink ribbon's origins. Some credit Charlotte Haley, a grandmother in Southern California who distributed postcards with peach-colored ribbons attached, with messages like this:

BREAST CANCER AWARENESS RIBBON!
B. C. A. R.
JOIN THE "GRASS ROOTS MOVEMENT!"
Help us to wake up our Legislators and America
by wearing this ribbon.
Not affiliated with any local, county, state, national,
or federal organizations.
(NO DONATIONS SOLICITED)
For further information or ribbons
please call: (805) 522–2071

Haley wasn't in the business of fundraising for charity; her mission was to drum up federal support for research. At sixty-eight, like many other cancer volunteers, her motivation was personal: Haley's grandmother had died from breast cancer at forty-five; her mother had died young from cervical cancer; her sister and daughter had breast cancer. If someone sent SASE's (self-addressed stamped envelopes) to Haley, she'd fill and return those with five postcards—each affixed with a peach-colored ribbon—for mailing to Congress.

After syndicated journalist Liz Smith mentioned Haley's "Peach Corps" and phone number in a column, requests for postcards escalated into the tens of thousands. In August 1992, the *Los Angeles Times* reported that Haley had put her husband, daughter, and ten-year-old grandson to work answering calls, applying glue, and cutting ribbons.[62-64]

A parallel awareness campaign was conceived by two powerful women over lunch at the 21 Club in Manhattan. As the story goes, that's where Alexandra Penney, editor of Condé Nast's *Self* magazine, chatted with Evelyn Lauder, senior vice president of Estée Lauder, the cosmetics giant, about ways to encourage screening by mammography. Evelyn, then in her fifties, was passionate about breast cancer research and care. Although she rarely spoke of it, she'd been treated for an early-stage tumor. As an executive at the multibillion-dollar cosmetics firm named for her mother-in-law—encompassing Clinique, Origins, and other brands—Evelyn understood marketing and had no qualms about exploiting the company's advertising clout to press editors for attention to this cause. In October 1992, *Self* sported a pink ribbon on its cover and Estée Lauder distributed 1.5 million pink ribbons over makeup counters in department stores around the country.[65-68]

Celebrity cancer disclosures were not yet routine. People cried upon hearing of actor Michael Landon's 1991 death, at fifty-four, from pancreatic cancer. After starring in two long-running TV shows, *Bonanza* and *Little House on the Prairie*, he was a beloved figure.[69-73] Before the glamorous actor Audrey Hepburn died at sixty-three, newspapers reported that she'd undergone intestinal surgery for cancer.[74-76] Frank Zappa died from prostate cancer at age fifty-two in December 1993, months after appearing on NBC's *Today* show. The usually edgy musician spoke with reserve about his condition. "I gather that yours was not caught early," journalist Jamie Gangel said during an awkward interview. Zappa seemed to avoid saying the c-word (*cancer*).[77,78]

In early 1994, Jacqueline Kennedy Onassis, the former first lady, disclosed that she was receiving chemotherapy for lymphoma.[79] When it became clear that treatment wasn't working, she chose to die at home. Newspapers publicized her decision. Doctors said further treatment would be fruitless, the *Washington Post* reported.[80] "Gravely Ill Onassis Goes Home After Halting Cancer Treatment," topped an Associated Press report in Salt Lake's City *Deseret News*.[81] Upon her death, the *New York Times* put cancer in the headline of a front-page obituary, "Jacqueline Kennedy Onassis Dies of Cancer at 64."[82] Her acceptance of comfort care at the end of life—palliative care, though newspapers didn't call it that—was important because, while people were starting to talk more openly about cancer in 1994, few were ready to discuss "hospice."

A confluence of interests—medical, philanthropic, commercial, and political—spawned an explosion of breast cancer fundraising and activism. The National Breast Cancer Coalition (NBCC) gained attention in Washington, DC. In 1991 breast surgeon and author Dr. Susan Love, National Alliance of Breast Cancer Organizations (NABCO) director Amy Langer, and the leader of an advocacy group for lesbians with cancer, Susan Hester, had formed this organization with two aims: lobbying and education. In 1992, NBCC president Fran Visco, a breast cancer survivor and trial lawyer, spoke before several congressional committees on the need to increase federal funding of breast cancer research.

NBCC developed one of the first programs to educate patient advocates, the idea being that—armed with knowledge—laypeople affected by cancer could more effectively sway public policy.[83–86] At its peak, NBCC involved hundreds of member organizations around the country. NBCC took a grassroots approach to fundraising for educational and lobbying programs, while the Dallas-based Komen organization expanded top down, with a national office and regional affiliates.

An alphabet soup of organizations emerged: Breast Cancer Action (BCA) based in San Francisco and Living Beyond Breast Cancer (LBBC),† based near Philadelphia, besides NABCO and NBCC. In 1993, Evelyn Lauder founded the

---

† LBBC would spawn at least two "daughter" organizations: breastcancer.org, initiated by LBCC founder, Dr. Marisa C. Weiss, to provide vetted online resources, in 2000; and MET UP, an activist organization, in 2014.

Breast Cancer Research Foundation (BCRF), adding to the mix. To the public, these acronyms—BCA, BCRF, LBBC, NABCO, NBCC—were confusing. Apart from Komen, which was growing enormous through its popular races, these groups may have seemed indistinguishable despite having varied agendas. BCA, for instance, took aim at cancer's environmental causes.[87] Although it wasn't yet evident, BCRF, focused on research, would eventually rival Komen; today these are the two largest breast cancer charities.

"Inspired by AIDS activists in the 1980s, women with breast cancer are turning scores of support groups into a national political advocacy movement," Susan Ferraro reported in the *New York Times Magazine*. She described a rally in Washington, DC, where around seven hundred NBCC advocates had demonstrated in May 1993. She compared the breast cancer rally to a larger gathering for another cause: "The week before, more than three hundred thousand gay and lesbian Americans, many of them AIDS activists, had jammed the Washington Mall." The August 1993 article, "The Anguished Politics of Breast Cancer," highlighted Sherry Kohlenberg, a thirty-seven-year old Virginia woman with a young son and terminal breast cancer. At the microphone, Kohlenberg said, "This year 46,000 women will die of breast cancer . . . I will probably be among these statistics. I will leave behind my husband and partner of 18 years, a motherless child, a devastated family and too many friends." There "is backlash" when women speak out, Ferraro wrote, but Kohlenberg didn't care. "I will not go silently," Kohlenberg said.[88]

The journalist's focus—a young woman dying from metastatic disease—countered the prevailing message of breast cancer's treatability. On that issue's cover, the *Times Magazine* ran a bold image of Joanne Motichka, a thirty-nine-year-old artist and model with these words: "You Can't Look Away Anymore." Matuschka, as she was known, wears a pale headscarf over a single-shouldered dress cut low on one side, revealing her irregular chest and mastectomy scar. She appears conflicted, possibly angry, and stands defiantly while turning her head from the camera, as if ashamed. This cover elicited cartloads of letters. While many *Times* readers appreciated the candid image of a woman's disfigurement, others were appalled. "I do not think women have to have an obnoxious voice or chronically display anger to push for a cure for breast cancer. Nor do I think that it is necessary to use 'shock therapy' on the cover of your magazine," wrote Margaret Richter of New York City (figure 8.1).[89]

This discussion mattered more than I realized as a young oncologist then reading the newspaper. Unlike today, when patients can view images on Facebook

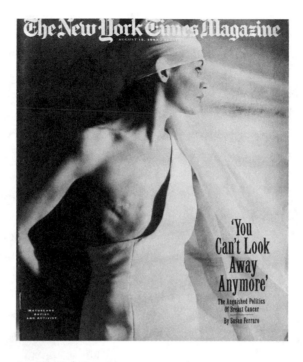

8.1 *New York Times Magazine* cover, August 15, 1993

and Instagram, photographs of mastectomy scars were seldom available. Women had little sense of how they'd look after an operation. And this was a common dilemma: of around 183,000 U.S. breast cancer patients that year, most were eligible for lumpectomy.[90,91] Apart from medical journals, there was almost no way to access such visual information. Doctors were paternalistic; even if they had a postmastectomy patient willing to show her scars, or a photograph, some would have hesitated for fear of scaring patients before surgery. Besides, many surgeons were not yet convinced that lumpectomy is sufficient in most cases; some wouldn't offer the smaller procedure to women with breast cancer. For these reasons, the photo was likely helpful though sensationalistic.

So much talking about breast cancer led to more openness about other cancers.

Days after Michael Milken was released from prison in January 1993, he received a diagnosis of aggressive prostate cancer. A doctor advised the disgraced financier, age forty-six, to put his affairs in order, that he had only months to live. After cooperating with investigators, Milken had served twenty-two months of his sentence, reduced from ten years to two, for federal crimes he'd committed at Drexel Burnham Lambert, an investment bank. The "junk bond king" wasted no time. In March 1993, he founded the Association for the Cure of Cancer of the Prostate (CaP CURE).[92-95] That November, Milken convened prostate cancer specialists, politicians, and philanthropists at the Virginia home of another billionaire, media mogul John Kluge, for a dinner at which Milken told experts, "Your job is to do the science. My job is to get the money."[96]

Milken's "venture capitalist" approach to cancer philanthropy differed from prior efforts in this way: there was no pretense of grassroots involvement or any educational aim. He would accelerate scientists' work—including risky, potentially high-yield projects—by streamlining the process by which investigators apply for grants and by promoting cooperative research through data-sharing. He asked his friends and former colleagues, among the wealthiest and most powerful men, to support this cause. In April 1994, News Corp. founder Rupert Murdoch, "corporate raider" Carl Icahn, casino magnate Steve Wynn, and others attended a CaP CURE dinner at New York's 21 Club where Milken sat between Calvin Klein, the clothing designer, and Dr. Howard Scher, a prostate cancer specialist at Memorial Sloan Kettering Cancer Center, and chatted with President Bill Clinton—who phoned in, the *Washington Post* reported.[97]

His story is an example of philanthropic reputation washing with an extra perk. After prison, Milken wanted to associate his name with a good cause. And he wanted to live! By directing funds toward research, he'd improve his image and help scientists discover better treatments for his cancer. Milken's past was "not a handicap, as far as I'm concerned, for someone trying to do good," said Senator Ted Stevens of Alaska. On Capitol Hill, he and Senator Bob Dole of Kansas, both prostate cancer survivors, advocated for prostate cancer research. "They call us the 'Prostate Pinup Twins,'" Stevens told the *Post.*[92]

Milken was impatient with the pace of research. In November 1995, CaP CURE organized the "first-ever National Cancer Summit" in Washington, DC. (It appears there was no second summit.) This conference was scheduled for a U.S. Senate building but because of a federal government shutdown, it took place at Washington's Grand Hotel. After planning an ambitious program, Milken and his PR team corralled oncologists, the NCI director, and representatives of other cancer organizations to attend. In a speech, Milken outlined his vision for collaborative research connecting scientists, clinicians, and "even laypersons." He likened his plan to the Manhattan Project, but for cancer, "set in the information age."

Americans shouldn't give up "war on cancer" but rethink it, Milken said, alluding to Nixon's declaration without naming that president. Progress against cancer had failed to keep up with technology, he recounted:

> In 1971 . . . Texas Instruments was developing the first pocket calculator. Intel introduced the microchip. . . . By 1976, five years later, the 'Viking I' spacecraft had beamed back detailed pictures of Mars' desert-like terrain. . . . [By 1993], personal computers were in 31 million American homes, 58 million households were wired for cable. . . . 25 years since the war on cancer was declared, Powerbooks have made those first Texas Instrument calculators seem like relics. . . . Yet victory still eludes us in our efforts to find a cure for cancer.

To convey urgency, Milken deployed emotion-loaded language: "We can sit back and wait . . . losing at least another ten to twenty million more American mothers, fathers, children, co-workers and friends. Or we can mobilize and find a cure now."[98]

His words harken to the recurring question raised by "war on cancer" critics of the 1970s and "moonshot" skeptics today, if cancer can be fixed like an engineering problem by devoting sufficient funds and resources to the task. His ideas were forward-thinking. Investments were needed in communications technology; robotics could be used to evaluate cancer drugs; and computers, with what today would be called artificial intelligence, would assist researchers working cooperatively, he suggested.[98–101]

While some snickered at Milken's attempt to "buy" a cure, many researchers and patients welcomed the infusion of CaP CURE funds. "Junk-Bond King Pours Millions Into Seeking a Cure for the Deadly Disease," headed a *Chronicle of Higher Education* story. "Participating scientists will pool such resources as tissue banks and will share data via computer," it reported. In 1995, among cancer researchers, these were radical ideas. Already Milken had invested $10 million in grants, planned to give another $15 million, and pledged $4 million for a prostate cancer research consortium.[102] Several years later, CaP CURE was renamed the Prostate Cancer Foundation.

In 2004, *Fortune* magazine celebrated Milken's philanthropy in a flattering story, "The Man Who Changed Medicine." It gushed, "Milken has, in fact, turned the cancer establishment upside down." By then the foundation had raised

$210 million, "making it the world's largest private sponsor of prostate cancer research." Milken's effort, "say numerous experts interviewed by *Fortune*, has been a significant factor in reducing deaths and suffering from the disease."[103]

A 1995 *Seinfeld* episode reveals that TV producers were becoming sufficiently comfortable talking about cancer to joke about it:

> "I got news," George tells Jerry. "Gary Fogel had cancer."
>
> "Yeah, I knew. . . . He told me a few months ago," Jerry responds.
>
> "Why did he tell you and not me?" George wonders.
>
> "Hey, believe me, you were better off not knowing. It's not easy to deal with someone in a situation like this. I was so nice to him I almost made myself sick," Jerry says.
>
> Their friend Elaine enters, interrupts, and asks what the men were discussing. They mention their acquaintance Gary, and she responds, "Oh, the guy with cancer?"

The storyline turns ugly. Months earlier, Jerry had given Gary a gift—a toupee store certificate—so that he might conceal hair loss from cancer treatment. The gang learns, however, that Gary was lying. He'd fabricated the diagnosis and that he was getting chemotherapy. George and Jerry express relief that they no longer have to behave nicely toward their acquaintance, because he doesn't have cancer.[104]

This plot anticipates what some call the "cancer card": mentioning a malignancy for advantage, to get one's way. And that some people will fake having cancer for sympathy or money. The fictional *Seinfeld* characters were notoriously self-centered, of course. Few individuals really mind helping acquaintances who are ill. But the screenwriters may have been on to something: the episode suggests that some people feel burdened by a perceived obligation to be supportive—to assist and be kind toward, to care about—acquaintances with cancer.

The other remarkable thing about this story is that it's about men talking.

In general, men are less open about their health than women. After its 1990 start, Us TOO, an Illinois-based support group for people affected by prostate cancer,

was expanding. Much as SHARE had begun in 1976 after a New York breast surgeon appreciated that his patients wanted to talk among themselves, Dr. Gerald
Chodak, a Chicago urologist, realized that people with prostate cancer sought
peer-to-peer communication. He sent a letter to patients about the initial meeting. Organizers selected the name Us TOO as a deliberate play on Y-ME, the
Chicago-based breast cancer organization known for its hotline, to make the
point that men get cancer and suffer from treatment, too.[105–108]

Us TOO spread to several hundred U.S. locations, the Bahamas, Australia,
and elsewhere, while a similar American Cancer Society (ACS) "Man to Man"
program became popular in Florida and other states. Us TOO exists today, providing in-person and online peer networks and education for people with prostate cancer and caregivers.[109–111]

"Prostate cancer is beginning to come out of the closet. Fifteen or 20 years
ago, you couldn't even mention the word prostate in polite mixed company,"
said urologist Dr. William Fair in an April 1996 *Time* story, "The Man's Cancer."
General Norman Schwarzkopf, a prostate cancer survivor, appeared on that
issue's cover (figure 8.2). The forthright piece by Leon Jaroff reported on progress and also complications, such as incontinence and impotence, that some-
time occur after prostate cancer surgery. He weighed potential benefits and
harms of screening for prostate cancer with a blood test for a protein called
prostate-specific antigen (PSA). Jaroff raised the concept of overdiagnosis, a
controversial issue today, without calling it that: "PSA readings sometimes
raise alarms that are misleading, fail to differentiate between fast-growing and
less threatening prostate cancer and can lead to debilitating treatment that
may not be necessary."[112]

Senator Bob Dole of Kansas, a prostate cancer survivor, was then running for
president. "What are the politics of prostate cancer?" asked Christine Gorman
in a companion *Time* piece. "Other political leaders—France's François Mitter-
rand and Jordan's King Hussein, for example—have suffered from the disease,
but none quite so publicly as Dole," she wrote. "Dole's candor is likely to help
him." At seventy-two, Dole's age may be a greater political liability than his
history of prostate cancer, she suggested.[113] Dole lost that election to incumbent
President Bill Clinton. His cancer history proved incidental over a long political career.

Other prominent men admitted having prostate cancer. Before his death
from prostate cancer, the *New York Times* book critic and author Anatole Broyard wrote candidly and forcefully about his experiences as a patient; his musings

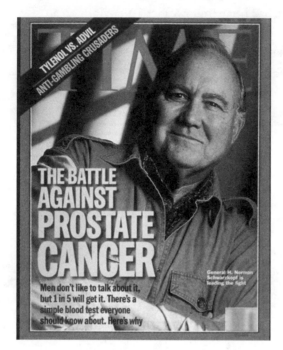

8.2 *Time* magazine cover, April 1, 1996

on cancer and medicine were compiled in a posthumous 1992 book, *Intoxicated by My Illness*.[114] Washington, DC Mayor Marion Barry Jr., shared his diagnosis in November 1995 at the time of Milken's summit;[115] golf legend Arnold Palmer was diagnosed in 1997, and New York Yankees manager, Joe Torre, in 1999.[116–119] Sir Roger Moore, the English actor who'd played James Bond, had prostate cancer in 1993 but he didn't acknowledge it then. (He did open up in a 2008 memoir.)[120–123] Perhaps Moore's Britishness, wanting to keep a stiff upper lip, contributed to his early silence.

The language of cancer is the subject of Margaret Edson's one-act play, *Wit*, about an English professor who's dying from ovarian cancer. The protagonist, Vivian Bearing PhD, is getting strong chemotherapy in an experimental trial. It's an intellectual piece: *Wit*'s title alludes to John Donne's seventeenth-century sonnets and Vivian's prior obsession, as a graduate student in literature, whether a semicolon or comma breaks the final line of "Death Be Not Proud." *Wit* ran off

Broadway from 1998 to 2000, was adapted into a 2001 film, and was revived on Broadway in 2012. Somehow it resonated.

This Pulitzer-winning drama, first performed in 1995, takes place in a hospital. An oncology fellow is assigned to Vivian's case. He was once her student, and he avoids talking with her. The senior oncologist, Dr. Kelekian, speaks in jargon. When Kelekian tells Vivian about her *carcinoma*, he and the patient talk simultaneously. To accentuate this point, Edson runs two vertical columns of parallel dialogue in the script. Both are speaking; neither is listening. Edson likens the complexity of words in metaphysical poetry to the language of medicine. Vivian recalls a student asking, "Why does Donne make everything so complicated?" The student continues, "Maybe he's scared, so he hides behind all this complicated stuff, hides behind this wit." The message is that doctors employ jargon to separate themselves from patients; they focus on details to avoid emotions.[124,125]

In the end, words prove inadequate to relieve Vivian's pain and isolation. Before dying, she shares an orange ice pop with a nurse. She retreats into memories and words of a children's book. What helps Vivian is human contact, the nurse's kindness at the end of her life.

Some experiences cannot be shared. In a work of fiction, "People Like That Are The Only People Here," Lorrie Moore tells the story of a mother of a baby with cancer. The Mother, a writer, struggles with narrating her experience. "A beginning, an end: there seems to be neither," it starts. "The whole thing is like a cloud . . . and everywhere inside it is full of rain." She reacts with disbelief to her child's diagnosis; the cancer cannot be the baby's; it must be hers. The Mother wonders if she's being punished, for too many babysitters and unmotherly thoughts. She writes, "Now her baby, for all these reasons . . . will be taken away." Most of the action takes place in the pediatric oncology ("Peed Onk") unit of a hospital. The title would be the mother's answer to a question posed by a visitor, her friend, about the "airy, scripted optimism" of most everyone on the Peed Onk ward.[126]

Moore's 1997 story, said to be semiautobiographical,[127] reveals an intimate knowledge of a pediatric cancer unit: catheters in bald boys, chemotherapy agents vincristine and actinomycin D, fluid-draining devices resembling toys. The Mother reflects on stages of feeling— "anger, denial, grief, and acceptance"—and her inability, or unwillingness, to stroll through. "Pulling through is what people do around here," she observes. "There is a kind of bravery in their lives that isn't bravery at all. It is automatic, unflinching, a mix of man and machine." The Mother does not feel cheerful, as others on the ward appear. She ponders "the whole conception of 'the story,' of cause and effect, the whole idea that people have a clue as to how the world works." (It's laughable.) She longs for a cigarette: "When a baby gets cancer, it seems stupid ever to have given up smoking. When a baby gets cancer, you think, Whom are we kidding? Let's all light up."

Inside the Peed Onk ward, the Mother is regaled with stories about what happens to families of kids with cancer: "Jobs have been quit, marriages hacked up, bank accounts ravaged." And what happens to the kids: "amputations, blood poisonings, teeth flaking like shale, the learning delays and disabilities. . . ." Their stories have "strangely optimistic codas," she notes. She's an ambivalent listener, but addicted: "Part of her welcomes and invites all their tales. . . . They are the only situations that can join hands with her own; everything else bounces off her shiny shield of resentment and unsympathy."

From the start, the Husband nudges the Mother to Take Notes. He's concerned they'll need money. She has reservations about this "nightmare of narrative slop" and "the moral boundaries of pecuniary recompense in a situation such as this."

Splintering charities eroded the ACS's dominance of cancer philanthropy. After 1989, when the society moved its national office to Atlanta, the ACS occupied a large, corporate-style building.[128,129] The "father" of cancer nonprofits faced competition from Komen, which was outpacing the ACS in its visibility regarding breast cancer and, by 1995, from Milken's CaP CURE for prostate cancer research. Among many legitimate new organizations from this era are the Ovarian Cancer Research Alliance (1994), Lustgarten Foundation for pancreatic cancer (1998), and Colon Cancer Alliance (1999). Each focused on a particular kind of malignancy.[130] During these years, the ACS extended its smoking cessation campaigns, nationwide statistical analyses of all cancer types, and studies of disparities in cancer's incidence and death rates, work that would be crucial for identifying and correcting inequities in cancer prevention and care.

Meanwhile the Cancer Fund of America, a lookalike, bogus organization, fed on the ACS's reputation. As the number of "for cancer" entities escalated, many with similar-sounding names, the Council of Better Business Bureaus cautioned consumers to donate by check and not by cash, to avoid getting scammed.[131,132]

Cause marketing—tying cancer charities to commerce—intensified. There are many examples from the 1990s. For instance, the Leukemia & Lymphoma Society gained dollars and publicity through Olive Garden ("Pasta for Pennies") and later Coinstar ("Pennies for Patients") collections. Milken's CaP CURE teamed up with Major League Baseball for the "Home Run Challenge." With Lee jeans, no purchase was necessary to support the cause: on Lee National Denim Day in October 1996, employees at over two thousand companies gave $5 for the privilege of wearing jeans to work, collectively raising $1.4 million for the Susan G. Komen Breast Cancer Foundation.[133–141]

The breadth of support for breast cancer stood out among health concerns. In May 1995, First Lady Hillary Clinton launched a mammography initiative with corporate support from FTD, the florists' network, and American Greetings, the card company. "'Mama' grams," tucked into Mother's Day cards and flower arrangements, contained messages like this: "Dear _____, Early detection saves lives. . . . Did you know . . . Medicare covers mammograms." The telegram-like notes included information on breast cancer screening. "A few florists expressed concern, common in the corporate world, that breast cancer was too depressing a subject to link with their product," the *Washington Post* reported. But Meg Whitman, the president and CEO of FTD, was keen on the plan: "I think the whole idea of a 'Mama' gram makes this a little less of a downer," she said.[142]

"Just yesterday, or so it seems, the ribbons were red and the cause was AIDS. Now, although money and empathy still flow to the AIDS cause, the pink team has pulled ahead in the philanthropic color war," Lisa Belkin wrote in the December 1996 *New York Times Magazine*.[143] From a marketing perspective, breast cancer had an advantage over AIDS. With breast cancer, there was no concern of turning off consumers because of lifestyle or sexuality connotations, Belkin wrote. "It comes with none of the potential baggage that support for AIDS may bring."

The journalist was already suffering pink ribbon fatigue: Belkin mentioned the "Fashion Targets Breast Cancer" campaign for which Ralph Lauren had "designed a T-shirt—no pink ribbon, thank you very much, but rather a bull's-eye logo."

∾

In the summer of 1999, cyclist Lance Armstrong stepped up to the Tour de France podium and delivered a potent message. At twenty-seven, he was the world's most famous cancer survivor and a hero to millions. Within three years of treatment for stage 4 testicular cancer, he took first place in an endurance sport. Armstrong gave hope to cancer patients around the world, not with words but by action—demonstrating that full physical recovery was possible after receiving chemotherapy for an advanced malignancy.[144–151]

Armstrong's course was incredible. Raised by a single mom in Plano, Texas, he was determined to succeed. After a disappointing finish at the 1992 Barcelona Olympics, he turned to professional cycling. He joined Motorola's team and enjoyed intermittent wins. The cancer diagnosis came in 1996, around his twenty-fifth birthday, when he'd sought medical evaluation for testicular pain and swelling, tiredness, and headaches. In his 2000 best-selling memoir, *It's Not About the Bike: My Journey Back to Life*, Armstrong tells of numerous metastases, some golf-ball-sized, rendering his chest x-ray "like a snowstorm." Two tumors lit up his brain scan. His prognosis was poor, but he was lucky. He received expert care and survived, seemingly unscathed, in phenomenal shape.[152]

In his book, Armstrong recounts reading about his condition. Long before "patient-centered" became a healthcare buzzword, Armstrong's oncologists adjusted his treatment—based on his preferences and needs as an athlete—by eliminating bleomycin from his regimen so as to minimize risk to the cyclist's lungs. Like other patients, he experienced nausea, baldness, weight loss, pain, extreme fatigue, and fear. He worried about losing his insurance and career. Upon recovering, in 1997 he founded the Lance Armstrong Foundation (later renamed "Livestrong").

Cancer patients admired Armstrong. Worshipped, almost. Everywhere, people wore yellow LIVESTRONG bracelets. To those of us working in oncology, Armstrong offered seemingly perfect testimony to the power of modern cancer care. He demonstrated a best-case scenario of what life might be after chemotherapy—and we lapped it up. In 1999, it was unusual to see anyone recover from such a widely metastatic tumor as he did with so much physical strength and stamina. "Fantastic!" was the consensus among doctors in my workplace. "Fabulous!" would have been more like it. Back then, few realized he was doping. For six more years, he came around each summer—a bit like an annual checkup—taking the top prize and reminding us of his successful treatment.

Testicular cancer is what killed Brian Piccolo, the *Brian's Song* namesake, in 1970. This uncommon malignancy tends to affect young men. Both he and Armstrong are reported to have had embryonal carcinoma, a rare and aggressive form of testicular cancer. After Piccolo's time, oncologists developed effective combination chemotherapy regimens, involving multiple drugs, to treat this condition. By the late 1980s, testicular cancer was one of the few solid tumors my teachers considered curable.[153,154]

Now we know Armstrong to be an unreliable narrator. He broke rules, not just by doping. He pressured his teammates to cheat and lied about all of it.[155–157] He was the most famous cancer patient alive, and he misled millions, duping everyone about his strength and looking terrific. The reality of cancer treatment is that it was often toxic, sometimes disabling, and frequently ineffective. Armstrong made having cancer seem too easy—like you could have your chemotherapy, recover, and pedal up a mountain.

Yet his cancer was real. For many patients and cancer professionals, coming to grips with Armstrong's deception was not easy. While many are angry about his lies, others are emphatic that he did good, that he's a flawed hero who encouraged many to LIVESTRONG.

It was a New Orleans cab driver who told me about the first precision oncology drug. "Did you hear?" he asked. "There's a cure for leukemia." I was on my way to the annual meeting of the American Society of Hematology in December 1999. He'd picked me up at the airport a day after the conference began. Dr. Brian Druker had presented results for STI-571, an experimental drug used to treat chronic myelogenous leukemia (CML). STI-571, or imatinib, now goes by the brand name Gleevec.[158] This pill targets an enzyme that's aberrantly turned on by a genetic switch that characterizes CML.

The buzz, reported in major news outlets, was that STI 571 worked.[159] Among thirty-one leukemia patients in the trial, all responded well and with minimal toxicity. This was a huge advance. In 1999, we were treating CML with allogeneic bone marrow transplant if patients were young and had a match, or with interferon, which involved daily shots and unpleasant side effects, and wasn't very effective.[160] Many died. Today, CML patients enjoy near-normal life expectancy.[161]

Gleevec didn't receive FDA approval until May 2001. Now, it's also prescribed for a rare stomach cancer and a few other conditions harboring genetic changes like those of CML. This was the beginning of precision oncology: the matching of cancer drugs to specific molecular abnormalities in tumors.

In *Fight Club*, the 1999 movie, the insomniac protagonist meets a woman at a testicular cancer support group. Neither has cancer. They attend to hear of others' pain and emotions, desperate to somehow make themselves feel better. These scenes reflect the ubiquity of cancer support groups, which peaked around this time, and portend a future of patients' overexposure: when sharing becomes routine, without protections or rules, patients become vulnerable; their openness might be abused.[162]

Soon, nothing about cancer would be off limits.

CHAPTER 9

COMPLICATIONS (2000–2010)

In March 2000, NBC's *Today* show aired footage of its cohost Katie Couric undergoing colonoscopy. The segment captures Couric prepping in her apartment, drinking cherry-flavored NuLytely, sucking a lime and pinching her nose to minimize unpleasant taste. Skipping the bathroom and diarrhea, the video cuts to the next morning. Couric heads from the TV studio to a hospital. She greets her doctor and soon appears on a stretcher wearing a hospital gown, getting an IV, and chatting under light anesthesia.[1]

Views of the inside of Couric's gut—projected on TV and over Times Square—were unprecedented. That evening on Comedy Central's *Daily Show*, Jon Stewart ribbed the chipper newscaster. While Couric's face, crosshairs, and words "Public Enema appear on-screen, Stewart winced, saying, "Perhaps next time Couric should try passing out a pamphlet" (figure 9.1). A *Washington Post* television critic, Lisa de Moraes, reacted with dismay: "NBC Tests Viewers' Intestinal Fortitude on 'Today.'" The show's executive producer, Jeff Zucker, had promised "they wouldn't show too much of his superstar's colon," she wrote. "He lied."[2,3]

After losing her husband to colon cancer, Couric was on a mission to encourage screening. Jay Monahan, a previously healthy lawyer, had died at age forty-two, nine months after doctors discovered his advanced case. Monahan left behind Couric and their two daughters.[4–6] And Zucker, *Today*'s thirty-four-year-old producer, was a young colon cancer survivor.[7,8]

That March, the first Colorectal Cancer Awareness Month, the U.S. Senate Special Committee on Aging held a session on this subject. Couric was invited to speak.[9] Senator Harry Reid, then age sixty, could hardly contain his enthusiasm for her visit. "It is not often we have a celebrity that we feel so close to that we can call them by their first name, but I think most of America feels that we know

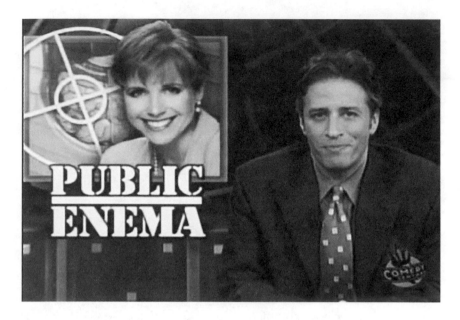

9.1 Jon Stewart talking about Katie Couric's on-air colonoscopy, *The Daily Show*, March 7, 2000.

you, Katie," he began. "I have had some experience with colons. My wife has a disease called ulcerative colitis," Reid shared. After a surgeon removed her colon, his wife no longer needed to worry about getting colon cancer. "My message to you today is one of thanks. By focusing attention on this disease, we will be able to get more money for research," Reid said. "This is a disease that isn't very fashionable. It is not easy to talk about colons and what needs to be done."

Couric told the senators her story. Like most people, she'd learned about colon cancer after it hit home: "I got a quick and painful education about this devastating disease." Colorectal cancer causes fifty-six thousand U.S. deaths annually, second only to lung cancer, she said. "But I also learned that it has a 90 percent cure rate, or better, if it is detected early." She invoked military language: "Colon cancer screening is a critical weapon in the fight against a disease no one needs to die from." She extolled benefits of public education: "Unfortunately, people are woefully unaware and uneducated about this killer. A lot of people simply don't want to talk about it. Colons, rectums, bowels—it is not exactly the stuff of cocktail party conversation." She continued, "Not that long ago people were hesitant and uncomfortable talking about breast cancer, and men rarely discussed their prostates. Now those cancers are routinely discussed. . . . We have to do the same for colon cancer."

Time put "Katie's Crusade" on its cover. "Katie Couric lost her husband to colon cancer," it said. "Now she's spreading the word: Get tested and save your life!" Physicians lauded Couric's effort and, in a 2003 medical journal, attributed higher colonoscopy rates to her televised procedure: "The Impact of a Celebrity Promotional Campaign on the Use of Colon Cancer Screening." They dubbed this "the Katie Couric Effect."[6,10]

Couric's openness, and journalists' willingness to challenge that, revealed a new dynamic in public cancer discussions. As awareness campaigns became extreme, critical views emerged. In this decade, dozens of public figures admitted having malignant diagnoses. As ordinary patients began using the internet to find information and express themselves, challenging perspectives gained visibility. Television shows depicted people with cancer as complex, nuanced, less idealized, and less heroic characters. Anger surfaced.

In her 2001 essay "Welcome To Cancerland," Barbara Ehrenreich offered one of the earliest critiques of "breast-cancer culture." After a mammogram and biopsy, Ehrenreich, a journalist with a PhD in cell biology, was thrust into a patient's position. She described a pink realm filled with "sticky sentiment" that distorts disease, overlooks death, and infantilizes women, and likened it to a religious cult. "Cancerland" alludes to Candy Land, the children's board game. Pink-beribboned teddy bears were sold by the tens of thousands for breast cancer patients, she noted. At a medical center, gift bags containing boxes of crayons were distributed to affected women. "Men diagnosed with prostate cancer do not receive gifts of Matchbox cars." Ehrenreich would not be pacified.[11]

Being a patient can diminish one's sense of self. You become a "thing," she suggested. "Unfortunately, there is a cancer," a surgeon informed her—as if "I, Barbara, do not enter into it." Burnout among oncologists had not yet received attention in news; if it had, she might have labeled the doctor's behavior as depersonalization, a well-described burnout manifestation. Here, it's worth comparing Ehrenreich's real-life encounter with the interaction of Dr. Budge and Emma in *Terms of Endearment*. In the novel, Dr. Budge "very kindly" says to Emma, "Old girl, you have a malignancy," and in the movie, he says, "Dear, you have a malignancy."[12,13] Ehrenreich, trained in science, sought humanness.

Pink-hued events tied to breast cancer were saturating America. Komen's Races "for the Cure" attracted around a million people each year. Some 2.2 million women at various stages of their "breast-cancer careers" and their relatives supported a breast-cancer "marketplace" stocked with themed clothing, jewelry, practical items like night-lights and banking "Checks for the Cure," and windchimes among other tchotchkes, Ehrenreich reported. Awareness was roping women in, swelling a "breast-cancer industry" of mammograms, surgical procedures, and chemotherapy infusions. AstraZeneca sponsored Breast Cancer Awareness Month, she noted. That company's parent, Zeneca, was spun from Imperial Chemical Industries, a producer of pesticides including acetochlor—deemed a "probable human carcinogen" by the EPA—she wrote, implicating the pharmaceutical firm in cancers from which it profits. "Breast cancer would hardly be the darling of corporate America if its complexion changed from pink to green," she wrote. "It is the very blandness of breast cancer, at least in mainstream perceptions, that makes it an attractive object of corporate charity."

Women were being deceived by so much positivity, Ehrenreich charged. "Beaming survivors, proudly displaying their athletic prowess, are the best possible advertisement for routine screening mammograms, early detection, and the ensuing round of treatments." Doctors, for their part, exaggerated benefits. Mammograms were overrated, yielding a "vanishingly small impact" on breast cancer mortality, she wrote. Treatment was not curative, and evidence for screening "equivocal." The pink culture served a patriarchal agenda: "Obedience is the message. . . . You are encouraged to regress to a little-girl state, to suspend critical judgment."

It should be noted that Ehrenreich, a critical thinker, had been persuaded—by data, by doctors, or by word of mouth. She did get a mammogram. She had cancer surgery. She took chemotherapy. And she did not take awareness for granted: "Fortunately, no one has to go through this alone," she wrote. "Thirty years ago, before Betty Ford, Rose Kushner, Betty Rollin, and other pioneer patients spoke out, breast cancer was a dread secret, endured in silence and euphemized in obituaries as a 'long illness.'" She credited the Women's Health Movement, in which she participated in the 1970s and 1980s, with legitimizing support networks and encouraging women to band together, share stories, and question doctors. "It is hard now to recall how revolutionary these activities once seemed," she wrote.

"This cheers me briefly, until I realize that if support groups have won the stamp of medical approval this may be because they are no longer perceived as seditious." This was a key observation. Support groups had become so mainstream, they abetted doctors in their mission and were complicit in favorably representing cancer and its treatment.

Cancer patients' disaffection rarely surfaced before 2001. "The equanimity of breast-cancer culture goes beyond mere absence of anger to what looks, all too often, like a positive embrace of the disease," Ehrenreich observed. The dominant survivorship narrative was transforming breast cancer into a "rite of passage," as if it were a gift, something construed as a positive experience, an ordeal though which one emerges a better person. "Unhappiness requires a kind of apology." Ehrenreich noted a post at breastcancertalk.org by "Lucy," who said her prognosis was "not good" and her story "not the usual one, full of sweetness and hope, but true nevertheless."

My breast cancer diagnosis came in October 2002, after a mammogram, ultrasound, and needle biopsy. In writing this book, I've appreciated how much has changed since then, when a forty-something woman's telling her kids, parents, friends, colleagues, and neighbors about a malignant diagnosis was unexpected, if not unusual. Sure, some acquaintances spoke openly about having cancer. But others in my community stayed mum. (Some still do.) Before Facebook existed, before blogs were a thing, telling someone you had cancer seemed like a big deal. It required a sit-down kind of conversation, or at least a phone call.

Fortunately, I had good health insurance. I knew the cancer specialists at my hospital, where I'd worked as a resident, fellow, and attending physician. I also knew the clerks, nurses, aides, and janitors, because I'd spent so many hours on the wards. (This was a perk of my employment. On the other hand, privacy was impossible.) The morning after I received my diagnosis, I set up appointments with a trusted surgeon and venerated oncologist. My physician colleagues treated me with respect and generosity.

I made decisions swiftly, first about surgery. I chose bilateral mastectomy. My decision was guided not by published evidence or genetic risk (I wasn't BRCA tested and had no family history), but by the particularities of my case. Because I have a curved spine, my doctors and I considered that I should avoid carrying unequal weights on my chest. My posture was poor; I leaned forward. Removing both breasts would help two problems: cancer and asymmetry. During surgery, a "sentinel" lymph node was removed from my armpit and checked; it was negative for malignant spread. My tumor was 1.7 centimeters in diameter. Pathologists also found spots of noninvasive, stage 0 disease—*ductal carcinoma in situ* (DCIS) and *lobular carcinoma in situ* (LCIS)—in my left and right breasts, respectively. In 2002, there was no more important determinant of prognosis than the presence or absence of malignant cells in nearby glands. With stage 1 invasive cancer, I felt relieved.

Not that I was out of the woods. My colleagues estimated that for a breast cancer with features like mine, the probability of relapse was around 15 percent over fifteen years. To lower my recurrence odds, I'd need additional treatment. After surgery, adjuvant chemotherapy would take my chances of recurrence down from 15 percent to 10 percent, approximately. That 5 percent long-term reduction—which another doctor might tout as lowering my risk by a third (5 out of 15), or 33 percent—seemed small at the time, small enough that I considered skipping those harsh drugs. But I was only forty-two. It seemed worth it, to lessen my chances of developing metastatic disease. I received four cycles of two intravenous drugs, Adriamycin (doxorubicin, aka "the red devil") and Cytoxan (cyclophosphamide), "AC," as we oncologists called this regimen, and worked through, wearing a wig. I recall painful mouth sores, nausea, and exhaustion. I fell on ice and broke my right arm. People sent gifts. Our apartment filled, briefly, with flowers.

A year after I finished chemotherapy, HBO aired the final season of *Sex and the City* in which Samantha—the most promiscuous of the foursome, portrayed by Kim Cattrall—contends with breast cancer.[14–16] Although plenty of TV series had included breast cancer storylines before 2004, none were so matter-of-fact about it. Samantha tells Carrie of her diagnosis while they're in a taxi on the way to Miranda's wedding. They plan not to mention the cancer, so as not to ruin Miranda's special day, but at the reception they tell Charlotte. Inevitably, Miranda notices something's wrong, and soon enough they're all in. "Hey, no tears," Samantha insists. This January 2004 episode offered an easy message about friends being supportive of friends who have cancer.

Then *Sex and the City* got deeper, exploring women's feelings of guilt and perception of blame surrounding breast cancer. In a loaded scene, Samantha visits Dr. Pinkner:

"I don't understand how this happened to me," Samantha says.

"It could be genetics, but since there's no breast cancer in your family, it could be a variety of factors—diet, lifestyle choices," Pinkner responds.

"Lifestyle choices?" Samantha questions. She's picking up on the implication that her behavior has caused her cancer.

"Some studies have shown women who haven't had children have an increased chance of getting it," Pinkner responds, not yet appreciating her anger.

"I see. So I brought this on myself?" Samantha's voice rises.

No, the doctor tries to tell her, he's talking about statistics.

"I think we're done here," she asserts. Wearing a flimsy gown, she storms out of the examining room.

Desperate for an appointment with a "woman doctor," after being told none are available, Samantha camps out in the waiting room of a sought-after oncologist. She confronts the receptionist: "Well, who do you have to fuck to get chemo around here?" The worker is not amused, and Samantha half-apologizes, saying, "I'm sorry, I'm upset. I'm dealing with cancer." The receptionist, inured and possibly burnt out, suggests that Samantha's predicament is so common that she can't be bothered, responding, "All of New York is dealing with cancer."

This series covered a subject about which oncologists typically say little: cancer and sex. When Samantha develops hot flashes, she attributes those to premature menopause from chemo. ("Chemo" was part of the lexicon by this time.) In one episode, her young boyfriend, Smith, watches Samantha practicing a speech for a foundation gala. She's wearing a leopard-print bra and red lace panties. He's turned on, and she can't deal with his arousal. Later, when Smith says he's getting therapy to cope with "all this cancer stuff," Samantha encourages him to sleep with others: "I'm not trying to push you away. I'm trying to keep you," she says. "If anyone knows how important sex is to a person, it's me. Correction. *Was* me" (emphasis added). Samantha feels that chemo has killed her sexuality.

At the black-tie dinner, Samantha experiences hot flashes while speaking from a podium, her face magnified on a Jumbotron. "If you want to see the face of breast cancer, look around you," she says. "It's the woman next to you at the dry cleaners, the nurse in pediatrics, the single mother picking her child up from school." Samantha perspires heavily. Her makeup runs. "Oh, the hell with it," she says, yanking the wig off her head and smiling. Around the room, elegantly dressed women pull off their wigs. The speaker tosses hers, as a bride might toss a bouquet of flowers, and everyone applauds.

Samantha gained viewers' respect. She's a woman with cancer, not its victim. When this episode aired, it took guts for an oncology patient to go bald. Doing so was tantamount to a two-part statement: I am getting cancer treatment, and I am not going to hide it.

A year after "Samantha" pulled off her wig, the musician Melissa Etheridge appeared bald on stage at the 2005 Grammy Awards. The *Chicago Tribune* covered her "Piece of My Heart" rendition: "It was startling to see a bald Melissa Etheridge, who was recently diagnosed with breast cancer, joyously ripping into a tribute to Janis Joplin by snarling the line, 'A woman can be tough.' She left no doubt."[17] Etheridge, who'd been receiving chemotherapy, discussed her decision—against a doctor's advice—to bare her scalp: "My surgeon literally said to me, 'You're going to want to get a wig because nobody wants to see a bald rock star,'" she told *Entertainment Weekly*. But actor Rosie O'Donnell and film director Steven Spielberg encouraged their friend to reveal her baldness. "No. You walk out there proud. You're beautiful," Spielberg told her.[18]

Etheridge was in good company. Thanks to awareness campaigns, many Americans perceived breast cancer as a "good cancer," beatable if caught early. Understanding it was neither a professional nor personal death sentence made it easier to disclose. The lengthening parade of celebrities out with breast cancer included other popular singers. Olivia Newton-John and Carly Simon were diagnosed in the 1990s,[19-23] Rockers Sheryl Crow and Marianne Faithfull would soon be diagnosed, as would Cynthia Nixon, who portrayed Miranda in *Sex and the City*.[24-28] Wikipedia, the crowdsourced internet encyclopedia, was notoriously unreliable in early years, after its 2001 launch.[29-31] Today, Wikipedia lists over two hundred notable individuals, catalogued by profession, living with or having died from breast cancer, with references.[32] White women constitute the vast majority of public cases. Robin Roberts, the Black *Good Morning America* anchor, and Peter Criss, the KISS band's drummer, were exceptions in that era.[33,34]

Cancer stories racked the music world. Punk rockers Joey and Johnny Ramone both died from cancer around this time.[35–38] The bandmates were unrelated. Lead vocalist Joey, née Jeffrey Hyman, died from lymphoma at age forty-nine in 2001; Johnny, the guitarist born John Cummings, died from prostate cancer at age fifty-five in 2004. The Ramones are said to have taken their adopted surnames from a pseudonym, Paul Ramon, that ex-Beatle Paul McCartney used for registering at hotels. In the intervening years, McCartney's wife, Linda, died from breast cancer.[39,40] In 2001, George Harrison of the Beatles died at fifty-eight from lung cancer, after a bout with throat cancer.[41,42] In 2005, the Rolling Stones drummer, Charlie Watts, talked of his recovery from early-stage throat cancer in a *Rolling Stone* Q&A.[43] In 2006, Phil Lesh of the Grateful Dead disclosed having prostate cancer.[44] It wasn't only rock musicians affected. For example, opera tenor Luciano Pavarotti underwent pancreatic cancer surgery and died the next year, at age seventy-one.[45–47]

As more people opened up, cancer stigma faded. Yet in some communities of color, orthodox Jewish neighborhoods, and elsewhere, whispering continued. Outside North America—in the Middle East, Africa, and other regions—women still hesitated to seek care for breast masses or gynecological tumors and, if they had cancer, hesitated to tell acquaintances. The 2019 Chinese–American film *The Farewell*, about a family that won't tell a grandmother that she's got cancer, suggests that, even now, old attitudes persist.[48]

Some tumors may be hard to discuss because they involve body parts deemed unmentionable, like the vagina or penis. And not everyone is inclined to share. For professional reasons, actor Kathy Bates didn't reveal her first cancer. "Back in 2003, when I had ovarian cancer, my agent told me not to tell anyone," she later admitted to WebMD. Her gynecologist warned of "stigma" in Hollywood. "But then I saw Melissa Etheridge doing a concert and just wailing on her guitar with her bald head, and I thought, 'Wow, I wanna be her!' So when the breast cancer diagnosis came, I knew I wanted to be honest about it." With breast cancer in 2012, Bates opened up.[49,50]

Behind the scenes at *The Sopranos*, Edie Falco dealt quietly with breast cancer in 2003. One of the producers, a friend in the know, arranged the show's filming schedule so the actor wouldn't be missed. "It was very important for me to keep my diagnosis under the radar, even from the cast and crew," Falco later told Health.com. "Well-meaning people would have driven me crazy asking, 'How are you feeling?'" she said. "With the cancer a secret, I bucked up, put on my Carmela fingernails, and was ready to work." In 2012, Falco discussed her preference for privacy with Anderson Cooper: "When Melissa Etheridge came out and did that concert, it was the most empowering, spectacular thing to see, and it was so not the way I do things," Falco said. "Everybody's different."[51,52]

The writer Nora Ephron famously plugged the aphorism "Everything is copy." Yet after being diagnosed with myelodysplastic syndrome, a preleukemic blood disorder, around 2005, she failed to mention it.[53,54] In her 2006 book, *I Feel Bad About My Neck*, she expounds on superficial subjects: designer purses, hair dye, a big apartment, strudel. Only in the final essay, "Considering the Alternative"— on aging—does Ephron get serious. "I am dancing around the D word," she wrote, cagily: "Death is a sniper. It strikes people you love, people you like, people you know, it's everywhere. You could be next. But then you turn out not to be. But then again you could be." She equivocates, then decides, "Let's not be morbid," and—after reflecting on the deaths of two friends—concludes with an ode to bath oil.[55,56]

Ephron enjoyed a lucrative screenwriting career, having penned *When Harry Met Sally*, *Sleepless in Seattle*, and other hits. Like Rachel Carson and Jacqueline Susann before her, she understood—and feared—negative consequences of disclosure. After her 2012 death, her son Jacob Bernstein wrote, "At various points . . . she considered coming clean to her friends and colleagues about her illness." If she revealed her disease, getting another film made would be "impossible," he indicated, because no media insurer would sign off on a deal. "Beyond that, what my mother didn't want was to have her illness define her, turning every conversation into a series of 'how *are* you?'s." Ephron struggled to represent preleukemia in a way that suited her. "You can't really turn a fatal illness into a joke. It is almost the only disclosure that turns you into the victim rather than the hero of your story. For her, tragedy was a pit of clichés," Bernstein wrote. "So she stayed quiet."[53,57]

While politicians and business leaders may be obligated to admit serious diagnoses, they're not necessarily forthright about it.[58,59] When John Kerry ran for president in 2004, a year after prostate cancer surgery, he said, "I am cured." At sixty, he deemed his health a nonissue, stating, "I am cancer-free, and the percentages of me being cancer-free 10 years from now are about as good as they get." While Kerry could become the first "cancer survivor" elected president, the candidate rejected the "survivor" term as "creating an unfair stigma," Lawrence K. Altman reported.[60]

Steve Jobs was CEO of Apple and Pixar when he underwent surgery in 2004 for a rare type of pancreatic cancer. Jobs informed Apple employees of his islet cell neuroendocrine tumor, that it "can be cured by surgery if removed in time," that his "was diagnosed in time," and that he wouldn't be needing chemotherapy or radiation, the *Wall Street Journal* reported. At forty-nine, knowing that Apple's value was tied to his health, Jobs projected a positive long-term outlook. He closed his memo in a "punchy manner," telling staff that he was using "his 17-inch PowerBook laptop" and wireless node to send the memo, the *Journal* noted. In 2004, a patient's posting to the web from inside a hospital was remarkable.[61]

Within a few years Jobs appeared gaunt, however. Investors speculated about recurrent cancer. In 2009, Jobs took a half-year medical leave and, without explanation or publicity, underwent liver transplantation. He died at age fifty-six in 2011.[62–64]

A tragic story involved Farrah Fawcett. In 2006, the former *Charlie's Angels* star and 1970s pinup suffered from anal cancer and a breach of her medical records. After details and lies ("Farrah Begs: 'Let Me Die' ") appeared in the *National Enquirer*, it turned out a UCLA Medical Center employee was selling information from Fawcett's hospital chart to tabloids. Paparazzi and sensational headlines made her cancer harder to deal with, Fawcett told the *Los Angeles Times*. She sued the hospital, hoping the case would inform future legal protections of patients' privacy.[65,66] With help of actor Ryan O'Neal, Fawcett's longtime partner and father of her son, and her friend Alana Stewart, Fawcett documented her experiences as a patient, including trips to Germany for alternative therapy, on video. (In a twist of reality, O'Neal, who starred in *Love Story* in 1971, had been diagnosed with chronic myelogenous leukemia.[67])

Fawcett was "forced to battle her cancer publicly," the *Los Angeles Times* reported in her 2009 obituary.[68] With Fawcett's permission, O'Neal's and Stewart's videos were edited to create *Farrah's Story*, a two-hour program that aired on NBC in May 2009, a month before she died. Americans were fascinated by Fawcett's travails. The documentary drew high ratings: nine million viewers in one night. "It was awful because it was an exploitative portrait of a celebrity's fight with cancer," Alessandra Stanley reviewed in the *New York Times*. "It was clear that Ms. Fawcett wanted to take back her story from the paparazzi and the celebrity magazines and have some control over its telling," Stanley wrote. "And like many cancer patients, she says she wants to find larger purpose to her suffering." O'Neal and Stewart were "both hailed and excoriated for abetting a project that many saw as ghoulish and voyeuristic, turning a harrowing death in progress into the ultimate reality show," Leslie Bennetts wrote in *Vanity Fair*.[69-72]

Progress against cancer was steady and subtle. Between 1991, when the U.S. cancer death rate peaked, and 2009, mortality from cancer fell from 215 to 173 per 100,000 population—nearly a 20 percent drop averaging over 1 percent annually.[73] Epidemiologists attributed much of this decline to smoking cessation.[74] Forty years after the surgeon general issued the landmark report, lung cancer, the leading malignant killer, was becoming less frequent. This improvement in cancer death rates was nearly invisible, however, because as the U.S. population expanded and aged, the absolute numbers of cases and deaths climbed. As before, public perception may have a "mortality bias" in this way: people disproportionately hear about deaths from cancer, because many who've had early-stage tumors don't mention it. Another limitation is the unevenness of progress: as detection, diagnosis, and cancer care improved for many Americans, disparities in survival rates—between Black and white people—became apparent.[75]

In 2003 researchers completed sequencing the human genome at a cost of around $300 million.[76] A year later, the FDA approved Tarceva (erlotinib), an oral medicine that blocks signals through the epidermal growth factor receptor (EGFR), for advanced, chemotherapy-resistant lung cancer. This was a big deal because chemotherapy for lung cancer was usually ineffective. Although erlotinib helps only a fraction of patients—generally those with tumors harboring EGFR mutations—it's often life-extending in those cases. When Tarceva was first approved in 2004, most doctors had no way to check for EGFR mutations, so oncologists prescribed this pill "blindly" to lung cancer patients. By 2010, clinicians had tools for evaluating selective DNA changes in lung cancer. These gene variants serve as *biomarkers*—indicators of which patients are likely to respond. Still most people with lung cancer could not yet be helped.[77,78]

Elucidating how human papillomavirus (HPV) causes cancer was another advance of this era. Previously, pathologists had identified HPV in cervical and other "squamous" tumors arising in the vagina, anus, penis, throat, and other body parts, but the molecular mechanisms by which HPV causes malignancy were unknown. With understanding of HPV as a carcinogen came realization that HPV-associated cancers could be prevented by vaccination. In 2006, the FDA approved the first vaccine (Gardasil) for immunizing girls and young women against HPV; in 2009, it was approved for boys and men. However, some parents and pediatricians were hesitant about this cancer prevention strategy, due to misinformation or confusion (the anti-vax movement was growing) or reluctance to mention a child's sexuality.[79–84]

Living with multiple myeloma, an incurable blood cancer, Geraldine Ferraro became an influential patient advocate. After her 1998 diagnosis, the former U.S. vice presidential candidate and congressional representative of New York learned that over half of myeloma patients died within four years of diagnosis. She sought advice from expert physicians and, notably, from Kathy Giusti, a peer patient who'd founded the Multiple Myeloma Research Foundation. In 2001, Ferraro disclosed her condition and that she'd been helped by thalidomide, an old drug notorious for causing terrible birth defects. After the *New England Journal of Medicine* published a 1999 study demonstrating thalidomide's effectiveness against myeloma, one of Ferraro's doctors prescribed it, and her malignancy was slowed. "Thank God for thalidomide," she said in a 2001 interview on NBC's *Today* show, at age sixty-five. She took thalidomide and later Velcade (bortezomib), which the FDA approved in 2003.[85–87]

"I feel great. I really do," Ferraro said in 2007, days before her seventy-second birthday. "I'm in remission now. I'm on a maintenance medication that really just allows me to continue my life and enjoy it, and it's fabulous," she told *Today*'s Jamie Gangel. "Ferraro owes her health to treatments developed since she was diagnosed that control the disease without the side effects of traditional chemo-therapy," *Today* reported. "It did not exist when I was first diagnosed," Ferraro said about Velcade. "This is what makes it a chronic disease now rather than a death sentence." She lived until 2011.[88,89]

The prospect of turning lethal cancers into chronic diseases appealed to oncologists, including me, who were accustomed to seeing our patients die within months or a few years of diagnosis. In 2008, longstanding *New York Times* health columnist Jane E. Brody picked up on this idea, citing an unpublished "hitchhiker model" for cancer care outlined by Dr. Michael Fisch of MD Anderson Cancer Center. The hitchhiker framework—buying time with one drug, then another—drew on physicians' experiences treating people with AIDS during the late 1980s and the 1990s. Starting with AZT, as new drugs came along, some patients taking early antiviral agents survived long enough to try the next. Similarly, some individuals with advanced cancer, periodically treated, are "living year after year with advanced disease, with cancers that have spread to the lung, liver, brain or bone," Fisch told Brody. "In 1997, we wouldn't have guessed this would be possible."[90,91]

As more celebrities shared their cancer stories, so did ordinary people. With software like Blogger or WordPress, most anyone could publish; you didn't need to know computer coding to "blog" (which was becoming a verb). Some early patient blogs remain at Blogspot, a Google platform. Still, only a small minority of people with cancer shared their diagnoses online.[92,93]

Between 2000 and 2009, the proportion of American adults with internet access climbed from less than half (46 percent) to three in four (74 percent) and the number of U.S. households with broadband connections rose from 5 to 57 percent. In these years, people became comfortable using the internet for email, shopping, and news. Individuals learned to search and find information. In 2006, the *Oxford English Dictionary* added "google" as a verb. Still many people were reluctant to use the web for sensitive matters like health. And as internet connections were not universal, a "digital divide" emerged as a source of disparate access to medical resources.[94,95]

The internet enabled quacks to sell bogus cancer "cures" as never before. One case involved Robert O. Young, a naturopath who falsified credentials and promoted alkaline ("pH Miracle") treatments for years before going to jail.[96–99] Some hoaxes were unobvious. For example, on her wellness website, CrazySexyCancer. com, Kris Carr recounted her 2003 Valentine's Day diagnosis of stage 4 epithelioid hemangioendothelioma and sold Goopish- "anti-cancer" products; she received favorable attention from the likes of Oprah Winfrey and Dr. Mehmet Oz and supportive write-ups in prestigious magazines like *Scientific American*.[100–102]

To counter misinformation, a handful of doctors began blogging at Science-Blogs.com, *Scientific American*'s blogging network, and elsewhere.[103–106] But the task of discrediting fraudsters was daunting, if not impossible, as the volume of conflicting and contradictory online information grew vast.

Breast cancer awareness campaigns grew bolder. Each year at more than a hundred U.S. sites, runners for the Komen foundation donned Pepto Bismol–colored tops and visors displaying corporate sponsors' logos. During Komen's 3-Day adventures, some participants walked sixty miles and camped in pink tents, dotting landscapes.[107–109] Avon, the cosmetics company, orchestrated 39-mile treks; each year at around a dozen U.S. sites, Avon Breast Cancer Crusade walkers donned pale pink hats, fanny packs, sunglasses, and other paraphernalia.[110,111] The ACS, for its part, developed the "Making Strides Against Breast Cancer" campaign, also pink-themed; its noncompetitive walks of three to five miles appealed to some older breast cancer survivors and families.[112,113] In sum, these activities periodically colored American cities, parks, and malls in rosy hues, blurring the sponsoring organizations' indistinct messages—and cause.[114]

Even the skies turned pink. Starting in October 2006, Delta employees painted ribbons on the outside of aircraft, wore pink uniforms, solicited contributions from travelers, and gave to the Breast Cancer Research Foundation (BCRF). In 2008, American Airlines, allied with Komen, painted images of giant pink ribbons on some planes, invited customers to wear pink while traveling, and encouraged donations.[115–117] The Estée Lauder Companies, closely tied to BCRF, arranged for monuments around the world—including the Empire State Building, Niagara Falls, St. Louis's Gateway Arch, the Eiffel Tower, Milan Cathedral, and Sydney Opera House—to be lit pink. Estée Lauder's breast cancer illumination initiative was so successful that in 2010, it broke the Guinness World Record for "Most Landmarks Illuminated for a Cause in 24 Hours." Not to be outdone, Komen turned pink the Giza pyramids in Egypt, a castle in Italy, and the mountaintop statue of Jesus in Rio de Janeiro. U.S. officials flooded the White House and some state capitols with pink lights, all for awareness.[118–121]

Breast cancer was so common, and awareness campaigns so ubiquitous, a person in North America could be challenged to forget about it. Pushback came from few sources. Starting in 2002, Breast Cancer Action's Think Before You Pink campaign encouraged consumers to ask questions before making purchases for the cause. Under Barbara Brenner's leadership, BCA called out companies for "pinkwashing." This term refers to the corporate practice of publicly supporting breast cancer charities all the while selling carcinogenic products. BCA has called out cosmetics and car companies, dairy producers, and others. In 2010, when Kentucky Fried Chicken ran a "Buckets for the Cure" promotion—that for each pink bucket of chicken purchased, KFC would give fifty cents to Komen—BCA responded: "What the Cluck?!" Obesity is a risk factor for breast cancer, Brenner told ABC News. "They are raising money for women's health by selling a product that's bad for your health . . . it's hypocrisy." "Pinkwashing" can also refer to the prettification of illness. The sociologist Gayle Sulik helped popularize this term in her 2011 book, *Pink Ribbon Blues.*[122–125]

Discomfiting perspectives surfaced. In *Weeds*, a Showtime TV series, Elizabeth Perkins portrayed Celia Hodes, a woman so unlikeable that upon her breast cancer diagnosis she gets no sympathy, even from her family. In a humanizing episode, her imperfectly reconstructed breasts are shown as she awaits the man who would be her lover, fearful he'll reject her cancer-treated form. Around 2006, fashion photographer David Jay began his photo essay *The SCAR Project** revealing disfigured young people with breast cancer in larger-than-life portraits. His work became the subject of an Emmy Award–winning documentary and showed in galleries around the world. Cartoonist Marisa Acocella Marchetto represented her breast cancer experience with humor in a graphic memoir, *Cancer Vixen*. S. L. Wisenberg, a fiction writer, converted her probing blog into a book, *The Adventures of Cancer Bitch.*[126–131]

Public appetite for realistic looks at breast cancer was limited, however. Pink breast cancer "culture" remained overwhelmingly popular. Many Americans

---

* SCAR is an acronym for "Surviving Cancer. Absolute Reality."

genuinely wanted to support breast cancer patients and research. People found it gratifying, and easy, to participate in awareness activities.

More and increasingly granular cancer charities formed, expanding the ways people could contribute and, essentially, divvying the "cause." In 2001, a group of Chicago-area lung cancer patients, horrified by their prognosis, established LUNGevity to support investigations into their disease.[132,133] Two new sarcoma organizations adopted complementary missions: the Sarcoma Foundation of America promoted research, while the Sarcoma Alliance sponsored awareness, peer support, and educational programs.[134,135]

Some cancer charities appealed to people in particular lines of work. The St. Baldrick's Foundation, for instance, began when a group of men in the insurance industry decided to support pediatric cancer research by shaving their heads. After an inaugural fundraising event at a New York City pub on St. Patrick's Day in 2000, St. Baldrick's (a fictitious name) took off among firefighters and police officers in New York, then elsewhere. So far it's raised and distributed over $322 million for childhood cancer research.[136–138] Meanwhile, the V Foundation ("V" for "Victory Over Cancer") became popular among professional athletes, executives, and media and sports figures. North Carolina State basketball coach Jim Valvano initiated this charity before his 1993 death from cancer; the V Foundation became Valvano's legacy.[139,140]

Niche agencies like the Inflammatory Breast Cancer Research Foundation and Triple Negative Breast Cancer Foundation gained reach on the web. The Metastatic Breast Cancer Network arranged educational conferences for stage 4 patients and caregivers, while Breastcancer.org vetted online information and managed message boards. The Pink Fund began providing financial support for patients' nonmedical expenses like rent or childcare. Some nonprofits targeted particular demographics. Sisters Network, based in Houston since 1994, Cierra Sisters in Seattle, and later Tigerlily, based in Virginia, center their advocacy on affected Black people and young patients. In California, Latinas Contra Cancer connect affected Hispanics. Later groups like the Blue Wave and, later, Male Breast Cancer Coalition, raise awareness of breast cancer occurring in men. Sharsheret, based in New Jersey, holds programs for Jewish cancer patients and caregivers. There are many examples.[141–152]

The biggest new player is Stand Up To Cancer (SU2C), an Entertainment Industry Foundation offshoot conceived by a few determined women in show business—Katie Couric, TV producer Noreen Fraser, former Paramount Pictures chair and CEO Sherry Lansing, and film producer Laura Ziskin, among others. On Friday evening of the 2008 Labor Day weekend, they held the first SU2C telethon in a Los Angeles theater. Thanks to the women's connections, all three major TV networks—ABC, CBS, and NBC—broadcast this event. In a simulcast performance, Beyoncé and others sang "Just Stand Up," a song crafted for the fundraiser, at a "Fashion Rocks New York" benefit. That weekend's telethon raised over $100 million, most of which was distributed to scientists through SU2C's partnership with the American Association for Cancer Research. The telethons have continued biennially, drawing superstar entertainers. During the 2012 telethon, Taylor Swift debuted a heartbreaking song, "Ronan," about a child with cancer; during an SU2C telethon in the United Kingdom, the actor Samuel L. Jackson plugged his "Love the Glove" campaign for prostate cancer screening.[153–155]

"Walt, is that you?" Skyler asks her husband in the final scene of the *Breaking Bad* pilot. They're in bed, she's pregnant, and he's come toward her in a new way. He's changed, and she doesn't yet know why. In this acclaimed cable TV series, a lung cancer diagnosis serves as a catalyst, transforming actor Bryan Cranston's Walter White—a modest, nonsmoking high school chemistry teacher in Albuquerque, New Mexico—into a ruthless drug kingpin. He starts cooking and selling methamphetamine, nominally to provide after his death for his wife, son, and unborn baby. *Breaking Bad* upturned the conventional idea of cancer patient as victim: Walter White is an antihero.

Breaking Bad elevated attention to cancer treatment's costs. With inoperable lung cancer, Walter hesitates before starting chemotherapy in season 1. The oncology practice requires a $5,000 deposit and estimates his out-of-pocket costs at $90,000, an out-of-reach sum for a high school teacher. In a memorable scene, Walter's family confronts him about his reluctance. Their discussion encapsulates many real families' deliberations and feelings about whether cancer treatment is worth taking. Seated in the living room, they pass around a "talking pillow" and share thoughts. Skyler is upset, she says, because Walt will die if he doesn't take the medicine. Walter Junior, their disabled teenage son, says he's angry; he thinks his father lacks courage to take chemotherapy. Hank, Walter's brother-in-law, speaks confusedly. Skyler's sister, a radiation technologist, says it should be Walter's decision to take chemo or not. She says she's known cancer patients who

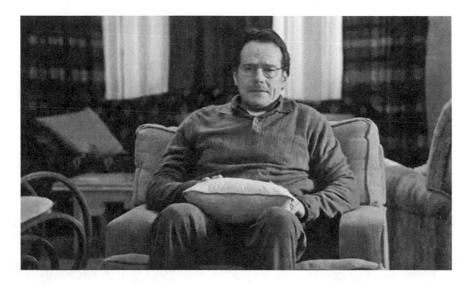

9.2 Walter White (actor Bryan Cranston) holds a "talking pillow" during a family meeting in *Breaking Bad*, Season 1.
Courtesy of Sony Pictures Television

took treatment only because their families wanted them to, while they would have preferred spending their remaining days away from doctors. Walter asserts that what he wants most is a choice. He's concerned about leaving his family with debt, and that treatment is unlikely to help much. He doesn't want to spend his final months of life feeling sickly (figure 9.2).[156]

If *Breaking Bad* were to begin today, the show's creator, Vince Gilligan, would probably assign his protagonist a different diagnosis, because Walter wouldn't be doomed by his lung cancer. In 2008 when the pilot aired, tumor DNA sequencing was not available except for research, targeted lung cancer treatment existed for only one gene, and immune agents were not yet approved. Since Walter's 2013 "death," the FDA has approved more than a dozen novel lung cancer drugs. Today, an oncologist would check Walter's malignant cells for changes in over a half dozen genes—*EGFR*, *ALK*, *ROS-1*, *MET*, *N-TRK*, *BRAF*, *RET*, and others— that confer sensitivity to nonexperimental agents. Or they might offer Walter an immune checkpoint inhibitor, an antibody drug that shrinks or stabilizes a significant fraction of lung cancers. However, the costs of Walter's cancer therapy would be exorbitant. As we'll consider, as treatments become more effective, financial toxicity becomes limiting and potentially lethal.

CHAPTER 10

CANCER EVERYWHERE (2010–2020)

Esther Earl was sixteen years old and dying from cancer when she posted one of her last vlogs. "I have scans tomorrow," she says at the video's start. Her head rests on a pillow. Her hair is messy and short. A cannula feeds oxygen into her nostrils. When she lifts her left arm, a catheter is visible. She's scared the scans will show her cancer isn't responding to chemotherapy. She feels lonely and tired and bored. "I feel sad about things that have happened in my life, and I feel happy that I'm still alive," she says. "I feel like I'm fooling you all. Because I'm not always amazing. . . . I'm not always this perfect person," she confesses. "I get pissed. I do stupid things. I get angsty. I cry. I hate my cancer. I judge people. I yell at my parents. I sometimes wish I've never gone through this, and then I realize that if that happened I wouldn't be who I am and then I get all like, oh, that's just confusing, but then sometimes I do wish it never happened, the cancer thing."

Four years after being diagnosed with stage 4 thyroid cancer, Esther Grace Earl (cookie4monster4) of Quincy, Massachusetts, managed a YouTube channel with thousands of subscribers, Tumblr and Twitter followings, and celebrity attention after meeting John Green, the young adult novelist, at a Harry Potter convention. The August 2010 video (figure 10.1) has been viewed nearly four hundred thousand times on YouTube. "I will see you guys tomorrow, probably," she closes.[1]

Earl died in Boston's Children Hospital on August 25, 2010. She was survived by her parents, four grandparents, and four siblings.[2]

Green's 2012 book, *The Fault in Our Stars*, was inspired by Earl's story. The teenage protagonist, Hazel Grace Lancaster, drags an oxygen tank wherever she goes because her lungs are compromised from thyroid cancer. She meets a handsome boy, Augustus (Gus) Waters, who'd had a "touch of osteosarcoma." They're

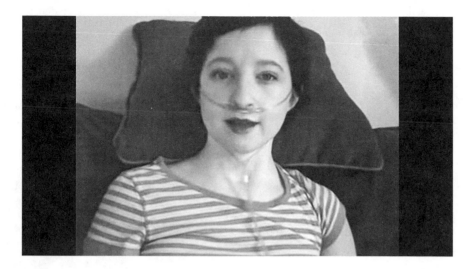

10.1 Esther Grace Earl in a YouTube video, August 2010

a prematurely wise pair. Hazel worries for her parents' grief, noting, "There is only one thing in this world shittier than biting it from cancer when you're sixteen, and that's having a kid who bites it from cancer." Gus lives philosophically. He's in the habit of pursing his lips around an unlit cigarette, explaining, "It's a metaphor, see: You put the killing thing right between your teeth, but you don't give it the power to do its killing." Predictably, they fall in love. Less predictably, one dies before the story's over.[3-6]

The *Fault* title, a Shakespeare reference,* alludes to the perpetual question cancer patients ask: *Why?* Or *Why me?* In Green's novel, Hazel is obsessed with a book," An Imperial Affliction" by a fictional Dutch author, Peter Van Houten. She reads it over and over, relating, "*AIA* is about this girl named Anna (who narrates the story) and her one-eyed mom . . . and they have a normal lower-middle-class life in a little central California town until Anna gets this rare blood cancer." Anna is honest about cancer as "no one else really is," Hazel declares. "Throughout the book, she refers to herself as *the side effect*, which is just totally correct.

---

* Julius Caesar, Act I, Scene II, Cassius to Brutus:

"The fault, dear Brutus, is not in our stars,
But in ourselves . . ."

Cancer kids are essentially side effects of the relentless mutation that made the diversity of life on earth possible," Hazel explains matter-of-factly.

In Green's tale, kids with cancer are unlucky, the fault in their stars. The book's popularity astonished publishers. In 2014, 20th Century Fox released a movie version. "'T.F.I.O.S.,' as fans call it, has been on a *Times* best-seller list for a hundred and twenty-four consecutive weeks," Margaret Talbot noted in the *New Yorker* around the film's release. "Whenever Green has appeared at a book signing he has been greeted by hundreds, often thousands, of screaming fans, mostly teen-age girls," she wrote. "The weirdness of this is hard to over-state. Green is a writer . . . 'Stars' is a novel about young people with a deadly disease."[7,8]

Hazel's wit rescues the kids-with-cancer story from sappiness. While snark was absent from prior cancer hits (see: *Love Story* and other "weepies"), in *Fault* it's abundant and on display—as a coping strategy when a cure can't be had. After attending a support group for teens with cancer, Hazel describes it unflinchingly:

> This Support Group featured a rotating cast of characters in various states of tumor-driven unwellness. Why did the cast rotate? A side effect of dying.
>
> The Support Group, of course, was depressing as hell. It met every Wednesday in the basement of a stone-walled Episcopal church . . .
>
> The six or seven or ten of us walked/wheeled in . . . and listened to Patrick [the adult leader] recount for the thousandth time his depressingly miserable life story—how he had cancer in his balls and they thought he was going to die but he didn't die and now here he is . . . divorced, addicted to video games, mostly friendless, eking out a meager living by exploiting his cancertastic past . . .
>
> AND YOU TOO MIGHT BE SO LUCKY!

Hazel's mindset enables her to absorb her circumstances realistically, to take some control. While attitudes can't save Green's fictional kids from cancer, it spares them from being pitied; they "own" their circumstances, however tragic.

Green video-chatted with affected high schoolers; some conversations were arranged by the Make-A-Wish Foundation, Talbot reported. She visited Green in Indianapolis and watched him during a Google Hangout with teens living with cancer, among others, in upstate New York, noting: "He set his laptop on the bed, positioning his chair close to it. His screen soon filled with an image of a dozen teen-agers, most of whom held copies of 'The Fault in Our Stars.'" Evidently, Green's novel—about a girl with cancer who wishes to meet the author of a book about a girl with cancer—centered in real discussions among teenagers living with cancer.

By blurring boundaries between online and fictional support groups, readers and authors, Green—and social media, more generally—brings audiences nearer to the Imperial Affliction, Hazel's truth. The "incurables" were no longer isolated in separate wards. Dying patients became visible. Their voices might be heard.

The internet was teeming with cancer stories in 2010. Blogs were the rage. I called mine *Medical Lessons* because it drew on my experiences as a patient and as a doctor, and because I was teaching-while-learning about medicine from a range of sources including patients. Among an informal network of cancer bloggers, a sense of community and mutual respect prevailed even when we disagreed, say, about an FDA decision. Blogs were a place for expressing concerns, putting ideas and questions "out there," sharing updates, and commiserating if someone's disease progressed or recurred. When a fellow blogger died, sadness spread. Gradually patients and advocates shifted to Twitter; many found the microblogging platform easy to use.

While doctors still discouraged patients from web-browsing about cancer, many ignored that advice. Patients "are no longer content to sit back, waiting for doctors to determine their fates," the 2010 Minneapolis *Star Tribune* reported, citing Dave deBronkart, a New Hampshire resident who'd been diagnosed with metastatic kidney cancer at age fifty-six. Patients "have access to the same information as their physicians—sometimes more—and many are playing a more active role in their medical decisions," the paper noted. DeBronkart had scoured the web for information which, he believed, was lifesaving, blogged about his experiences as "e-Patient Dave," and became a popular speaker. DeBronkart, an MIT graduate, had "'credibility' as a cancer patient," it was said, because he's "a really smart guy who can speak the scientific language of doctors." Together with his primary care physician, Dr. Danny Sands, deBronkart founded the Society for Participatory Medicine, accelerating an "e-patient" (empowered, engaged, equipped, and enabled) movement.[9-11]

As usual, breast cancer led the way in public cancer conversations. In July 2011, patient advocates Jody Schoger and Alicia Staley chose the hashtag #bcsm, signifying "breast cancer social media," to label an open Twitter discussion, or "tweetchat." The #bcsm tweetchat became a weekly event, Mondays at 9 P.M. eastern time. An inchoate community—including early- and late-stage breast cancer patients, caregivers, physicians, and others, lurkers—coalesced around #bcsm. At the organizers' request, a few doctors got involved to steer the discussion from hype and misinformation.

Twitter might seem an unlikely place for a cancer support group, Liz Szabo wrote in *USA Today* in 2012. Yet "the online chat, known as BCSM . . . has a growing following of men and women looking to share war stories, empower patients and change the national conversation on breast cancer," she reported. By 2013, hundreds were participating. The leaders met in person and in 2014 spoke about their online community at the South by Southwest (SXSW) festival in Austin, Texas.[12–14]

Soon advocates for people with other malignancies started tweetchats: brain tumor social media (#btsm), lung cancer (#lcsm), adolescent and young adult cancers (#ayacsm), and gynecologic cancers (#gyncsm) organized early. Preexisting hashtags, like #lymphoma and #myeloma gained followings. Because most tweets are public, newly diagnosed patients could readily connect with others.

Gradually, cancer conversations on Twitter turned from awkward to no big deal. In 2011, when journalist Xeni Jardin posted her breast cancer diagnosis to Instagram and Twitter, that made news. Six years later, when actor Julia Louis-Dreyfus shared, "1 in 8 women get breast cancer. Today, I'm the one," and plugged for universal health care, that she divulged her diagnosis on social media wasn't remarkable; comments centered on her message, not the medium. By 2019, when *Jeopardy!* host Alex Trebek revealed having pancreatic cancer in a YouTube video tweeted by the official *Jeopardy!* account, people were saddened about Trebek's condition but not shocked by this way of sharing. In 2020, the tragic death of actor Chadwick Boseman from colon cancer was announced on Twitter; that post became the most "liked" in the platform's history.[15–22]

Although relatively few doctors used social media in 2010, within a few years many signed up. Some physicians used social media to promote their practices or research. Stodgy professional societies like the American Association for Cancer Research and American Society of Clinical Oncology began using Twitter for announcements and disseminating reports. During conferences, organizations promoted panels of tweeters to spread messages, a bit like the cancer control propaganda printed by the ASCC in the Progressive Era, but on a larger and digital scale.[23–26]

At the start of his 2010 book tour for *Hitch-22*, a memoir, Christopher Hitchens was diagnosed, at sixty-one, with inoperable esophageal cancer. In his remaining eighteen months, he penned essays for *Vanity Fair* magazine that were compiled in a final book, *Mortality*.[27] In an "Afterword," his wife, Carol Blue, wrote that initially Hitchens had been "ambivalent" about reporting his cancer, but felt obliged: "He had made a pact with his editor and chum, Graydon Carter, that he would write about anything except sports, and he kept that promise."[28]

While exercising a "short-lived campaign of denial," concealing his illness, Hitchens realized, "This is what citizens of the sick country do while they are still hopelessly clinging to their old domicile." With cancer, Hitchens found himself in a welcoming "new land." Surely this is a reference to Sontag, who opened *Illness as Metaphor* with these words:

> Illness is the night-side of life, a more onerous citizenship. Everyone who is born holds dual citizenship, in the kingdom of the well and in the kingdom of the sick. Although we all prefer to use only the good passport, sooner or later each of us is obliged, at least for a spell, to identify ourselves as citizens of that other place.

Hitchens dubbed this place "Tumortown," alluding to Ehrenreich's "Cancerland," and joined the chain of writers on cancer who report from an insider's view. In Tumortown, cancer is considered from the vantage of someone affected.

Hitchens grappled with the perennial issue of cancer and blame, if patients are at fault for their illness. Long ago, doctors had linked esophageal cancer to alcohol and tobacco. Old medical texts described a synergistic effect: heavy drinking combined with smoking amplifies risk. Esophageal cancer treatments were rarely effective. Hitchens knew all this. Yet he admitted "taunting the Reaper" after his father died "swiftly" from esophageal cancer. He professed having "no regrets for a lifetime of heavy smoking and drinking," the *New York Times* mentioned in its 2011 obituary.[29] In a posthumous foreword to *Mortality*, Graydon Carter, Hitchens's pal and editor, doubled down on the hard-drinking image: "I can recall a lunch in 1991. . . . Pre-lunch tumblers of scotch were followed by a couple of glasses of wine during the meal and then a couple of post-meal cognacs."

Well known for his atheistic views, Hitchens was not surprised that some attributed his cancer to divine retribution. On a website "of the faithful," he found discussion of his case: "Who else feels Christopher Hitchens getting terminal throat cancer [sic] was God's revenge for him using his voice to blaspheme him?" The post continued, "It's just a 'coincidence' [that] out of any part of his body, Christopher Hitchens got cancer in the one part of his body he used for blasphemy? Yeah, keep believing that, Atheists. He's going to . . . die a horrible agonizing death, and THEN comes the real fun, when he's sent to HELLFIRE forever to be tortured and set afire."

Hitchens rejected the notion that a "vengeful deity" caused his cancer. God's arsenal would be "sadly depleted" if "all he can think of is exactly the cancer that my age and former 'lifestyle' would suggest," he wrote, arguing further, "If you maintain that god awards the appropriate cancers, you must also account for the numbers of infants who contract leukemia."

On an emotional roller-coaster—of possibility and disappointment, familiar to many cancer patients—Hitchens wrestled with hope, if it's worth trying standard or experimental treatments. He was simultaneously optimistic about medical science and realistic about his fate: "This is both an exhilarating and a melancholy time to have a cancer like mine," he wrote. "New peaks of medicine are rising and new treatments beginning to be glimpsed, and they have probably come too late for me."

The Komen organization was everywhere and huge in 2011. Many Americans knew it as "the" breast cancer charity. Through corporate philanthropy, plus millions of small contributions connected to its races, Komen's annual receipts exceeded $400 million. Its broad mission included cancer education, research, screening, and treatment. By this time, Komen had given more money for breast cancer research and community programs—$75 million that year; $2 billion since 1982—than any private agency.[30–32]

In January 2012, Komen announced it would sever its grants to Planned Parenthood. Behind this decision was Karen Handel, a conservative "pro-life" politician and Komen's senior vice president for public policy. She and some

Komen donors objected to the women's health provider's pro-choice services. The amount at issue, around $680,000 annually for cancer screening, represented a small fraction of Komen's $54 million screening budget and tiny bit of Planned Parenthood's yearly revenue. Komen reversed its decision within days. But the outcry was extreme and damaging.[33–39]

The 2012 "fiasco" unleashed fury about the Komen organization, the politics of women's health, and, more generally, cancer awareness. Thanks to social media, patient advocates' differences were aired publicly—like a giant pink "catfight" that bled all breast cancer charities, potentially diminishing support for numerous organizations and sympathy for those affected. Many individuals who'd previously supported Komen—who'd appreciated its elevation of breast cancer as a concern, but questioned its priorities—felt betrayed. "Komen's decision to wade into a politically charged issue had made the largest breast cancer nonprofit in America its most hated charity," Kate Pickert, a journalist and breast cancer survivor, later wrote in *Radical*.[40]

On Twitter, criticisms of Komen and pinkwashing tended to track with anger over mammography and view that the prevalent message—of early detection saving lives—was wrong, that screening had failed to prevent breast cancer deaths. Some physicians had become disaffected with mammography, writing that it resulted in overdiagnosis of harmless tumors and overtreatment in many cases. Lay books and op-eds highlighted harms and costs of screening.[41–43] This counternarrative appealed to journalists and advocates, for reasons including that many knew women whose mammograms had failed to detect cancer or whose tumors recurred after supposedly successful treatment of early-stage disease.[44] As news became increasingly opinion-based on cable TV and social media, arguments followed political leanings. Nancy Brinker had deep Republican ties, and the Planned Parenthood issue set left-leaning women's health advocates heading elsewhere—to other organizations, away from ribbons and anything "pink," as if the color—and what it represented—were radioactive.

The next spring, Peggy Orenstein's "Our Feel-Good War on Breast Cancer" appeared as a *New York Times Magazine* cover story.[45] Editors framed her widely read piece with mockable images: a pink teddy bear with Komen's trademarked pink ribbon, cheerleaders raising pink pom-poms, a pink baking oven and apron. "I used to believe that a mammogram saved my life," Orenstein opened coyly, sixteen years after her first breast cancer, about which she'd also written in that *Magazine*.[46] After having a second breast cancer diagnosed and treated, and seeing friends "die anyway" after early detection, Orenstein was no longer convinced. She questioned the mantra: "Study after study revealed the limits of screening—and the dangers of overtreatment," she wrote, citing mammography critics. "Women are now well aware of breast cancer. So what's next?"

A staggering number of journalists reported having breast cancer. Robin Roberts led a string of affected ABC *Good Morning America* (*GMA*) anchors: Roberts in 2007, Amy Robach in 2013, diagnosed by a Couric-style on-air mammogram, and Joan Lunden, a previous long-standing host, in 2014. Hoda Kotb, an NBC *Today* host, had received breast cancer treatment around the same time as Roberts, her morning TV colleague and competitor. Andrea Mitchell, another NBC TV journalist, shared her case in 2011.[47–51] After an early-stage diagnosis in 2002, Cokie Roberts, a well-known national political reporter, experienced a long-term remission; her tumor recurred, however, three years before she died in 2019 from complications of breast cancer. "She didn't want people to know she was sick," Cokie Roberts's friend Nina Totenberg said on NPR.[52,53]

In June 2012, *GMA* host Roberts told viewers that she had myelodysplastic syndrome (MDS). At fifty-one, her preleukemic blood disorder likely stemmed from her breast cancer treatment, she indicated. Roberts's MDS—a potentially lethal complication of chemotherapy and radiation—gave opportunity, perhaps underutilized, to talk about cancer treatment's toxicity and why more therapy is not always better. On TV, the chipper newscaster discussed preparing for a bone marrow transplant from her sister, a perfect match.[54,55] After taking five months' medical leave for the transplant—by all accounts successful—Roberts returned in February 2013. On air, she received a gift basket from "neighbors," the cast of NBC's *Today* show.[56,57]

Roberts, who is Black, used her platform to educate the public about bone marrow registries and the need for more diverse donors. A CNN feature highlighted disparities: While Caucasians had a 93 percent chance of finding a bone marrow match through a national registry, among African Americans and other minorities the chances were only around 66 percent, CNN reported. "I am very fortunate to have a sister who is an excellent match, and this greatly improves my chances for a cure," Roberts stated.[58,59]

In March 2013, actor Valerie Harper appeared on *GMA* by video in conversation with Roberts.[60] The two celebrities chatted patient-to-patient about their cancer experiences. At seventy-three, Harper had advanced lung cancer. She didn't smoke. Nor had her mother, who'd died from lung cancer. Harper had just published a memoir, *I, Rhoda*. After 2009 surgery for stage 2 disease, doctors had told her she was in remission. "The book ends with me saying I'm cancer free," Harper told Roberts. Weeks before the *GMA* interview, in January 2013, Harper had been hospitalized with numbness and slurred speech. It turned out she had leptomeningeal carcinomatosis, she told *People* magazine; her lung cancer had spread to the brain's lining (figure 10.2).[61,62]

Harper understood her stage 4 condition as incurable. Still she wanted "to live every moment to the fullest," she told Meredith Vieira of NBC. She sought multiple doctors' opinions and tried alternative approaches including acupuncture and Chinese tea. Harper's condition improved with cancer medicines. By September 2013, she was sufficiently well to enter ABC's *Dancing with the Stars* Season 17 and last four episodes. (She was eliminated from the competition after missteps in a Viennese waltz.) She testified before a U.S. Senate committee on needed research, and lent her name to charities.[63–65]

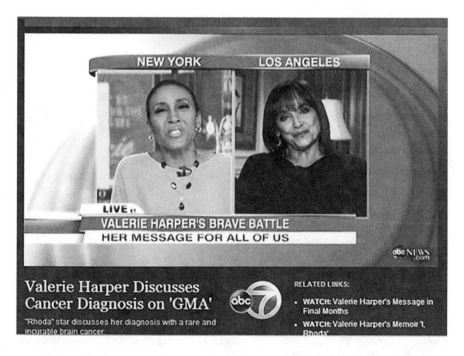

10.2 *Good Morning America* anchor Robin Roberts speaks patient-to-patient with actor Valerie Harper, March 2013.

Harper outlived doctors' expectations—surviving ten years after her initial lung cancer diagnosis and six years with known metastases. She was not immune to cancer's financial toxicity, however. Weeks before her death at age eighty, Harper's out-of-pocket expenses became so burdensome that her husband, Tony Cacciotti, set up a GoFundMe page. "Valerie has been grateful over the years for the medical breakthroughs along this difficult journey but insurance doesn't cover everything," he posted.[66,67]

Cancer appeared in popular culture. Even in comics. Take Deadpool, a figure originating in Marvel's "New Mutants" series and resurfacing in the film *X-Men Origins: Wolverine* (2009). Only later did fans learn of Deadpool's cancerous backstory: his human counterpart, Wade Wilson, in desperation with incurable cancer, agreed to receive an experimental therapy. The treatment, administered in a horrific scene, gives Wilson phenomenal energy healing and martial powers, but disfigures him and only stalls the cancer. He becomes a hideous, initially mouthless mercenary, "Merc," and then evolves. In 2016, actor Ryan Reynolds portrayed Deadpool's pained, powerful, and sad character in the first of two eponymous movies.[68–72] This character's cancer and side effects of therapy, however "comical," reinforce view of oncology care as scary and disabling.

Doctor Jane Foster, another Marvel figure, is diagnosed with stage 4 breast cancer in the recent "Thor: God of Thunder" series. Foster declines "magical" remedies and accepts chemotherapy. When she wields Mjolnir, the hammer of Thor, it has two effects: it perpetuates the cancer and gives her superhuman strength. Actor Natalie Portman has cameoed as Foster in Marvel's *Thor* (2011), *Thor: The Dark World* (2013), and *Avengers: Endgame* (2019) films. She stars—as a hero with stage 4 cancer—in the latest feature, *Thor: Love and Thunder* (figure 10.3).[73–75]

Several movies and TV series centered on cancer stories. In the 2011 film *50/50*, Joseph Gordon-Levitt convincingly portrays a young man with a rare cancer and uncertain survival.[76,77] Showtime's *The Big C* featured Laura Linney as a middle-aged mom and schoolteacher with advanced melanoma and lasted four seasons, from 2010 to 2013.[78–80] ABC Family's *Chasing Life* depicted the complicated circumstances of a young journalist with leukemia and survived only two seasons, 2014 to 2015.[81,82] In each of these programs, cancer did not necessarily overwhelm

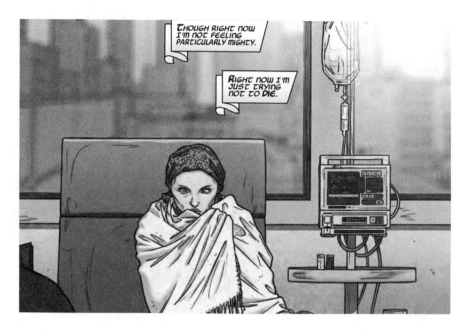

10.3 Jane Foster image, *The Mighty Thor: Thunder in Her Veins*
© *MARVEL (with permission)*

other issues, such as family and relationships, in the characters' lives. In contrast to *Love Story* forty years earlier, in *Chasing Life* the protagonist, a young woman with acute leukemia, has a chance of surviving; she is not doomed by cancer.

Cancer has affected so many characters on TV and in film, more than can be considered in these pages. By this time, fictional representations of malignant conditions, cancer treatments, and outcomes are so varied and numerous, it's impossible to know how they influence viewers' consciousness and medical decisions.

The public was bombarded by cancer stories. Each day delivered a new tale of woe—or triumph.

Not surprisingly, reality TV stars got cancer. Ethan Zohn, a handsome *Survivor: Africa* winner, had been diagnosed with Hodgkin's lymphoma in 2009. His disease recurred in 2011. After stem cell transplants and treatment with a novel drug, Zohn entered a long-term remission, as covered by *People*, *Parade*, and *Entertainment Weekly*.[83–92] Tamra Barney, an Orange County *Housewife* and fitness guru, disclosed having cervical cancer in 2012 and, later, melanoma.[93–95] After departing *Housewives*, Camille Grammer of Beverly Hills underwent surgery for endometrial cancer; she has Lynch syndrome and spoke about it on *The Doctors*.[96–98] Other "Real" cases followed.[99]

Actor Michael Douglas had a talked-about case. In 2010, just before a promotional tour for *Wall Street*, a movie in which he starred, Douglas shared a "throat cancer" diagnosis on David Letterman's *Late Show*. In May 2013, he created a stir when he said his HPV-associated tumor was caused by oral sex. Months later, Douglas clarified that he'd actually had stage 4 tongue cancer but opted to call it "throat cancer" for professional reasons. "Let's just say it's throat cancer," a doctor suggested, Douglas told the *Guardian*. "And I said OK." Otherwise surgery involving removal of part of the jaw and tongue would be considered necessary, a surgeon had advised, Douglas said. It wasn't "going to be pretty."[100–105]

A strange episode involved Venezuelan President, Hugo Chávez. After undergoing emergency surgery in Cuba in 2011, Chávez was open about having cancer, but he didn't disclose the type.[106–109] In tweets, he occasionally expressed appreciation for the medical care he received.[110] After Chávez's 2013 death, then interim President Nicolás Maduro raised the possibility that the leftist leader's cancer had been caused by his enemies: "We have this intuition that our Commander Chávez was poisoned by dark forces that wanted to get rid of him." Maduro indicated that Chávez's tumor had behaved in a very unusual way. Maduro noted that the United States and other countries "developed programs in the 1940s and 1950s to experiment with intentionally causing cancer," the *New York Times* reported.[111]

Cancer patients and caregivers increasingly bypassed traditional sources of medical facts. Surfing the web, watching TV, or listening to podcasts, people gleaned information, sometimes true, and advice—about genetic dispositions, preventive strategies, and cancer treatments—shared on Facebook, Reddit, YouTube, you name it.

In May 2013, Angelina Jolie wrote of her decision to undergo a preventive double mastectomy and breast reconstruction in the op-ed pages of the *New York Times*. The beautiful actor detailed her reasoning. Considering her mother's premature death from cancer and that she'd inherited a cancer-disposing *BRCA*

(BReast CAncer) gene mutation, she was at high risk. Two years later, she had her ovaries removed for the same reason. Jolie's case—and the enormous publicity surrounding her choice—raised awareness of BRCA and hereditary cancer syndromes.[112,113] Many people didn't realize that inheriting BRCA-1 or -2 mutations not only elevates a person's risk for breast cancer, but also predisposes to developing ovarian cancer, pancreatic cancer, and prostate cancer.[114,115]

"Previvor" is a phrase some individuals who've inherited cancer-linked genetic variants use to describe their status—of being at high risk but not yet having disease.[116,117] As more people learned they have BRCA or less famous mutations—of PALB-2 or ATM, mismatch repair genes in Lynch syndrome, TP53 in Li-Fraumeni syndrome, and others—at-risk communities formed. AliveAndKickn, an advocacy organization founded by colon cancer survivor Dave Dubin, sponsors HEROIC, a hereditary cancer patient registry, and promotes educational events including Lynch Syndrome Awareness Day.[118,119] FORCE (Facing Our Risk of Cancer Empowered) includes people with hereditary breast and ovarian cancer syndromes, among others.[120,121] At FORCE conferences, affected individuals hear updates from expert physicians, researchers, and advocacy leaders; some enjoyed the opportunity to chat about screening, prophylactic medicines, and surgical options with other previvors.

Kayleigh McEnany, a Harvard-educated lawyer who later became White House press secretary under President Donald Trump, calls herself a previvor. In 2018, she tweeted, "I did it!!! I'm officially a Previvor! #PreventativeMastectomy," with a photo of herself, thumbs up and smiling in a hospital bed and gown. Fox News covered McEnany's story: a published image shows her revealing a mastectomy drain, otherwise hidden under her shirt, while attending a Tampa Bay Lightning NHL hockey game.[122,123]

As more patients shared their stories, more people questioned the merits of doing so. The issue percolated until January 2014, when the internet blew up around the case of Lisa Bonchek Adams, a forty-four-year-old mother of three who blogged and tweeted about her life with metastatic breast cancer. Adams was constantly posting updates about her condition while receiving care, including palliative care, at Memorial Sloan Kettering Cancer Center and, when I met her, participating in a clinical trial of a then-experimental kind of drug called a PI3 kinase inhibitor. With recurrent breast cancer after mastectomy and chemotherapy, she knew she was dying. She tweeted engagingly, with humor, and often. "Okay, fine, you asked for it: I'm going for one million tweets," she'd shared in 2012. (Which led me to wonder, first, Why? And second, Would she make it?)[124,125]

A journalist, Emma G. Keller, triggered the uproar with a *Guardian* column titled, "Forget Funeral Selfies. What Are the Ethics of Tweeting a Terminal Illness?" She charged Adams with oversharing: "Adams is dying out loud," Keller wrote. "She's in terrible pain. She knows there is no cure, and she wants you to know all about what she is going through." The women had exchanged messages when Keller organized a 2013 *Guardian* chat about cancer and DNA. Keller became obsessed with Adams:

> A few weeks ago I noticed she was tweeting a lot more. . . . The clinical drug trial she was on wasn't working. Her disease seemed to be rampaging through her body. She could hardly breathe, her lungs were filled with copious amounts of fluid causing her to be bedridden over Christmas. As her condition declined, her tweets amped up both in frequency and intensity. I couldn't stop reading. . . . I felt embarrassed at my voyeurism. Should there be boundaries in this kind of experience?

Keller reported Adams's said mission—educating others about life with metastatic breast cancer—and added her two cents: "Tweeting makes her less lonely, it gives her a purpose, it distracts her from her pain, and the contact it brings clearly comforts her." Further, the columnist analyzed, "It's clear that tweeting as compulsively as Lisa Adams does is an attempt to exercise some kind of control over her experience."[126]

The story exposed disagreements over cancer patients' visibility and, also, their vulnerability to journalists. Keller had previously written on breast cancer. In a first-person 2012 *Guardian* post called "Double Mastectomy: My Brutal 40-Day Breast Cancer Cure," Keller recounted being diagnosed with ductal carcinoma in situ (a noninvasive, stage 0 form) and undergoing mastectomy with reconstructive surgery in a twelve-hour $250,000 operation. Perhaps she was discomfited reading Adams's tweets because she herself feared recurrence. Regardless of her motivation for writing it, Keller's 2014 piece was criticized for its callous tone and misleading statements. Days later, the *Guardian* took the unusual step of removing the column, which can still be read on the "Wayback Machine," an internet archive.[127,128]

Meanwhile Bill Keller, Emma's husband and a former executive editor of the *New York Times*, escalated the situation with an op-ed titled "Heroic Measures" in which he used Adams's case to question merits of aggressive oncology care. That's a reasonable question, in itself. But Bill wrote hurtfully and without caring to understand his forty-four-year-old subject's situation or views. His article contains substantive mistakes: about Adams's attitude toward palliative care (she favored it); and on "battling" cancer (she loathed the term). Bill linked to his 2012 op-ed, commandingly titled "How to Die," in which he reflected on the peaceful death of his father-in-law from cancer at age seventy-nine in a British hospital. "There is something enviable about going gently," he suggested. After mentioning his wife's "brush with cancer," Bill compared his father-in-law's "calm death" with a (mistaken) version of Adams's course: "She is all about heroic measures," Bill wrote of Adams. "She is constantly engaged in battlefield strategy with her medical team. There is always the prospect of another research trial to excite her hopes. She responds defiantly to any suggestion that the end is approaching."[129,130]

Reactions were harsh. "FORMER NYT EDITOR MANSPLAINS TO CANCER PATIENT TO SHUT UP AND DIE THE RIGHT WAY" topped a Feministing.com post by Katie Halper. "It is bizarrely tone-deaf, ghoulish, & lacking in empathy all at once," tweeted Xeni Jardin. In a *Nation* post, "No Shame: Bill Keller Bullies Cancer Patient," Greg Mitchell wrote that Bill Keller "between the lines, suggests that Lisa Adams just die, already." Zeynep Tufekci, who studies the intersection of technology and society, had been following Adams for her own reasons; she was interested in how social media renders previously isolating conditions, like terminal cancer, visible. "Lisa Adams is doing one heck of a job educating people," Tufekci wrote on *Medium*. She called the couple's behavior "cancer-shaming."[131–134]

Margaret Sullivan, the *Times* "public editor," covered some aspects of the disagreement. She mentioned that some readers reacted favorably to Bill Keller's column for his advocacy of palliative care. He responded, "By living her disease in such a public way, by turning her hospital room into a classroom, she invites us to think about and debate some big, contentious issues."[135]

Needing money, some cancer patients turned to the web for personal fundraising. Start-ups like YouCaring.com and GiveForward.com made asking easy: "It takes only a few keystrokes for a family to set up a Web page, where they tell their story and state a fundraising goal," *Kaiser Health News* (*KHN*) reported. "They can spread the word on social media sites such as Facebook. Donations can be made with credit cards or via PayPal." *KHN* highlighted the story of a thirty-two-year-old Alexandria, Virginia, man with stage 4 lung cancer whose friends and family contributed $56,800 to defray medical expenses uncovered by insurance. Since its 2008 start, GiveForward had raised over $47 million for patients and, by skimming a small percent from each donation, profited significantly, *KHN* reported in 2013.[136,137]

"Go Fund Yourself" titled a later piece in *Mother Jones*. "The crowd may become the insurer of last resort," wrote Stephen Marche. Tech-enabled platforms can exacerbate racial, economic, and educational divides because people of lower means tend to have less wealthy social networks, he explained. Most online campaigns fail to meet fundraising targets, so patients need be savvy "marketers of their own tragedy." Crisis narratives—a sudden diagnosis or accident—are more effective fundraisers than chronic conditions. Posting good images and a frequent stream of updates can enhance revenue. "People want to come back to the story, to find out what happens . . . to see how their money has changed somebody's life," a marketing director told Marche. "The story people want to hear is that they're giving you money and you'll get better right away and return to being a contributing member of society."[138]

On social media, patients aired appeals for off-label medicines and genetic tests their insurance wouldn't cover. Heartbreaking stories, such as the plight of Nathalie Traller—an Oregon teenager whose rare sarcoma had progressed through chemotherapy—grabbed attention. Traller's doctors recommended a checkpoint inhibitor, a then-new kind of monoclonal antibody that can unleash the immune system against cancer. By 2014, several pharmaceutical companies had FDA-approved or in-the-pipeline checkpoint inhibitors, but none were yet available for people with Traller's condition or young age. Her family contacted Genentech, Bristol-Myers Squibb, and Merck, pleading for this kind of drug to be made available on a compassionate use basis. They campaigned on Facebook, YouTube, Instagram, Twitter (#4Nathalie), and a blog. As reported in an obituary, Genentech did make an exception, enabling Traller to receive an immunotherapy agent starting in August 2014, and this helped for a while. Traller died at age sixteen in late 2015.[139,140]

Some people faked having cancer for financial gain. While the incidence of "Münchausen by internet" can't be known, even rare episodes breed distrust. In a well-publicized case, Marissa Marchand joined a breast cancer Facebook group and pretended to be a single mom with terminal disease, eliciting kind words and gifts from strangers. When Marchand stopped posting, group members worried that she'd died. She was arrested in Colorado for feigning a cancer story and taking thousands on GoFundMe. Sadly, it's not only strangers who deceive in this way. Jenny Flynn Cataldo, an Alabama woman, bilked GoFundMe contributors of $38,000 and, from her friends and parents, nearly a half million dollars.[141-144]

In Columbus, John Looker charmed leadership of Pelotonia, an annual bike ride supporting Ohio State's cancer center, for several years. Pelotonia featured Looker, who claimed brain cancer, in promotional videos. He became an influencer: people gave him cash and checks, wore "Looker's Hookers" T-shirts, and bought "Lookies" cookies. Suspicions surfaced about the veracity of Looker's story, but patient privacy protection laws precluded Pelotonia's CEO, Doug Ulman, who'd previously led the Livestrong Foundation, from investigating. In 2018, Looker admitted inventing his condition. In 2019, the Ohio attorney general announced a settlement regarding his "misrepresenting a cancer diagnosis to solicit and subsequently misuse charitable donations."[145-147]

Money isn't the only reason people lie about having cancer. Some seek attention, sympathy, or an excuse. The novelist Dan Mallory told colleagues that he had brain cancer, when he did not, and later attributed his cancer fabrication to delusions from a bipolar disorder. Netflix has distributed two series in which central characters pretend to have cancer. In *Sick Note*, after receiving an esophageal cancer diagnosis, a young man finds that people are nicer to him; when he learns there's been an error, that he doesn't have cancer, he struggles to inform coworkers and friends for fear they'll stop treating him well. In *Mythomaniac*, a French drama, a woman feigns having cancer so that her husband and children will give her the attention she feels she deserves.[148-151]

While the breast cancer community—patients, advocates, and charity supporters—was tearing itself apart in public arguments, the tiny Metastatic Breast Cancer Network had been directing attention toward the unmet needs of those living with stage 4 disease and, in October 2013, establishing the Metastatic

Breast Cancer Alliance. The Alliance involved the "big pink" charities, Komen and the Breast Cancer Research Foundation (BCRF), a dozen smaller agencies, and pharmaceutical companies. With a cooperative tone, the Alliance set goals of raising awareness of metastatic breast cancer (MBC), documenting how many are affected (no one knew), and promoting research on metastases.[152–155]

In April 2015, a new group was born in Philadelphia, where several hundred patients and advocates had traveled for a Living Beyond Breast Cancer (LBBC) "metastatic summit." Some arrived on scholarships distributed by LBBC and funded by pharmaceutical companies. After hearing statistics about their condition during an advocacy workshop, two attendees—Jennie Grimes, thirty-four, of Los Angeles, and Beth Caldwell, thirty-nine, a Seattle mom and civil rights lawyer—decided to emulate ACT UP, the AIDS activist organization, by holding a "die-in." With life expectancies under three years, they were angry about the slow pace of research. In the hallway of the Loews Philadelphia Hotel on a Sunday morning, over a hundred MBC patients and advocates lay down as an act of protest. Some summit registrants elected not to participate in the die-in; they weren't comfortable with such a dark demonstration. Before leaving Philadelphia, a core group formed MET UP, the METastatic Exchange to Unleash Power.[156]

That October, Caldwell led a die-in on the West Lawn of the Capitol in Washington, DC. "We feel a strong kinship with AIDS patients," she told me. "At the height of the AIDS crisis, there were about forty thousand deaths per year in the United States, and that's how many people die of metastatic breast cancer every year in the United States." Metastatic breast cancer "is terminal," Caldwell said. "The die-in captures the effects of the disease, what's happening to women I know, who are dying." MET UP appealed to individuals, including me. who recalled ACT UP's role in the AIDS crisis or who simply appreciated its gravity. But this group failed to attract members; around its 2016 peak, MET UP involved a few dozen women and men. It held a few more die-ins, sparsely attended. Caldwell died at age forty-one, in 2017.[157–160]

Americans were becoming aware of MBC. In response to criticisms, Komen upped its grants for stage 4 research and organized dozens of educational conferences for MBC patients and caregivers. Meanwhile METAvivor, an organization focused on stage 4 breast cancer research, grew almost exponentially. By the decade's end, METAvivor was raising millions of dollars through "Metsquerade" balls and fashion shows, along with donations from industry including Allergan, a breast implant manufacturer. Its lay-led board distributed millions in grants to scientists studying metastatic disease (figure 10.4).[161–165]

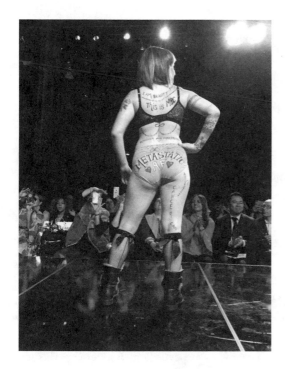

10.4 Model with metastatic breast cancer in a fashion show benefiting METAvivor, a nonprofit organization, New York City, February 2019

Photo by Elaine Schattner

Lines separating pharma, patient advocacy, and advertising blurred as drug manufacturers engaged with patients more directly—by organizing dinners and paying for some travel. At several patient-oriented events I've attended, companies set up videography stations, making it easy for people with MBC to speak on camera and post stories to the web, effectively showcasing their survival. Pfizer produces Ibrance (palbociclib), the first cyclin-dependent kinase (CDK) inhibitor approved for treating breast cancer. Pfizer's *A Story Half Told* photography project, which I first viewed in a New York City gallery in 2015, depicts MBC patients' lives.[166–169] In 2018 Lilly, which sells a competing CDK inhibitor for breast cancer, launched a "Thriver Movement." Lilly notified investors it was enlisting advocates; it was understood that patients' involvement could lift sales.[170–172] Eisai manufactures Halaven (eribulin), a drug approved for MBC, and "partnered" with METAvivor in a #ThisIsMBC campaign; photos and videos of patients appear on an Eisai-run website.[165,173] These are just a few instances of industry-initiated "advocacy" programs; campaigns are underway, or being developed, for other cancers.

"In April 2015, five patients with metastatic lung cancer sat together in a Washington DC bar and shared their longing for a cure." These words open an astonishing *Nature Reviews Clinical Oncology* paper about the *ROS1*ders—an advocacy group to which the authors belong—and a new style of cancer patient activism. Among 175 people attending a nearby LUNGevity "Hope Summit," an educational meeting for patients and caregivers, those five shared a rare condition: lung cancer driven by *ROS1* gene fusions. As they told their story four and a half years later, while most oncologists had "never even met a patient with *ROS1*-positive disease," they'd become experts.

The *ROS1*ders reported a thriving Facebook group with over five hundred *ROS1*-positive cancer patients and caregivers in thirty-six countries. Their group expanded to include people with any of eight cancer types, such as melanoma and pancreatic cancer, with *ROS1* gene variants.[174]

As some people with cancer are living longer, they are taking control not just of cancer conversations, but of research priorities. Aiming to speed development of more accurate diagnostic tests and effective treatments for *ROS1*-driven tumors, the *ROS1*ders collaborate—as partners—with academic and industry scientists. Other molecularly-defined patient advocacy groups have emerged, such as the EGFR Resisters, Exon 20 Group, and KRAS Kickers. These modern cancer "volunteers" don't simply offer time or money to the cause. They contribute their knowledge, experience, and perspectives, besides biological samples and medical records, to the research endeavor.[175–178]

The crush of public cases continued. Politicians developed cancer and disproportionately, it seemed, they developed brain cancer. In 2008, Massachusetts Senator Edward (Ted) Kennedy was diagnosed with brain cancer; he died the next year.[179,180] In July 2017, Arizona Senator John McCain, a survivor of melanoma, was diagnosed with glioblastoma, an aggressive form; he died the next summer. These true stories serve as a collective reminder that research is still needed into rare tumors against which progress lags.[181,182]

When Vice President Joe Biden's son Beau died from brain cancer in May 2015, Joe grieved terribly. At forty-six, Beau had been a husband and father. He was a Bronze Star veteran who'd served in Iraq, a lawyer with political aspirations. The vice president was no stranger to tragedy. In 1972, his wife and daughter had been killed in a car crash. After Beau's 2013 diagnosis until his death, the vice president was reticent about his son's brain tumor, saying little in public before October 2015 when he announced from the White House Rose Garden that he wouldn't then run for president; he wasn't ready. There is no "timetable" for the grieving process, Joe knew from experience.[183,184]

During his final State of the Union address in January 2016, President Obama announced a U.S. cancer "moonshot" and charged Biden with "mission control." To bipartisan applause, Obama said, "Let's make America the country that cures cancer once and for all." This was an emotional moment in the Capitol, powered by feelings of the two men, months after Beau's death.[185–187]

Biden was intensely motivated to help people affected by cancer. He got right to work touring labs, meeting with investigators, and listening to patients. A Cancer Moonshot task force and Blue Ribbon Panel involved scientists, clinical trial and health disparity mavens, patient advocates, and biotech executives, among others. The cancer community was energized by all this activity—along with an anticipated $1 billion lift to the federal research budget. Other heads of state took an interest, reportedly asking Obama about Biden's program. With passage of the 21st Century Cures Act in December 2016, the cancer "moonshot" was slated to receive $1.8 billion in funding over seven years.[188–190]

The U.S. cancer moonshot fizzled, however, after President Donald Trump took office. With private funding in 2017, Biden created the Biden Cancer Initiative. That organization suspended operations when Biden campaigned for president.[191–193] After his 2020 win, cancer research remained a priority for President Biden.

A public lesson of progress against cancer came by way of former President Jimmy Carter. At age ninety, Carter was diagnosed with and treated for metastatic melanoma, a lethal form of skin cancer, that involved his liver and brain. After surgery in August 2015, he held a press conference and spoke directly of his condition. Doctors had prescribed radiation and immunotherapy with a drug called pembrolizumab, which he mentioned. Carter said he expected to keep teaching Sunday school in Plains, Georgia, and expressed regret that he might not travel to Nepal with Habitat for Humanity as planned.[194–196]

By 2015, openness was such that Carter received calls from world leaders; former and current presidents George H. W. Bush and Barack Obama tweeted their good wishes.[197,198] That December, Carter updated congregants at his church: he was cancer free. In March 2016, Carter no longer needed the immune drug; he'd be monitored, that's all. Months later, Carter and his wife, Rosalynn, volunteered with Habitat for Humanity in Memphis, Tennessee, constructing homes.[199–203]

An expanding range of celebrities shared personal experiences and images of cancer. In 2016, the Black Eyed Peas musician Jaime Gomez, known as Taboo, announced he'd undergone surgery and chemotherapy for testicular cancer. Gomez sought to raise awareness—and lessen stigma—of cancer in Mexican and Native American communities. In 2016 the ACS named Gomez a "global ambassador."[204,205] Another American musician of color, Beyoncé, shattered norms by including a Mississippi woman who'd undergone a double mastectomy, topless, in the film version of her acclaimed album *Lemonade*.[206–208]

Doctors told their stories. Dr. Paul Kalanithi, a brilliant neurosurgeon, wrote a memoir before dying from lung cancer. At thirty-seven, he left behind a wife, a child, and best seller, *When Breath Becomes Air*.[209–211] The neurologist and popular author Dr. Oliver Sacks revealed having melanoma and why he decided to forgo chemotherapy, before he died at age eighty-two. Recent additions to the crowded subgenre of cancer books by doctors who've had breast cancer include works by Drs. Trisha Greenhalgh and Liz O'Riordan, a British GP and breast surgeon; Dr. Beverly Zavaleta, a Harvard-educated family physician in Texas; and Dr. Uzma Yunus, a Pakistan-born U.S. immigrant, psychiatrist, and mother who died from the disease in 2019.[212–214]

Supreme Court Justice Ruth Bader Ginsburg experienced several bouts of cancer in these years. With balance of the Supreme Court at stake during Trump's presidency, many people hoped Ginsburg might somehow overcome these maladies. She'd had cancer previously: colon cancer in 1999, while in her sixties, and early-stage pancreatic cancer, treated in 2009, while in her seventies. By 2018, she'd become a cultural icon, the "notorious RBG," when she suffered broken ribs. Doctors found two malignant lung nodules; surgeons removed part of her lung. The Court issued occasional statements about Justice Ginsburg's health. In 2019, doctors identified a tumor "on her pancreas." She received radiation. Next, cancer involved her bile duct; doctors placed a stent. At age eighty-seven, Ginsburg received treatments including chemotherapy. She continued working until she died in September 2020, weeks before the U.S. presidential election.[215–221]

When Chadwick Boseman died from colon cancer in August 2020, the world was stunned. He'd chosen to keep his diagnosis private. At only forty-three, the beloved actor was well known to audiences around the world; he'd portrayed prominent Black Americans Jackie Robinson, James Brown, and Thurgood Marshall in biopics and, not long before his death, Marvel's Black Panther superhero.[20,222,223]

In her 2018 book, *Everything Happens for a Reason (and Other Lies I've Loved)*, Kate Bowler, a historian, circles the Why Me? question from the perspective of someone diagnosed at thirty-five with incurable stage 4 colon cancer and responding, so far, to immune therapy. For her PhD thesis, she'd studied the prosperity gospel: the religious idea that god's believers will be rewarded with health and wealth. When her malignancy was discovered, she was a young mother with a promising academic career. Bowler's condition makes people uncomfortable, she perceives, because it reminds them of human fragility. When acquaintances and strangers offer "reasons" for her illness, she wonders, "What if everything is random?"[224]

The issue of fate—if cancers arise due to chance or might be averted—figured into one of the most heated scientific arguments of this decade. In 2015, Johns Hopkins researchers Cristian Tomasetti and Bert Vogelstein reported that most mutations in cancer stem from random errors, genetic "typos" that occur during normal DNA replication.[†] Most tumors can't be explained by environmental exposures, behavior, or inherited genes, they determined. Rather, "bad luck" is usually a contributor.[225,226] The paper received heavy press—"Most Cancer Types 'Just Bad Luck'" (BBC), "Cancer's Random Assault" (*New York Times*), etc.—and a flood of criticism. Commentators faulted the analysis, and a 2017 follow-up paper,[227] on methodological grounds, that it was mathematical (and not empirical); some mistook their results to suggest that most cancers can't be prevented; others objected to Vogelstein's view that since many cancers can't be avoided, early detection is a key strategy.[228–231]

The findings were so charged that two outlets ran pointedly distinct headlines over the same article: "Most Cancer Mutations Due to 'Bad Luck,' but Many Cases Still Preventable" at *Stat News*, "Most Cancer Cases Arise from 'Bad Luck'" at *Scientific American*.[232,233] "This story reveals less about why people do or don't get cancers, and more about how hard it is to talk or think about these diseases," Ed Yong wrote in the *Atlantic*.[234]

---

† The scientists' words closely resemble Hazel's comments about the "The Imperial Affliction" in the *The Fault in Our Stars*, a work of fiction.

I'd been puzzled by the fierceness of the debate—why journalists, among others, were so worked up about this largely abstract paper on cancer's roots. Scientists often disagree. Then I realized, what drew the outcry was not the analysis itself but the matter of cancer's origins—if it might be prevented, if people are to blame for their malignancies.

This is a fraught subject. Many cancer patients and families, searching for reasons, resent any insinuation that they are somehow responsible for their illness. Even today, some individuals feel guilty about developing cancer, believing it a consequence of misbehavior or flawed psyche. This issue bugged Sontag, it irritated Samantha in *Sex and the City*, and it worried me. Around my diagnosis, I wondered if I was to blame for my cancer for having spent too many hours at the hospital and lab, away from my family.

Of course, no one deserves to get cancer.

When I entered medical school, few of cancer's causes were understood, and patients were "victims." Since then, doctors have acquired knowledge of disposing conditions—genetics, environmental and behavioral factors—that play a role, besides chance. Scientists say that approximately half of cases might be avoided, as we'll consider in a final chapter. Yet a 2019 Harris poll found that one in four Americans "believe if they are going to get cancer, they are going to get it, there is nothing they can do."[235]

Such a fatalistic view warrants public education so that individuals might lessen their personal risk, and that society would support more research into cancer's causes and prevention. Cancer will take over six hundred thousand American lives this year, and over nine million globally. The physical and financial costs of treating cancer are great. Despite progress, many cases cannot be cured. I believe that discerning cancer's causes and improving treatments are not competing aims; they are complementary. By reducing cancer's occurrence, more funds would be available to provide optimal care for those seeking relief.

PART III

CANCER'S FUTURE

In this section, we'll consider the ramifications of openness about cancer for modern patients. We'll look at oncology's costs, the downside of skepticism, and the possibility of preventing cancer.

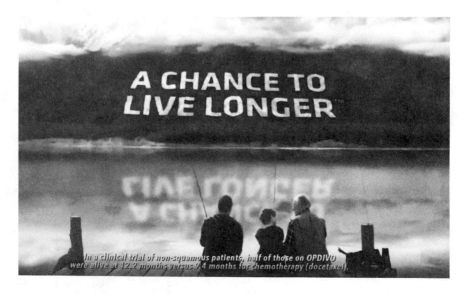

Advertisement for Opdivo, a cancer medication

CHAPTER 11

THE MODERN PATIENT'S BURDEN

A century ago, cancer facts were delivered unidirectionally: doctors told patients what's best. Experts penned pamphlets for distribution by women, no questions asked, and journalists helped spread the word. Samuel Hopkins Adams—a muckraker, no less—cooperated with specialists when he set out to inform the public about cancer. His 1913 *Ladies' Home Journal* feature came with a physician's stamp of approval.[1] Messages were simple: cancer is curable if caught early; surgery, not medicine, is proper treatment; cancer is neither contagious nor heritable; avoid quacks selling bogus cancer "cures."

Fast-forward: the web democratizes medical knowledge. Today, most anyone can share the experience of having cancer or its treatment, post articles, and offer advice peer-to-peer. Overall this trend is helpful. For someone facing a malignant diagnosis, it's never been easier to find information and connect with others. The internet can reduce patients' vulnerability to local doctors' biases and imperfect knowledge.

But in some ways, being a cancer patient or caregiver is harder than ever. Amid a surplus of conflicting reports—and modern style of practicing medicine that teaches and demands respect for patients' preferences—the onus of responsibility for oncology decisions has shifted. "It's up to you" is the new doctor's mantra, which leaves many people with cancer seeking guidance.

In principle, modern patients are empowered and engaged; in reality, many are ill-equipped to navigate diverse sources, conflicting data and recommendations. Sorting through loads of jargon-riddled reports before a life-or-death decision can overwhelm a person to a point of paralysis, of becoming stuck. For this reason, some of the most educated patients I've known still prefer following a trusted doctor's recommendations. But they are lucky to have a knowledgeable physician who listens and cares for them. Not everyone does.

This book celebrates openness about cancer. Public cancer conversations are not always benign, however. I attest to the dangers. Previously, editors served as gatekeepers to news, limiting cancer reports and commentary. Journalists cited experts and fact-checked. But the current situation—cancer information chaos—cannot be reduced to a complaint about social media. That's because discerning what's correct or even a legitimate opinion about cancer isn't straightforward when medical journals publish conflicting studies and doctors argue, publicly, about statistics and trial results. On Twitter and in podcasts, oncologists debate merits of novel agents, journalists offer different takes on the same, and patients air their own ideas, oftentimes valid. Dozens of cancer charities, competing for donations, sponsor distinct and contradictory messages. Deception can be subtle, misinformation hard to spot.[2]

Online cancer chatter encompasses a huge, confusing, and conflicting range of viewpoints. Often, seemingly credible sources provide partial or self-serving information. Top cancer centers, for instance, run slick websites with educational links and videos detailing—i.e., advertising—what expertise and clinical trials they happen to offer. Too often, experts' financial and academic conflicts of interest go unstated on social media. Clinical investigators may engage with patients online while recruiting subjects for their research. Some doctors say they're using Twitter to educate or learn, when their real aim is to attract patients to their practices. Patient influencers and advocates receive payments for posting to Instagram or Twitter, but they don't necessarily mention it. Journalists lurk, seeking stories. Anonymous posts and fake cancer stories spin doubt.

The plethora of pharmaceutical advertisements for name-brand cancer treatments—on television, radio, the web, and elsewhere—annoys many physicians; it irritates medical ethicists who complain about marketing false hope to desperate patients. It might surprise a reader, here, but I don't mind seeing commercials for new cancer drugs and diagnostic tests. That's because too many people with cancer haven't been offered or prescribed appropriate evaluations or medications by their physicians. I believe that patients—the public—have every right to see these commercials so long as they're clearly labeled as advertisements, that they might then ask their doctors something along the lines of: "I saw an ad on TV for a new lung cancer drug, might it be helpful in my case?"

As recently as 2010, it wasn't uncommon for doctors to instruct cancer patients, "Don't go on the internet." I had acquaintances whose surgeons issued those very words. Many oncologists of my generation and older genuinely but paternalistically wanted to spare their patients dismay upon reading hard statistics. Some didn't have the patience for hearing what "Dr. Google" suggested. And if patients discovered helpful information—a drug to consider or clinical trial for which they'd be eligible—not all physicians appreciated the enlightenment. From a doctor's point of view, practicing medicine was easier, and faster, when patients didn't challenge their knowledge and authority. But reverting to paternalism—when doctors decide without informing patients of options, what advocates like Rose Kushner fought against in the 1970s—is inconceivable. Those days are over.

In writing, I've wondered, would survival and quality of life of people with cancer be better if all patients simply accepted their oncologist's advice—or if everyone affected sought information, asked questions in an open community as can be found on the web, and chose among reasonable FDA-approved or in-trial treatments, or observation, with or without palliative care? While there can be no randomized trial to answer this question, I am confident that unrestricted discussions lead to better outcomes.

Years ago, I taught in an ethics course for medical students. A key concept was patient autonomy: the capacity, and right, of people to make treatment choices based on their preferences and values.[3-6] Cancer patient autonomy was a pipe dream, I considered, because most people don't sufficiently understand human physiology, biology or statistics to appreciate risks and benefits of treatments. In my experiences rounding on oncology wards, few patients wanted to read the fine print about randomized studies or chemotherapy before signing on. The language in those documents was daunting, besides that clinical decisions were pressing and the situations intense.

If there's one message in this book, it's that better education of most everyone particularly in math and science would serve people with cancer. Being educated is the only way people can effectively interpret news about cancer, make truly informed decisions, and, should illness arise, control their fates in ways that align with their values. Because even if good cancer treatments were available and affordable, individuals would still need be persuaded those are worth taking. This point hearkens to the early cancer society and Adams, the journalist who in 1913 asked expert surgeons and physicians, "What can we do about cancer?" and reported their unanimous response: "Educate the people to save themselves."

Consider vaccines. When I was a child in the 1960s, polio and measles became diseases of the past, no longer a worry. Forty years later, many Americans questioned the benefits of immunizations; they were misled by distorted or false information, persuaded by charming speakers, or simply confused. After a time, adults had no memory of how polio can be crippling or measles lethal. As anti-vax views spread and gained believers, measles outbreaks returned to North America, endangering schoolchildren and adults. More recently, the Covid-19 pandemic has uncovered profound rifts in people's willingness to accept vaccines and, underlying those, uneven trust in medical science. Some differences fall along U.S. political party lines: in 2021, Democrats were much more likely to receive Covid-19 vaccines than Republicans.[7,8] After vaccines against the virus became available, Covid-19-related deaths were higher in red states and tracked with Trump support by county.[9,10] During the pandemic, rampant misinformation became such an obstacle to public health that in 2020 the World Health Organization declared an "'infodemic' crisis."[11,12]

After a century of medical advances, ignorance and distrust of doctors remain lethal. Misinformation and wariness of mainstream physicians, exacerbated in some communities by the legacy of medical racism, by some doctors' intolerance toward people who identify as LGBTQ+, by language barriers, and by poverty, in itself, drive patients to off-grid practitioners and quacks. As in the early twentieth century, fear leads some people with early-stage, curable tumors to choose alternative care or reject medical interventions entirely, until it is too late. For these reasons, education would help reduce disparities in cancer prevention, screening, and survival.

Learning biology, simple concepts like cells, should begin in elementary school. There's no reason, short of low expectations, why most high school students don't study cell biology, immunology, and genetics. That way most everyone would know or at least be familiar with terms like "monoclonal antibodies" and "variants of uncertain significance" long before they might need consult an oncologist or search the web after a loved one's malignant diagnosis. If statistics were part of the curriculum, patients and caregivers might participate meaningfully in discussions and make treatment decisions based in reason, not fear.

Doctors, too, would be better equipped to interpret forthcoming torrents of information—about clinical trials, cancer biology, new medicines, diagnostic tools, and who-knows-what future technology—if they arrived at medical school having strong backgrounds in math and science, along with good communication skills. While it's trendy to admit nonscience majors into medical schools and to offer writing and arts-oriented courses for students once there, the volume of scientific knowledge physicians need grasp for clinical practice today, besides essential humanities like medical ethics, is greater than ever.[13,14] As things stand, the lack of knowledge of some practicing physicians about cancer tests and treatments leads many patients to seek information elsewhere. There is nothing more frustrating than consulting a doctor who can't answer questions. Greater education of physicians would position them to recognize statistical aberrations and other problems in published medical reports, and to discern hype from valid claims about new cancer treatments.

Education won't in itself cure anyone of cancer. But it will enable patients to make better choices. People for whom effective treatments exist will be more likely to choose those, and people with terminal disease might suffer less. For those affected, having knowledge of their doctors' reasoning—being active participants in medical decisions—will, in itself, be an advance.

CHAPTER 12

CANCER IS NOT AS IT USED TO BE

When I completed my residency in internal medicine, I took a standardized exam. We were asked to classify tumors—as curable or incurable. I darkened ovals in either of two columns: some types of lymphoma, early-stage colon and breast cancers were curable; follicular lymphomas, advanced melanoma, and lung cancers were incurable. The examiners' point—why we were asked about cancer's curability—was twofold: first, that we'd advise patients with treatable tumors to consult with specialists, because they'd likely benefit from oncology care; and second, that we wouldn't offer false hope, that we'd convey to those with incurable cancers that, apart from trials of experimental treatments, palliative care was best and aggressive care futile. Today, these distinctions blur.

Cancer has never seemed less formidable to seasoned oncologists. After decades of incremental progress, advances in a constellation of interrelated fields—biology, molecular pathology, pharmacology, and informatics—are shuffling tumor categories and changing the outlook for many affected. An exploding volume of data on malignancy in its myriad forms is enabling scientists to develop better medicines and doctors to prescribe those with increasing granularity, to eradicate tumors with less toxicity. It's hard to know, or say, which cancers may be treated effectively.

The central idea of precision oncology is to match drugs to specific abnormalities, such as genetic mutations or protein changes in tumors.[1-4] Precision oncology has its critics, sure. Skeptics are vocal.[5,6] Valid concerns include prohibitive costs and disparities of access. Many tumors still can't be cured. Some doctors, lacking sufficient background in science, don't understand precision oncology; they may be uncomfortable interpreting molecular assays and prescribing medicines accordingly. In my view, however, the naysayers have their heads in sand. The issue is not hype—precision oncology already benefits many cancer patients, and will continuously improve—but whether society is willing to pay for relevant diagnostic tests and treatments.

Oncologists' understanding of cancer has matured since I entered the field. Thirty years ago, we were practicing in the dark. We lacked tools to identify tumor subtypes or predict treatment responses. Since 2003, when the human genome was sequenced, innovations like next-generation sequencing permit fast and affordable evaluation of many genes ("genomics"). Now, pathologists at cancer centers routinely check specimens for DNA mutations, amplifications, switches, and fusions. Using robotic machines, they can evaluate many proteins ("proteomics") and RNA ("transcriptomics"). Scientists assess epigenetics, chemical aspects of DNA that influence gene expression. Novel techniques for examining cancerous cells, DNA, and particles in blood by "liquid biopsy" permit monitoring of some tumors in exquisite detail without subjecting patients to invasive procedures.[7-9]

A new way of looking at cancer is tumor agnostic, meaning that malignancies can be classified, and medicines prescribed based on cancer's molecular properties, or biomarkers, and not necessarily on the body part such as "prostate" or "esophagus." In 2017, the FDA issued its first tissue-agnostic cancer drug approval for Keytruda (pembrolizumab), an antibody that unleashes the immune system, as treatment of malignancies with either of two biomarkers: high microsatellite instability (MSI-H) or mismatch repair deficiency. A clinical trial of this agent against metastatic colorectal cancer—a hopeless condition until recently—demonstrated responses in 44 percent of tumors with MSI-H; four in five of the responding patients experienced durable remissions.[10] In 2018, the FDA issued its second tissue-agnostic approval for Vitrakvi (larotrectinib) in advanced cancers harboring fusions of the N-TRK oncogene. TRK fusions are rare, occurring in fewer than 1 percent of malignancies.[11] But for those whose tumors harbor this biomarker—and doctors don't always check—larotrectinib is a wondrous drug. In clinical trials of patients with TRK-rearranged tumors, three-quarters of patients with previously refractory cancer experienced remissions after taking this oral agent. In 2019, the FDA approved another medication for tumors with N-TRK gene fusions. This trend continues.[12,13]

The breadth and therapeutic potential of modern oncology drugs is fantastic. Since 1985, over thirty monoclonal antibodies have been approved by the FDA as cancer treatments; dozens are in the pipeline now. Some of the most effective old monoclonals, like rituximab for lymphoma and trastuzumab for HER2-positive breast cancer, have been reformulated to be given by quick injection rather than by intravenous infusion, adding convenience. Novel drug conjugates, cancer-targeting antibodies bearing tumoricidal toxins, represent an emerging class of powerful medicines; the FDA has approved a half-dozen of these "smart bombs." While I was reporting on biotech between 2014 and 2018, "living" biological therapies like CAR T cells (chimeric antigen receptor T cells) received loads of attention in press conferences, and investments. Those individualized treatments, prepared for each patient by removing and editing genes of their immune cells, are technically challenging and expensive to manufacture, but have curative possibility.

While I'm not enthusiastic about old-style chemotherapy—anthracyclines, platinum-based drugs, taxanes, etc.—I acknowledge their continued role. Those harsh medicines shrink many kinds of tumors and, in some instances, work better than available targeted agents. However, when I hear of patients receiving traditional agents in clinical trials, I cringe. These are not the future of cancer care. While some academics insist that randomized studies include standard-of-care chemotherapy, in some circumstances the old drugs are so ineffective and toxic that I question the ethics of including them in control arms. I look forward to the day when better treatments have been found for every cancer type and insurers will pay for those up front, so that patients needn't suffer through and "fail" several cycles of chemotherapy before they're eligible for a new drug.

A common misconception is that precision oncology involves matching one drug to one tumor, like Gleevec (imatinib) for chronic myelogenous leukemia. It's unlikely that a single medicine will suffice for most cancers. As with HIV, for which medicines like AZT weren't curative, combinations of anti-cancer agents—medication "cocktails" tailored to each patient's tumor—may prove most effective. Designing unique regimens based on thorough tumor profiling, accounting for heterogeneity and molecular changes over time, wasn't feasible fifteen years ago. It is today.[3,14,15]

Many of the latest cancer medicines come as pills. In theory this is hugely advantageous for patients; many no longer need spend their days hooked up to intravenous devices. (It's also a safety advance, as intravenous catheters carry risks of infection.) There are numerous examples. Since 2014, the FDA has approved at least three cyclin-dependent kinase inhibitors, four PARP inhibitors, and several Bruton's tyrosine kinase inhibitors. Other pills block production of hormones and are used to treat breast or prostate cancer. A powerful agent, Venclexta (venetoclax), promotes death signals inside cells; it was first approved for chronic lymphocytic leukemia treatment in 2016. When I read about this drug, I was thrilled because it pertains to my former lab's work on BCL-2 and other prosurvival molecules in B lymphocytes.

Many insurance plans don't cover oral medications as they do intravenous agents, however. Patients wind up with huge bills or choose old drugs to avoid out-of-pocket expenses. These financial and policy glitches can and should be fixed, as we'll consider in the next chapter.

Precise cancer therapy is not more cancer therapy. Rather, it enables patients to skip chemotherapy that's unlikely to help, and to try matching agents sooner—when benefit is more likely. And if someone doesn't respond to treatment or their tumor profiling indicates a poor prognosis, they and their families might accept hospice care knowing they've explored all reasonable options, that they're not prematurely "throwing in the towel." Studies demonstrate the benefits of incorporating palliative care—which aims to relieve symptoms—in treatment plans for patients with advanced cancer; it extends survival. Knowing this, cancer specialists should encourage pain relief, treatments for nausea, and other palliative measures soon after diagnosis. There is no contradiction between providing palliative care and precision oncology.[16–18]

Not to be overlooked in any discussion of progress against cancer is the field of computational oncology, one of the most exciting areas of modern medicine. Today, investigators can scan tumors for thousands of potential molecular aberrations, store zettabytes of data, and sort through all that information.[19,20] These technical advances permit physicians to provide more accurate diagnoses and, as trials data and real-world evidence—regarding survival, toxicity, and quality of life after specific treatments—are collected faster, match cancer patients to optimal therapy. Eventually this can happen in real time.

When I was a clinical faculty member at Cornell in the 1990s, I developed a practice centering on lymphomas and blood conditions. I was conservative about giving chemotherapy, especially for patients with advanced solid tumors like lung or breast cancer, for the simple reason that I thought it cruel to give treatments that were unlikely to extend life and likely to cause unpleasant side effects. I rarely billed for infusions. My division chief said I was a therapeutic nihilist.

Today I feel differently about treating patients with advanced cancer. One reason is that through my work as a journalist, I've interviewed many individuals who've benefited from new treatments. The patients I've encountered at meet-ings represent a skewed sampling, I realize; they're healthier, wealthier, and better-informed than those who don't travel. But I cannot deny how much they've influenced my thinking about oncology care. The other reason is that in recent years I've attended national conferences where cancer researchers presented updates and I was awed, blown away, by advances since 2006, when I stopped practicing. Yet the news I read after those sessions often downplayed findings and emphasized costs. Perhaps it takes time away from a field, an interval of years, to appreciate how much has changed for the better.

After a century of scientific and clinical advances against cancer, progress is evident. Effective treatments exist for many forms, and better ones are nearing readiness including medicines for historically hard-to-treat tumors like pan-creatic and liver cancers. Thanks to science, the proportion of cancer patients who might be helped is constantly rising. The big picture—of progress rendering malignancies treatable and possibly curable—warrants balanced and careful consideration.

CHAPTER 13

IS CANCER TREATMENT A LUXURY?

"The longer I live, the more I cost @fepblue. But this is how insurance works: we pay premiums and we get health care. #SaveBeth."

My late friend Beth Caldwell, a mom, civil rights lawyer, and MET UP founder, tweeted this message when her insurer, BlueCross BlueShield's Federal Employee Program, declined to pay for a combination of targeted treatments prescribed by her doctor for her widely metastatic neuroendocrine form of breast cancer.[1] Weeks later, Caldwell received the off-label meds from the manufacturers, Genentech and Novartis. Her tumor progressed, and she died in 2017, at forty-one.[2-6]

Since 1975, the number of U.S. cancer survivors has climbed from 3.6 million to over seventeen million. This success—a research triumph!—is tempered by costs and disparities; as cancer diagnostics and treatments improve, many Americans can't afford them. In 2015, oncology costs amounted to $183 billion—around 5.7 percent of all U.S. health care spending. Prescription drugs accounted for "only" $18 billion (11 percent) of that year's tab; most (89 percent) cancer-related expenses were attributed to medical services such as surgery, scans, and infusions. However, as more people are living longer on new anticancer drugs, medication expenses are rising disproportionately. Based on growth and aging of the U.S. population alone, the overall annual cost of oncology care in the United States is projected to reach $246 billion by 2030.[7-9]

What inspired me to write this book, my motivation, is that I don't believe that modern cancer care should be a luxury. As a society we provide best available remedies to individuals with all kinds of illnesses—diabetes, high blood pressure, depression, HIV and AIDS, arthritis, epilepsy, most everything for which treatments are available. Cancer should not be considered differently.

Insurers bear the cruel calculus that as cancer patients live longer, they cost more. For this reason, some plans won't pay for genomic cancer testing. Consider this math: in 2021, commercial pathology labs charged around $6,000 for molecular profiling of a clinical tumor sample.[10] That's less than half the price for a month's supply of a typical new cancer medicine. The "problem" is that if molecular evaluation uncovers a treatable finding for which FDA-approved drugs are available, the insurer needs to pay for that prescription. If the treatment works and the patient lives for months or years, the insurer's costs escalate. In 2020, U.S. spending on cancer drugs reached $71 billion. Analysts ascribed that steep increase over five years in large part to proliferating use of checkpoint inhibitors and small-molecule drugs against a widening variety of tumors.[11] As precision oncology matures and novel agents help a wider net of people with more kinds of cancer, these expenses will rise even further.

The term "financial toxicity" refers to harms from treatment—akin to side effects like baldness, nausea, anemia, neuropathy, or infertility—attributable to costs. Over half of working-age cancer survivors suffer money problems such as job loss and debt as a consequence of their diagnosis.[12] Being "cancer poor" results in lost money for food, leisure, and travel; it causes hardship, stress, and even personal bankruptcy. To save money, patients skip and divide prescribed medication doses.[13,14] It's an old concern. Recall Dr. Albert Soiland, the Los Angeles radiologist who in 1930 alerted colleagues that 80 percent of cancer patients couldn't afford cancer surgery or radiation.[15]

Consider Gleevec. When this drug (imatinib) was approved for chronic myelogenous leukemia (CML) in 2001, its life-extending potential was unknown. Before then, allogeneic bone marrow transplantation was considered the best treatment for a young person with CML. Novartis, the manufacturer, set Gleevec's monthly price at $2,200 and gradually increased that to $12,000 in 2015, when the patent expired. Today, people with CML on Gleevec or similar agents enjoy near-normal life expectancy. Generic forms sell for $8,000 monthly and Novartis has lowered the brand's price. Without discount coupons, a year's supply of this "old" anticancer pill costs around $100,000. So if someone is diagnosed with CML at age fifty and lives to be seventy, the cost of their CML treatment would approximate $2 million.[16, 17] Since 2018, pharmaceutical companies have set prices for some new targeted oral cancer meds in the range of $18,000 monthly, the equivalent of $216,000 per year, or more.[18] These figures are plainly unaffordable and would break budgets of private and public insurers, raising premiums for all.

To ensure profitability in this context, private insurers may limit which FDA-approved drugs are included in their formularies or cap payments per insured person. Payers often require patients' tumors to progress through old treatments, like chemo, before approving newer medications; this practice delays patients' receipt of newer drugs. In general, Medicare and Medicaid cover FDA-approved tests and medications. However, some states, including Massachusetts, have eyed restrictions on Medicaid formularies.[19,20] As more treatments for more cancer types become available, budget concerns may lead additional states to try restricting coverage. Although Medicare is required by law to cover tests and treatments that are "reasonable and necessary," that agency's recent decision not to cover a controversial medicine for Alzheimer's disease, or possibly to require drug-receiving patients to enroll in phase 4 trials, indicates Medicare's willingness to say no.[21]

The subject of lowering costs extends well beyond this book's scope. However, from my experiences practicing oncology and as a patient, I do have some suggestions. First, that we might approximately halve the need for treatments by adopting early detection and preventive measures, as will be considered in the last chapter. Second, that cancer drugs and procedures can be rendered more affordable through better policy. Third, oncologists should be educated to avoid overtreating patients with harmless tumors and excessively treating others.

As things stand, payments for oral medications are variably carried by patients depending on their insurance, often with high copays. That coverage gap should be fixed by oral parity laws as have been enacted in some states requiring insurance companies to cover pills as they do intravenous medicines. In recent years, some pharmaceutical firms have hiked medication prices by around 9 percent annually.[22,23] While the companies merit earnings—what's said to motivate innovation—their gains might be shaved if not slashed. If medications could be considered essential, and their prices negotiated by the U.S. federal government, more people might receive them.

Another possibility is for manufacturers to package cancer drugs in more and varied doses, to reduce wastage.[24,25] I remember an episode nearly twenty years ago, when I got into minor administrative trouble for giving one of my patients only a half-vial's worth of Neulasta (pegfilgrastim). She needed this drug to maintain a safe white blood cell level during lymphoma treatment. Previously this agent, a commonly prescribed growth factor, had caused her to experience significant aches and pains and, also, her white cells to rise excessively. The half-dose worked like a charm in her case, without those side effects. But pharmacy rules dictated that we discard the remaining half vial, around three thousand dollars' worth of medicine. Last I checked, that drug still cannot be ordered in smaller doses. Perhaps, also, costs of producing and shipping medications should be considered in drug pricing: if it's cheaper to manufacture and distribute pills than biological agents (such as antibodies), those prices could be lowered and companies would still profit.

An overhaul of the way physicians are compensated—valuing cognitive work—would help. Payment systems should be changed so that doctors and hospitals including academic centers don't profit by giving infusions rather than pills or quick shots that patients could take at home. The business of "infusion centers" is rife with conflicts of interest; the costs of paying oncology nurses to supervise infusions and other expenses—catheters, monitors, chairs, even rent—should factor into considerations of cost-effective treatments.

Improved training of doctors would lower costs by reducing diagnostic errors. Cognitive mistakes result in patients undergoing unnecessary procedures and receiving inappropriate medications, all of which is physically and financially costly. Better postgraduate medical education would reduce cancer's overtreatment, as physicians would be less likely to overprescribe therapy for slow-growing tumors. And as cancer biomarkers ("companion diagnostics") improve—and more accurately predict which tumors will respond to a medicine—treatment costs should drop. If oncology drugs were not given indiscriminately but only to patients with molecularly matched tumors, prescriptions would decline.

There is no doubt that Americans overwhelmingly support cancer research. In 2015, 87 percent of Democrats and 63 percent of Republicans—74 percent overall—responding to a poll commissioned by the American Association for Cancer Research favored increasing federal funds for cancer investigations.[26] Paying for oncology care, however, is another story. "Medicare for All" and Medicaid expansions are deeply divisive issues. A 2019 Gallup report found that "although more Americans have warmed to the idea of a greater government role in paying for health care, it remains the minority view in the U.S."[27,28]

You might wonder, as I have many times, about the purpose of the cancer research enterprise: What's the point of so much effort—huge sums, and careers, dedicated to scientific investigations—if patients can't benefit from advances? I considered this problem in 1987 while in medical school and traveling through Bolivia, where doctors used outdated equipment and administered old antibiotics, and back in New York City I worked in a modern lab, hoping to discover clues for better medicines. That separation—of medical progress from people needing care—is the reason some wealthy Americans in the nineteenth century traveled to Europe, where treatments were more advanced, and established the New York Cancer Hospital.

That same separation—of top-notch health care from communities—exists today. It is evident in U.S. regions like Appalachia, where poverty, low education, and limited health care promulgate a cycle of high cancer rates, deaths and fatalism, and in Indigenous American communities, including reservations, where malignancy is fostered by distance and distrust. Even in Chicago in 2015, when a sixty-year-old Black woman presented to the emergency room of a "safety net" community hospital she received archaic evaluation and care for a cancerous breast mass. In that city's South Side and elsewhere, structural racism has positioned many American College of Surgeons–accredited medical centers apart from poor Black communities and, disproportionately, people of color away from expert care.[29-32]

A reader might consider, as I once did, that disparities in cancer mortality could be explained by differential care access and social determinants of health, like education and poverty. But it's not as simple as that: evidence points to disparities in what treatments patients with the same insurance are provided by their physicians. In one study of women, all with Medicare and HER2-positive breast cancer, 74 percent of white and 56 percent of Black women with stage III disease received trastuzumab as indicated to reduce the high risk of recurrence with that otherwise oft-lethal subtype. Similarly, oncologists are less likely to order tumor genomic tests for Black patients with lung cancer; as a result, many don't receive FDA-approved, life-extending targeted treatments.[33-37]

Attitudes and, in some circles, resentment toward cancer patients—as being "expensive"—weigh into public discussion and policy. Some people still blame cancer patients for being sick and for that reason don't think treatments should be covered. Old tropes, considered in earlier chapters, tie cancer to affluence. Unfortunately these have not disappeared, a disservice to patients of any income level. As has always been the case, cancer affects those who are poor and less educated, and is more likely to kill people without access to well-trained doctors.

Ultimately, whether a community is willing to help those affected depends on sympathy and perception of whether cancer is worth treating. In her 2019 book, *The Undying*, Anne Boyer wrote, "The cost of one chemotherapy infusion was more money than I had then earned in any year of my life." In midlife, the author needed to convince herself—a single mom, no less—that her life was worth saving, that she should take treatment for an aggressive case of triple-negative breast cancer. Indeed. Perhaps we—all of us—have to consider ourselves worthy, as better cancer treatments emerge.[38]

CHAPTER 14

HAS AWARENESS BACKFIRED?

In my study, a wide four-tiered shelf holds books about cancer. Memoirs are arranged by tumor type—breast cancer or other cancer; autobiographies and essays by journalists, doctors, celebrities, activists, or "ordinary" patients, organized by authorship category; other sections support cancer fiction, cancer science, cancer handbooks, cancer history, cancer plays, cancer poetry, and cancer humor. For lack of space, I've resorted to stacking some cancer books in neat piles on the floor. Some I've given away.

This book reports cancer's growing visibility. A central thread is patients' voices. At the start of the twentieth century, patients rarely lived long and, if they did, had no way to publicize their experiences. Survivors were invisible to society. How much has changed! Today, many affected advocate for themselves on social media and elsewhere—posting photos, detailing their lives, asserting viewpoints. Many thrive. Their vitality might be celebrated. Yet the emotional, physical, and financial problems faced by cancer patients so frequently appear in news and social media feeds, they might seem a burden to others. Perhaps the parade of public cases is more than most of us can handle or want to hear—that for lack of time, money, or emotional bandwidth, we tune it out.

Awareness may have backfired in this way: a downside of so much talk of cancer is that we risk becoming inured to patients' needs. If people tire of hearing about cancer, reading about cancer, paying for cancer, and maybe even knowing about cancer—that's the opposite of what was hoped for one hundred years ago by specialists and progressive thinkers.

I call this social phenomenon, an acquired indifference, "community burnout." Burnout is a syndrome characterized by emotional fatigue and lost enthusiasm for goals. Physician burnout is common in oncology, said to affect a third of practitioners. When doctors and nurses experience burnout, they depersonalize patients who need them, "processing" them as objects, avoiding feeling. To protect themselves, to get through their days and home to dinner and sleep, they stop caring. Many become numb. Once idealistic physicians turn cynical.[1-4]

Community burnout is hard to gauge, as few individuals will state publicly that they "don't care." Signs of burnout include waning sympathy and cynicism about oncology. Burnout is a close relative of nihilism. Regarding cancer, it traces to 1921, when some doctors called out the cancer society's "flash in the pan" educational drives. In 1939, the ASCC's publicity director fielded swipes about its "most irritating" informational campaigns. Sixty years ago, journalist Richard Carter depicted cancer volunteers as insufferable. By the 1980s, declining concern over carcinogens, after so many alarms that it seemed "everything causes cancer," suggested a collective resignation, or shrug: the cancer problem is so vast and complex, attempting to solve it is a hopeless enterprise.

Journalists play an outsized role in perception of cancer's curability; their "burnout," or plain cynicism, influences what many people think. As told in earlier chapters, relationships between journalists and cancer experts evolved in the last century—from collaborative to testy. A hundred years ago, when progressive writers sought to enlighten the public, they cooperated with specialists in doing so. The early cancer society cultivated relationships with editors and reporters. In the 1950s, the ACS sponsored travel-by-train tours during which journalists of the National Association of Science Writers visited labs and toured hospitals around the country. Communications were cordial: "Dear Mrs. Lasker: For myself and for the other science writers who are making the American Cancer Society research centers tour, I must thank you for the beautiful send-off that you gave us last Sunday at your home," wrote Marguerite Clark of *Newsweek* after a 1952 reception at Lasker's New York City apartment.[5,6]

It took a while for skeptical views—challenging priorities of cancer agencies and what progress they claimed—to receive mainstream attention. A turning point came in 1975, when the *Columbia Journalism Review* (*CJR*) and *Washington Post* published a critical piece by Daniel S. Greenberg, a credible journalist and *NEJM* contributor. Contrary to popular reports, progress against cancer was minimal and mainly attributable to surgical advances before 1955, Greenberg maintained. A "passive lay press" was responsible for "transmission" of hopefulness conveyed by "statistic-studded literature" handed out by the ACS, he suggested. Cancer research, while costing the government, and taxpayers (implicit), enormous sums, "has its own politics, vested interests, warring factions, and public-information apparatus."[7,8]

Writing for *CJR*, a magazine about journalistic integrity, Greenberg quoted anonymous sources. While "there is no conscious intention to mislead the public . . . there is a desire to sustain public support and federal appropriations by conveying a picture of an immensely difficult problem that will slowly yield," he wrote. "Optimistic" claims are harmful, an unnamed researcher told Greenberg, "because as long as the establishment is persuading the public that results are being achieved, there isn't going to be any pressure for supporting alternatives to these dead-alley lines of research."

Negative reports—alleging a lack of headway against cancer, that progress was hyped—fed alternative, skeptical views that the ACS and NCI exaggerated advances to keep their budgets replete. While working to lessen tobacco use in North America, those agencies failed to investigate environmental carcinogens; the "cancer establishment" was caving to industry and political concerns, Greenberg and others, notably Dr. Samuel S. Epstein, charged. Epstein, a British-born American academic, public health maven, and 1978 *Politics of Cancer* author, wrote extensively on industrial toxins, ACS failures, and, later, against mammography.[9–13] I consider this argument—that leading cancer organizations failed to prioritize cancer prevention—an origin of oncology's divergence from the field of public health.

The *NEJM*, for its part, published hard-hitting analyses: "Progress Against Cancer?" (1986) and "Cancer Undefeated" (1997), by Dr. John C. Bailar III, a physician with a PhD in statistics. The first, coauthored by Elaine M. Smith, PhD, an epidemiologist, revealed that from 1950 to 1982, U.S. cancer case and death rates had tracked upward—the wrong direction. They called for a shift in focus of the federal anticancer effort, from treatment to prevention. A decade later, Bailar and Dr. Heather L. Gornik, then a medical student and future cardiologist, extended the analysis of cancer stats through 1994. "The effect of new treatments for cancer on mortality has been largely disappointing," they concluded.[14,15]

One problem with trumpeting these dour assessments today is that a quarter-century has passed. Progress against cancer—the fruition of a century's research—is finally reaching clinics. Only since 2010 have some of the hardest-to-remit malignancies, like advanced lung cancer and melanoma, become treatable. The pace of advances is not necessarily linear, as some insist.[16] My impression, mainly as a journalist now, is that progress is accelerating. Oncology is at an inflection point.[17–21]

Unfortunately for the reading public, disputative media reports on cancer became most frequent almost precisely as progress picked up, led by complaints since 2009 regarding news and charity messages promoting mammography. Controversy over breast cancer screening is not this book's subject. (I have written on that elsewhere.) But it pertains. The screening issue is what drew me to the larger problem—of distrust, suspicion of doctors' intentions amid conflicting information, and fear—and how those feelings discourage people from seeking oncology care.[22,23]

By downplaying benefits of cancer care, while emphasizing toxicity and costs, journalists may, with good intentions, dissuade people from choosing helpful treatments. There are many examples. At annual meetings of the Association of Health Care Journalists over years, hundreds of medical reporters and editors heard from Gary Schwitzer, a media "watchdog." His philanthropically funded website, https://www.healthnewsreview.org, provided critiques of health care news and, for an audience of journalists, cited experts who consistently dismissed positive reports about cancer screening and treatments.[24,25] John Horgan, a self-declared "grouchy skeptic" who directs the Center for Science Writings at the Stevens Institute of Technology in Hoboken, New Jersey, blogged until 2020 at *Scientific American*'s *Cross-Check* with posts like "Cancer Medicine Is Failing Us."[26]

Physicians may be sources of cynicism about oncology. In 2014, Dr. Richard Smith posted to the *BMJ* blog that "dying of cancer is the best death." Smith, a former editor of that British medical journal, cautioned readers: "Stay away from overambitious oncologists, and let's stop wasting billions trying to cure cancer." (His words echoed those of another influential man, Bill Keller, the former *New York Times* executive editor, that same year.)[27,28] Starting around 2015, takedowns of reports on precision oncology and the pace of FDA cancer drug approvals turned Dr. Vinay Prasad, an oncologist and author, into a Twitter sensation. His opinions, tweets, and podcasts proved popular, evidencing that hyper-skeptical views about oncology, that many cancer drugs are too expensive and don't help patients, appealed to many; his message resonated.[29–31]

Backlash, not against a particular story but against the very goal of "curing cancer," became most acute after President Obama announced the U.S. Cancer Moonshot initiative to be led by then Vice President Joe Biden. Predictably, journalists criticized the project as naive: "The very notion of a single cure . . . is misleading and outdated," the *New York Times* informed readers. (This obvious point was understood by the vice president and most everyone involved in the project.) In a *Times* op-ed titled "We Won't Cure Cancer," Dr. Jarle Breivik of Oslo argued that cancer is an inevitable consequence of aging. Trying to cure it is foolish, he suggested, writing, "Every time we cure a person of cancer, we produce a person with an increased probability of getting cancer again. It is the Catch-22 of oncology." Elsewhere, physicians complained of déjà vu. Or called for a "Cancer Groundshot" focused on prevention and public health measures.[32–36]

These are not academic debates. Skepticism, to the point of denying progress, harms people with cancer. It is negative hype—and a disservice to those affected. Disbelief and distrust of oncologists is the reason why, in the twenty-first century, we need awareness of cancer's treatability.

Awareness should not be taken for granted. It is a privilege. In well-educated communities like mine, we mock awareness campaigns even though there remain places, even here in North America, where people are reluctant to get checked for cancer and, if diagnosed, feel embarrassed. Although it's rarely documented, cancer patients still experience shame for needing medical care, for carrying a malignant diagnosis, for "marking" their family, for costing too much. I know this because as a journalist, I've interviewed people who've expressed each of those concerns—the very feelings described by Lorna Doone Burks in her 1940s journal, *I Die Daily*.

A key idea in this book is cancer awareness as a constructive force—an influence that encourages affected individuals to seek timely care, without shame. In preparing this manuscript, I stopped at the U.S. border knowing that in other areas of the world, cancer stigma and fear remain pervasive. A survey of women with breast cancer in India, for instance, demonstrated their frequent embarrassment: 90 percent avoided social engagements because of disfigurement. In Hunan, China, a young pharmacist with stomach cancer apologized to his parents for adding to their burdens, then disappeared. In South Africa, most cancer patients experience stigma, and cancer is perceived as a death sentence.[37–39]

Overcoming cancer fatalism will take time. What'll help most, I suspect, will not be doctors' statistics or journalists' words. It will be the increasing visibility of real people in communities who are living longer—and well—with conditions that until recently would have been terminal. Much as Dr. Anna Palmer formed the Cured Cancer Club in 1938 to show, by example, proof of cancer's treatability, modern patients declare their aliveness: I'm still here! #NotDeadYet. Another birthday :) Etc.

CHAPTER 15

CAN WE PREVENT CANCER?

"It is only within the last few years that cancer has been considered a public health problem," Dr. James Ewing wrote in 1929. "I suppose that the old attitude was due to the fact that cancer is not an infectious disease; also largely because of the popular notion that it is not preventable; and probably also, to a large extent, to the feeling . . . that the disease is incurable." Ewing was the brilliant pathologist who directed research at New York's Memorial Hospital. Doctors understood little of cancer's causes in Ewing's day. Yet he believed that many cancers could be prevented and, because most cases—even those diagnosed early—could not be cured by surgery or radiation, that prevention should be prioritized.[1,2]

Before writing this book, I'd nearly forgotten about the roots of cancer control in public health, a field that focuses on the well-being of people in communities.[3] That's because oncologists in general don't prioritize cancer screening or prevention in their practices or their research; they focus on *treating* malignancy. As a journalist, I perceived tension between the oncology and public health communities—the concern being that as cancer tests and treatments become increasingly expensive and numerous, fewer resources are available for primary and maternal care, pediatric vaccines, and other "basics." Because cancer therapy is so costly and toxic (and ineffective, some say), prevention would be better. I agree! And so I've returned to this crucial topic in the final chapter.

Many people don't realize that a significant fraction of lethal cancers—estimates range from 30 percent to 70 percent—can be prevented.[4] Scientists have uncovered a host of modifiable risks. Experts now appreciate that carcinogens include natural substances arising within our bodies, such as food metabolites and hormones, and from the outside, like radon.[5,6] Infections, many preventable or treatable, account for 13 percent of malignancies worldwide.[7] Tobacco use still contributes to nearly 30 percent of U.S. cancer deaths.[8,9] (Elsewhere in the world, where cigarettes still are promoted, this proportion is likely higher.) Excessive exposure to ultraviolet radiation, including sunlight, causes melanoma. Yet tanning salons remain legal.[10] Obesity factors into nearly 4 percent of cancers.[11–13] As for the growing body of evidence that alcohol is a carcinogen, many people including doctors are unaware or in denial.[14–16]

"The goal of curing the victims of cancer is more exciting, more tangible, more glamorous, and more rewarding than prevention," Rachel Carson noted in 1962, quoting the NCI's Dr. Wilhelm Hueper.[17,18] Then as now, a lack of incentives stymied environmental oncology research. Cancer's long latency—typically years or decades—renders it hard to establish causative exposures. Malignancy can arise from toxins absorbed by diet, from air or through skin; in the womb, during childhood, or later; from sequential and unknown chemicals absorbed in uncertain amounts. Ethics preclude testing of putative carcinogens in humans, so scientists carry out less-definitive studies in lab dishes and rodents.[19,20] While doctors receive little money or recognition for preventing cancer, treating disease is lucrative. Pharmaceutical industry support for studies in environmental oncology is essentially nil, and opposition from chemical, food, and other industries can be career-stifling. Although many patient advocates like the idea of preventing cancer, most advocacy organizations seek "cures."

Despite these obstacles, the science of cancer prevention is advancing. Just as new laboratory tools and computational systems speed delivery of precise cancer treatments, they accelerate knowledge of cancer's causes. In the past decade, investigators have identified patterns of genetic damage—molecular "fingerprints"—that can flag cancer specimens for past exposures to ultraviolet light, DNA-damaging medicines such as alkylating agents (a class of chemotherapy), polyaromatic hydrocarbons in cigarette smoke and other fumes, alcohol in liver cancer, and other mutagens. Previously only a few hundred of the tens of thousands of chemicals to which humans are exposed in daily life had been tested for their cancer-causing potential, but that's changing as researchers employ high-throughput machines to efficiently assess how chemicals affect human cells and genes, and how toxic substances may act in concert.[21–25]

The question of whether malignancy stems from an exposure—or behavior—that might be avoided, or arises from bad luck, is a scientifically, personally, and politically contentious issue. Scientifically, because it's hard to prove cause and effect for many carcinogens. Personally, because patients are sensitive to being scrutinized for having illness. And politically, because lawmakers decide if extant knowledge will be implemented, such as by taxing cigarettes or regulating pollution, to reduce our collective risk and prevent disease.

Since Carson's time, the pendulum of scientific consensus on carcinogens has shifted—from concerns about the environment, to focus on oncogenes and genetics in the 1980s, to current emphasis on the complex interplay of environmental (including behavioral) and genetic risks, in addition to chance.[26,27] A key idea is that disease-linked genes are not necessarily determinative. For instance, most but not all women who inherit pathogenic *BRCA1* or *BRCA2* gene variants, around 70 percent (estimates vary), will develop breast cancer by age eighty. As doctors learn about factors influencing an inherited cancer disposition, an individual's risk may be lowered.[28] Still there will always be an element of randomness—as in Tomasetti and Vogelstein's "bad luck" result.[29,30] What this means is that all the preventive measures in the world won't stop cancers entirely. Unfortunately, some children will get leukemia; some individuals who've never smoked will have lung cancer; some people will develop brain cancer, inexplicably. But preventive measures could significantly lower cancer's incidence.

What's rarely discussed is the economic argument for cancer prevention—that screening for premalignant and early-stage disease might reduce the financial burden of late-stage oncology care. In her 2019 book, *The First Cell*, Dr. Azra Raza argues that treating advanced cancer is both costly and futile; efforts to prevent disease, or detect it early, would be wiser.[31] Overall, there are two ways to prevent cancer. *Primary prevention* stops cancer before it forms—by eliminating its causes. *Secondary prevention* stops cancer from causing illness or death—by catching and treating it early. In general, screening for cervical, breast, prostate, colon, lung, and skin cancer reduces deaths from cancer by secondary prevention.

Primary cancer prevention—what I consider true prevention—can't be accomplished by physicians alone; it involves convincing people including lawmakers that cancer is indeed preventable, and motivating them to take action to lessen personal and societal exposures.

Infectious carcinogens are among the most preventable of cancer's causes. These include viruses, bacteria, parasites, and fungal and mold particles.[7,8,32] Many cases of liver cancer, a lethal condition, could be prevented with vaccines against hepatitis B or medicines for hepatitis C. Both viruses are liver carcinogens. Many stomach cancers are caused by infection with *Helicobacter pylori*, a bacterium that's easily treated with antibiotics. The fluke *Schistosoma haematobium*, common in north Africa and the Middle East, causes bladder cancer; other treatable worms, consumed in raw fish, cause bile duct cancers. Aflatoxins—fungal contaminants affecting corn and other crops in sub-Saharan Africa, Central and South America, and southeast Asia—cause malignancy.[7,33–38]

Scientists have known for decades that human papillomavirus (HPV) causes cancers of the cervix, anus, throat, and other organs. Before the 1960s, cervical cancer was a common cause of death in middle-aged women; after the Pap smear was introduced, deaths declined. Today, with HPV vaccination and inexpensive screening, mortality from cervical cancer might be close to zero. Yet cervical cancer remains a common killer of middle-aged women in Africa, parts of South America, and the Caribbean.[39] In England, implementation of a national HPV immunization program has reduced the incidence of cervical cancer in young women.[40] By contrast, in Alabama, a "red" U.S. state where Medicaid has not been expanded, cervical cancer rates are rising.[41] Our sad failure to control cervical cancer—a lethal malignancy for which inexpensive screening tools have been available for sixty years, caused by a virus for which preventive vaccines are available, demonstrates how hard is the task.

Reducing humans' exposure to possible, likely, and established chemical carcinogens challenges policymakers. Consider PFAS, a large group of human-made compounds deemed "forever chemicals" because they don't disintegrate.[*] Starting in the 1940s, DuPont developed one such substance, PFOA, for use in Teflon coating of nonstick cookware; another large company, 3M, used PFOS in Scotchgard, a fabric protectant.[42,43] By the 1970s, DuPont and 3M were sufficiently concerned that they began testing employees' blood for these compounds, *ProPublica* has reported.[44] After thousands of lawsuits were filed regarding cancers and other illnesses in people living near factories, military bases, and other spots where high PFAS levels were detected in groundwater, U.S. companies stopped using PFOA and PFOS; some switched to alternative PFAS, Chemours's GenX.[44–48] Eighty years ago, these "chemicals barely existed; today, they can be detected

*Perfluorinated and polyfluoroalkyl substances (PFAS, "pee-fahs"), also known as perfluorinated compounds (PFCs), comprise thousands of chemicals including perfluorooctanoic acid (PFOA or C8) and perfluorooctanesulfonic acid (PFOS).

in the bloodstream of nearly every human being," Ted Alcorn wrote in *Lancet Oncology*, a British journal.[49] All Americans are affected, and those with occupational exposure have higher levels.[50] Studies demonstrate the ubiquity of PFAS in human blood samples around the globe.[51] The World Health Organization deems PFAS as possible carcinogens; on a website, the U.S. National Institute of Environmental Health Sciences reports ongoing studies.[50,52]

Yet the U.S. Environmental Protection Agency (EPA) has been slow to regulate PFAS contaminants in public drinking water such as by setting maximum safe levels. Given the lack of federal guidance regarding health effects of PFAS and other possible human carcinogens, some state governments may wind up interpreting data and setting limits to protect their communities. Ultimately, states' varying regulation of industrial pollution will contribute to and compound disparities in cancer's incidence.

"Poverty is a carcinogen," stated the NCI director Dr. Samuel Broder in 1991, when I was a fellow in oncology.[53] Like many doctors then, I realized that people without means lacked money for copays, or insurance altogether, and so they were less likely to be screened and, if they had cancer, get treatment and recover. But I didn't fully realize the history—or depth—of the problem: why people living in poverty were more likely to develop cancer in the first place.

"Often, the heaviest exposures are among people who are forced by limited income to live in close proximity to pollutants and polluted sites," said Dr. Samuel H. Wilson of the NIH's Institute of Environmental Health Sciences at a 1997 session on "Cancer, the Environment, and Environmental Justice."[54] He spoke of damaging health effects in people living near Wisconsin's Milwaukee Estuary, where the Kinnickinnic River meets other waterways as it enters Lake Michigan. After a century of pollution from tanneries and other industry contaminated the Milwaukee estuary sediment with heavy metals, cancer-causing polychlorinated biphenyls (PCBs), and polycyclic aromatic hydrocarbons, the EPA had designated the estuary an "Area of Concern" in 1987. After then, the EPA and NIH funded a community health center and environmental health clinic that primarily served nearby Hispanic, Asian, and Black communities, providing healthcare, education, and disease surveillance with particular attention to environmental risks such as radon levels and water pollution.[55-58]

Disparities in exposure to environmental toxins, and therefore in cancer risk, are widespread, longstanding, and known. Katsi Cook, a midwife and researcher, also spoke at the 1997 meeting. She outlined health effects, including cancers, experienced by people of the Akwesasne Mohawk Nation who live by the St. Lawrence River, whose ancestral land was contaminated by PCBs.[59] The presence of environmental poisons in New Jersey's Newark Bay, California's Central Valley and other regions, disproportionately affecting Hispanic people and others of color, is well-documented.[60]

Today, the most notorious example of environmental racism is "Cancer Alley" along the lower Mississippi River where a toxic mix—of poverty, local residents' powerlessness, corporate tax perks encouraging industry, and Louisiana's lax regulation of polluters—has contributed to high rates of cancer and deaths from cancer. Despite local activists' wanting to clean up the area, construction of new petrochemical plants was permitted until recently. In 2020, international attention to how systemic racism affects Americans' health led the United Nations to call for an end to environmental racism in Cancer Alley.[61–64] In 2021, with President Biden in office and a Democratic administration controlling the EPA, construction of a multibillion-dollar Formosa Plastics plant was paused for scientific review.[65,66]

Cancer Alley is not singular. Rather, the situation in Louisiana demonstrates how vulnerable are some communities, in the absence of federal oversight, to industrial pollution of chemicals including carcinogens.

Of all cancer prevention strategies, reducing risk by modifying lifestyle is, for many cancer patients and families, hardest to swallow. I know this from my experiences among breast cancer patient advocates who, understandably, resent hearing from physicians that they shouldn't drink wine, that they should avoid stress and exercise more. It would be self-defeating, however, for advocates to deny evidence. To the extent that what we eat, drink, and do elevates our risk for cancer or its recurrence, we should be aware of that information. Although ways by which lifestyle and dietary factors may cause cancer are not entirely understood, research is ongoing. There are plausible mechanisms. For instance, it's known that fat cells produce estrogens that can spur growth of some breast and womb cancers.[67] Binge drinking may result in buildup of acetaldehyde, a carcinogenic metabolite.[68,69] These "unpopular" findings remind me of how doctors and other people denied the link between cigarettes and cancer sixty years ago.

In the early years of the AIDS crisis, as told by Larry Kramer in *The Normal Heart*, gay men argued about whether or not bathhouses should be closed because shutting them implied that their behavior was causing disease.[70] Ultimately, AIDS activists supported closure because they wanted to reduce spread of the virus. Similarly, cancer patients and advocates will need to face facts and act accordingly. It would help, of course, if doctors were nonjudgmental about lifestyle and cancer risks, whatever those turn out to be. Fat-shaming or selectively questioning women, and not men, about how much they drink, exactly, or exercise, or work, or feel stressed, is counterproductive.

Rachel Carson extolled cancer prevention but, perhaps with her own case in mind, also called for discovery of better treatments: "Efforts to find cures must, of course, continue," she wrote. That tension—between prevention and remedies—remains at the heart of debates over research priorities and cancer costs today. Arguments arise between patients with metastatic disease, desperate for better medicines, and advocates favoring prevention and better detection strategies. This division relates to the separation of "incurables" from patients with treatable cancers in wards of New York's earliest cancer hospital, considered in chapter 1 of this book. That separation should no longer be.

Through science and education, our society can accomplish both prevention of avoidable cancers and better treatments, even cures, for those tumors that still arise. These dual aims are complementary. As prevention will lower cancer's incidence, more resources will become available for care of people with advanced cases. I believe this can happen—if we recognize that it's possible, and if we choose this shared goal.

EPILOGUE

In early February 2022, President Joe Biden moved to "reignite" the U.S. Cancer Moonshot. He spoke midday at a White House ceremony attended by prominent cancer scientists, clinicians, organizational leaders, patient advocates, and press. The project is dear to Biden. In 2015, he'd lost his son Beau to brain cancer at age forty-six. Chances are, you didn't hear of the relaunch. We were two years into the Covid-19 pandemic.

As I write these words, over a million Americans have died from a novel virus that has swept the globe since 2019, killing over 5.7 million people worldwide, and counting. The pandemic is not over; its toll—in human lives, interpersonal relationships, education, businesses, culture—creeps upward. Covid-19 upturned the order of medical priorities: Surgeries were postponed. Screenings were delayed. Cancer conferences went virtual and received less attention in news.

Cancer's relegation to a less pressing concern is not entirely a consequence of Covid-19, however. Thanks to science—and increased awareness of cancer's treatability—malignancy is less scary than it was when I became a doctor. Consider these trends: between 1991 and 2018, the U.S. death rate from cancer fell by 32 percent. While much of this steep and reportedly accelerating drop stems from smoking cessation's leading to fewer lung cancers, progress in screening and better treatments factor significantly.[1,2] Sixty years ago, less than half of patients lived long after a cancer diagnosis; for U.S. patients receiving a cancer diagnosis in 1975, overall five-year survival was only 48 percent; for those diagnosed in 2013, it was 69 percent.[3] This statistic reflects meaningful progress: cancer is no longer a death sentence. Yet there is work to be done. Inequities of access to expert evaluation, and to best treatments, contribute to lower survival rates among Black, Indigenous, and other marginalized peoples.[4]

The urgency of cancer needs no explanation to the six hundred thousand Americans and nearly ten million people around the world who will die this year from a malignant disease, or to their loved ones. Here in the United States, over 1.9 million people will learn they have cancer; around the globe, twenty million will receive a diagnosis in the next year alone. Millions of deaths—besides toxicity and costs of treatment—might be averted with extant knowledge if we adopt preventive measures, provide modern diagnostic tests and treatments to all affected, and continue research. But the likelihood of that trifecta being implemented is slim to none; each measure depends on the public's willingness. Research is the easy part.

From the Covid-19 pandemic, two lessons for oncology stand out. The first is scientific. Within weeks of its emergence, the virus's genetic composition and structure became known; laboratories quickly developed relevant tests. Within just a few months, several pharmaceutical companies produced highly effective vaccines, some based on mRNA technology, which has potential (yet investigational) applications in cancer prevention and treatment. What's evident from all of this, and the rapidity of these technological breakthroughs, is that—if insurers would cover the costs, which needn't be inordinate—every cancer patient's tumor could be sequenced and monitored for key mutations, recurrence, and genetic drift.[5-7] It's no longer a stretch to suggest that cancer therapy might be designed with computational support to optimize treatment in each case and be adjusted periodically based on genetic, protein, and other features.

The second lesson pertains to communication and the unfortunate politicization of medical information. A doctor might think, naively, that "facts are facts," that most educated people would accept scientific findings and make choices accordingly. But as we've seen during the pandemic, divergent interpretations of data, counterfactual arguments, and misleading misrepresentations get shared by individuals on social media, podcasters, celebrities, network-platformed journalists, politicians, and even by some physicians. The constant questioning and berating of dedicated scientists is harmful because it casts doubt, by extension, on all medical research. Openness and debate are essential to scientific advances, of course, but there needs be a way for ordinary people who are not doctors to discern credible from unvetted sources.

As considered in earlier chapters, there are many reasons people with treatable cancers don't get effective therapy: distrust of mainstream doctors and medical institutions, lack of money for what insurance doesn't cover or not having insurance altogether, geographical distance from cancer specialists, fear of side effects from treatment, and other circumstances. Doctors, for their part, may fail to prescribe appropriate treatments. This happens because of some physicians' ignorance about cancer tests and drugs, their lack of time to consider each patient's case, and their biases including racism. These failures by physicians and the health care systems employing them result in inequitable or delayed molecular testing of some patients' cancers and, consequently, disparate outcomes. Each of these "social" inadequacies—inadequate funds, and lapses in trust, knowledge, time, or empathy—may be equally consequential to a cancer patient's survival as the pace of their tumor's growth; these merit oncologists' attention, and remedy.

Here I should add a final note on words surrounding cancer. Understandably, some patients and caregivers object to the use of military words in context of illness. In particular, whether battle metaphors are appropriate—if it's OK to say you're "fighting cancer" or hope to "beat this"—sparks debate. Some advocates and doctors point to the flip side of invoking strength to eradicate cancer: that if someone succumbs to illness they may feel as though they've failed, that they didn't try hard enough to overcome their malignancy. These are valid points, and practitioners need be sensitive to this issue. However, when I was practicing medicine, I observed that what helps, what comforts, one person may be unhelpful to the next. So while my personal preference is to avoid terms I associate with war or violence of any kind, I don't object to angry or pugilistic language so long as it's not applied to humans, but to disease. If someone with cancer wants to say or feel that they're "fighting it," I wouldn't argue about this point. As told in these pages, styles of advocacy—favored colors (pink or black?), emblems, and words—have shifted over decades. In my view, patients are best served by a culture of tolerance.

At the end of *Illness as Metaphor*, Susan Sontag wrote about advances in chemotherapy and, with remarkable prescience, the power of immunotherapy to bring about cures. "Cancer will be partly de-mythicized; at it may then be possible to compare something to a cancer without implying either a fatalistic diagnosis or a rousing call to fight by any means whatever a lethal, insidious enemy," she wrote. "The cancer metaphor will be made obsolete, I would predict, long before the problems it has reflected so persuasively will be resolved."[8]

Indeed. As cancer becomes known in its myriad forms and grows increasingly treatable, the metaphor fails. The Dread Disease, the Emperor of All Maladies, has been transformed into a spectrum of diseases, sometimes but not always fatal. As new therapies emerge, cancer will in many cases be managed—and experienced—as a chronic disease, not necessarily curable but treatable, like other conditions, ordinary. It will no longer be so feared.

ACKNOWLEDGMENTS

Writing a cancer book could be depressing, you might think. But thanks to many individuals—patients and activists, caregivers, clinicians, scientists, statisticians, journalists, librarians, CEOs, strangers on the internet and others, neighbors who've shared thoughts, words, and time, it's been the opposite. Over and over, people have demonstrated generosity. The experience leaves me hopeful.

To my dear friend Elaine Soffer, I am grateful for more than her detailed notes on chapters; she responded unfailingly to my ups and downs, angst, and emails even when, I am sure, she had other things to do. Debbie Glasserman helped a million times and then some, in little ways over years, besides answering my unending questions about publishing. When I see this book in print, I'll think of Katherine O'Brien, a wonderful writer and patient advocate who, early on, encouraged me to report on this subject and, before dying from metastatic breast cancer, offered comments and helpful feedback on this book's first draft.

One pleasure in doing research for this project was meeting people who care deeply about information, chiefly librarians and archivists. I thank Arlene Shaner of the New York Academy of Medicine Library, staff at the Patricia D. Klingenstein Library of the New-York Historical Society who helped a while back, the late Nancy Cunningham of the Mirand Library at Roswell Park Cancer Institute in Buffalo, Mary Ann Quinn of the Rockefeller Archive Center, Kathy Brennan of Memorial Sloan Kettering Cancer Center, Amber Dushman at the AMA Archives in Chicago, Stephen Greenberg at the National Library of Medicine in Bethesda, Micaela Sullivan-Fowler at the University of Wisconsin in Madison's Ebling Library, and Jessica Murphy at Harvard's Countway Library in Boston.

The New York Public Library is a phenomenal resource through which I accessed a wealth of databases including America's Historical Newspapers, American Periodicals, Historical African American Newspapers (ProQuest), JSTOR, the Women's Magazine Archive, and more. During the Covid-19 pandemic, the NYPL system proved indispensable, enabling me to complete the research and fact-checking process. Many scientific papers were accessed through the library of Weill Cornell Medicine.

I am grateful for many conversations informing this book including those with Nancy Brinker, Rick Davis, Susanna Fox, Janet Freeman-Daily, Cindy Geoghegan, Dr. Marshall Glesby, the late Jessie Gruman, Juan Hindo, Karuna Jaggar, Amy Schiffman-Langer, Susan Leigh, Dr. Anne Moore, Cathy Ormerod, James Patterson, Andrew Schorr, and Fran Visco. Becky Siegel and Robert Smith of the ACS, and Rick Buck of the American Association for Cancer Research, helped variously and repeatedly. There are several academics who, a while back, were kind enough to meet with me about this project. Although it would be presumptuous to mention those scholars at this point, if they are reading they should know that I am thankful for their suggestions and advice.

To Patrick Fitzgerald, the editor who acquired this book for Columbia University Press, I am forever appreciative. I thank my literary agent Jessica Papin for the confidence she placed in me and for her persistence in getting this book to contract. I am grateful to Anne Ekstrom, a thoughtful editor and neighbor who perused an early version of the manuscript and helped me rethink this book's premise. And to James Yoder, my son's friend and wordsmith who reviewed early chapters with a critical mind. I thank Amanda Grooms for her careful assistance with fact-checking.

To everyone at Columbia University Press, thank you for making this real! To my editor Eric Schwartz, who listened and listened patiently, and thoughtfully answered so many questions, I am beyond appreciative. To Lowell Frye, I am grateful for your attention to details, and for your kindness throughout this process. To Marielle Poss, thank you for directing this to completion. To Ben Kolstad and Kara Cowan at KGL, I am indebted for the fine-tooth combing you gave to the manuscript.

I am incredibly proud of my sons, Aaron and Ethan. And grateful: they each provided sharp, analytical, and, true to their distinct personalities, entirely different critiques of some early book chapters followed by infinite encouragement and, later, nudges to hit "send," to get this done.

Paul, thank you for your watching and discussing *Love Story* and *Brian's Song* in one weekend, and *Terms of Endearment* in the next. And for everything.

NOTES

ABBREVIATIONS

ACS	American Cancer Society
ACT UP	AIDS Coalition to Unleash Power
AMA	American Medical Association
ASCC	American Society for the Control of Cancer
ASCC Bulletin	Bulletin of the American Society for the Control of Cancer
ASCC Campaign Notes	Campaign Notes of the American Society for the Control of Cancer
CDC	Centers for Disease Control (after 1992: Centers for Disease Control and Prevention)
EPA	U.S. Environmental Protection Agency
FDA	U.S. Food and Drug Administration
GFWC	General Federation of Women's Clubs
JAMA	Journal of the American Medical Association
Komen	Susan G. Komen Breast Cancer Foundation
NCI	National Cancer Institute
NEJM	New England Journal of Medicine
NIH	National Institutes of Health
NYC Cancer Committee	New York City Cancer Committee
WFA	Women's Field Army

1. CANCER, KEPT APART (BEFORE 1900)

1. "For a New Hospital," *New York Herald*, April 8, 1883.
2. "Kermis," *Oxford English Dictionary*, online edition (Oxford: Oxford University Press), www.oed.com/view/Entry/103017. "In the Low Countries, parts of Germany, etc.: a periodical (properly, annual) fair or carnival, characterized by much noisy merry-making."
3. "Gossip of Gotham," *St. Paul Daily Globe*, April 15, 1883.
4. "Amusements: Kirmess" *New York Herald*, April 22, 1883.
5. "A Quaint Dutch Festival," *New York Times*, April 29, 1883.
6. "The Kirmess, or Dutch Fair, Given in New York, by the 'Upper Ten,' for the Benefit of the Hospital for Cancer and Skin Diseases . . ." *San Antonio Light*, May 25, 1883.

7. "The Kirmess. Brilliant Success of the Charity Festival at Delmonico's," *New York Herald*, April 29, 1883.

8. "The Kirmess at Delmonico's," *New-York Tribune*, April 29, 1883.

9. F. R. Sturgis, "Surgical Cases Occurring in the Massachusetts General Hospital, Service of Dr. Samuel Cabot," *Boston Medical and Surgical Journal* 76, no. 18 (June 6, 1867): 365–68, https://doi.org/10.1056/nejm186706060761801.

10. Samuel W. Gross and Henry C. Boenning, "Some Points in the Life and Diagnosis of Carcinoma of the Mammary Gland, Based Upon a Study of One Hundred Cases," *Boston Medical and Surgical Journal* 102, no. 13 (March 25, 1880): 289–93, https://doi.org/10.1056/NEJM188003251021301.

11. Francelia Butler, "Some Social Aspects of Cancer History," in *Cancer Through the Ages: The Evolution of Hope* (Fairfax: Virginia, 1955), 32–40.

12. "Blackwell's Island (Roosevelt Island), New York City," National Park Service, accessed May 5, 2022, https://www.nps.gov/places/blackwell-s-island-new-york-city.htm. The island had a "hospital for 'incurables.'"

13. Hayes Martin, Harry Ehrlich, and Francelia Butler, "J. Marion Sims—Pioneer Cancer Protagonist," *Cancer* 3, no. 2 (March 1950): 189–204, https://doi.org/10.1002/1097-0142(1950)3:2<189::AID-CNCR2820030202>3.0.CO;2-1.

14. Seale Harris, *Woman's Surgeon: The Life Story of J. Marion Sims* (New York: Macmillan, 1950).

15. Francelia Butler, "James Marion Sims: Pioneer Cancer Fighter," in *Cancer Through the Ages*, 45–60.

16. Harriet A. Washington, *Medical Apartheid: The Dark History of Medical Experimentation on Black Americans from Colonial Times to the Present* (New York: Anchor, 2006). In this remarkable book, Washington raises global questions about the history of medicine and research, asking, "Why should we give the physicians' medical narratives more credence than the numerous contentions of slaves, sharecroppers, and contemporary African Americans that they have been subjected to abusive medical research?" (p. 9).

    Washington's rebuke of Sims and his legacy is fierce and appropriate. She has documented a brutal side of Sims that was unknown to many physicians. She focuses on Sims in this book's introduction, asking: "Was Sims a savior or a sadist?" (2) and in a section on "antebellum ethics" (61-70).

17. Jeffrey S. Sartin, "J. Marion Sims, the Father of Gynecology: Hero or Villain?," *Southern Medical Journal* 97, no. 5 (May, 2004): 500–505.

18. J. Marion Sims, *The Story of My Life*, ed. H. Marion-Sims (New York: D. Appleton, 1884), "a little hospital of eight beds," 230.

19. J. Marion Sims, "Removal of the Superior Maxilla for a Tumour of the Antrum: Apparent Cure. Return of the Disease. Second Operation. Sequel," *American Journal of the Medical Sciences* (April 1847): 310–14.

20. J. Marion Sims, "Osteo-sarcoma of the Lower Jaw. Removal of the Body of the Bone Without External Mutilation," *American Journal of the Medical Sciences*, no. 28 (October 1847): 370–73.

21. Harris, *Woman's Surgeon*, 152–56.

22. Uncle Dudley, "Health Is Their Business," *Boston Daily Globe*, September 13, 1951.

23. "Reports on the Woman's Hospital of New York," box 2, folder 72, Hayes Martin Papers, Memorial Sloan Kettering Cancer Center Archives, Rockefeller Archive Center, Sleepy Hollow, NY. Copies of typed sheets detailing history of the Woman's Hospital refer to an anonymous offer of $185,000, presented by Mr. J. E. Parsons, which was declined. Only later was that offer attributed to John J. Astor (III).

24. J. Michael Straughn Jr., Roy E. Gandy, and Charles B. Rodning, "The Core Competencies of James Marion Sims, MD," *Annals of Surgery* 256, no. 1 (July 2012): 193–202, https://doi.org/10.1097/SLA.0b013e318249ce3b.

25. J. Marion Sims, *The Woman's Hospital in 1874. A Reply to the Printed Circular of Drs. E. R. Peaslee, T. A. Emmet, and T. Gaillard Thomas, Addressed "to the Medical Profession, May 5, 1877"* (Kent, 1877).

26. "A Cancer Hospital Wanted," *New York Times*, March 8, 1884,

27. *The New York Cancer Hospital First Annual Report* (New York: G. P. Putnam's Sons, 1885), "Letter from the late Dr. J. Marion Sims," 23–24.

28. "Unveiling of the Sims Statue," *Medical Record* 46 (October 27, 1894).

29. "The Statue of Dr. J. Marion Sims in Bryant Park," *JAMA* 23, no. 18 (November 3, 1894): 689–90, https://doi.org/10.1001/jama.1894.02421230029003.

30. J. C. Hallman, "Monumental Error: Will New York Finally Tear Down a Statue?," *Harper's Magazine*, November 2017.

31. William Neuman, "City Orders Sims Statue Removed from Central Park," *New York Times*, April 16, 2018.

32. "Dr. Duncan Bulkley Publishes Memoirs; Founder of Skin and Cancer Hospital Tells of His 56-Year Practice Here," *New York Times*, January 18, 1925.

33. "Rich Women Begin a War on Cancer; Mrs. Sage, Mrs. F. W. Vanderbilt, and Mrs. Speyer Helping to Plan National Campaign," *New York Times*, April 23, 1913.

34. "Mrs. James Speyer Dies at 12:45 a.m.," *New York Times*, February 23, 1921.

35. Charles R. Hearn, "Speyer, Ellin Leslie Prince Lowery," in *Notable American Women, 1607–1950: A Biographical Dictionary*, ed. Edward T. James, Janet Wilson James, and Paul S. Boyer (Cambridge, MA: Belknap, 1971), 3: 336–37.

36. "William R. Travers Dead; Final Rest of a Man Universally Popular. Dying at Bermuda After a Long and Languishing Illness—Sketch of His Career," *New York Times*, March 28, 1887.

37. "William R. Travers's Will," *New York Times*, April 7, 1887.

38. Geoffrey T. Hellman, "Banker, Old Style," *New Yorker*, February 27, 1932.

39. "Interments Listed by Vault," New York City Marble Cemetery, New York, NY. Vault 89, John A. Lowery, interred August 23, 1890, accessed May 5, 2022, https://www.nycmc.org/intermentvaults.html.

40. "Ready for the Trout Streams; Anglers Preparing for the Opening of the Season," *New York Times*, March 29, 1883.

41. "It Is Growing Steadily," *New York Times*, January 11, 1891.

42. *First Annual Report of the New-York Skin and Cancer Hospital* (New York Theo L. De Vinne, 1884).

43. "General Grant's Health. Why He Quit Smoking—Rumors of a Cancer," *Philadelphia Inquirer*, January 12, 1885.

44. "Gen. Grant in Better Health; An Affection of the Tongue Which Is Yielding to Treatment," *New York Times*, January 12, 1885.

45. Stefan Lorant, "Baptism of U. S. Grant," *Life*, March 26, 1951, 90–102.

46. James T. Patterson, prologue to *The Dread Disease: Cancer and Modern American Culture* (Cambridge, MA: Harvard University Press, 1987), 1–11.

47. "Sinking Into the Grave; Gen. Grant's Friends Give Up Hope," *New York Times*, March 1, 1885.

48. "General Grant's Cancer. The Life History of Epithelioma of the Tongue," *Philadelphia Inquirer*, March 20, 1885.

49. "Gen. Grant Not So Well; His Throat Honeycombed with Cancer Cells," *New York Times*, April 26, 1885.

50. Ron Chernow, "Taps," in *Grant* (New York: Penguin, 2017), 928–58.

51. Ulysses S. Grant, *The Best Writings of Ulysses S. Grant*, ed. John F. Marszalek (Carbondale: Southern Illinois University Press, 2015), 194.

52. *Second Annual Report of the New-York Skin and Cancer Hospital* (New York: Styles & Cash, 1885).

53. *Thirty-Sixth Annual Report of the New York Skin and Cancer Hospital* (New York: New-York Skin and Cancer Hospital, 1918).

54. "In the Cause of Charity. Great Success of the Kirmess at the Metropolitan Opera House," *New York Herald*, April 30, 1884.

55. "Booths of Every Nation; The Pretty Spectacles to Be Seen at the Kirmess," *New York Times*, April 30, 1884.

56. "Profits of the Kirmess," *New-York Tribune*, May 9, 1884.

57. "To Give a Kirmess. The Event the United Workers Will Undertake at Union Armory," *New Haven Register*, September 28, 1885.

58. "The Coming Kirmess. Extensive Preparations Being Made for an Elaborate Affair. The Names of the Various," *Cleveland Plain Dealer*, February 14, 1886.

59. "Miscellaneous," Chicago *Inter Ocean*, May 14, 1887.

60. "In True Dutch Style. An Open Air Celebration of the Festival of the Kirmess," *New York Herald*, May 23, 1886.

61. "A Most Attractive Kirmess; The Projected Entertainment for the Skin and Cancer Hospital," *New York Times*, May 25, 1886.

62. "All Ready for the Kirmess. Brilliant Prospects of the Open Air Festival at Vanderbilt Park," *New York Herald*, May 27, 1886.

63. "Chelsea Park Transformed; A Most Successful Opening of the Kirmess Yesterday," *New York Times*, May 28, 1886.

64. "Success of the Out-Door Kirmess. Brilliant and Picturesque Scenes in the Thirty-Fourth-St. Park," *New York Tribune*, May 28, 1886.

65. "Second Day of the Kirmess. Fashionable Society Thronging to the Picturesque Grounds," *New York Herald*, May 29, 1886.

66. Miss Lookabout, "Fashionable Women. New York Dress and Manners in a Big Crowd. Dutch Blood Quickened in Young Veins. Miss Lookabout's Observations at the Kirmess," *Boston Sunday Herald*, May 6, 1883.

67. "In Place of the Kirmess. A 'Festival of the Year' for the Skin and Cancer Hospital," *New York Herald*, April 8, 1887.

68. "The Festival of the Year," *New York Times*, April 26, 1887.

69. "The Festival of the Year: From Which Some Hints May Be Gleaned for the Arrangement of Bazaars," *Art Interchange* 18, May 7, 1887.

70. "Obituary Notes," *New York Times*, June 28, 1887.

71. "Note and Comment," *Springfield Republican*, June 29, 1887.

72. "Charity's Fair Apostles. Their Visit to the Country Branch of the Skin and Cancer Hospital," *New York Herald*, October 30, 1887.

73. It's likely that Elizabeth Cullum was Dr. Sims's patient. She had been a member of the Ladies' Auxiliary of the Woman's Hospital, and he was the most prominent gynecologist in New York City before his death in November 1883.

74. Bob Considine, *That Many May Live: Memorial Center's 75 Year Fight Against Cancer* (New York: Memorial Center for Cancer and Allied Diseases, 1959). The meeting about the need for a cancer hospital took place at Elizabeth Cullum's home, 261 Fifth Avenue, on February 7, 1884, 22–23.

75. *History of the Causeries du Lundi, 1880–1912* (New York: Knickerbocker, 1912).

76. Dinitia Smith, "A Drawing Room of Their Own," *New York Times*, June 12, 2005.

77. "The New-York Cancer Hospital; Laying the Corner-Stone of a Much-Needed Institution," *New York Times*, May 18, 1884.

78. *The New York Cancer Hospital Second and Third Annual Report*. (New York: New York Cancer Hospital, 1886–87)

79. Francelia Butler, "Bastille on Central Park," in *Cancer Through the Ages*, 79–91.

80. "Obituary. Mrs. George W. Cullum," *New York Tribune*, September 17, 1884.

81. "The Late Mrs. Cullum," *Baltimore Sun*, September 20, 1884.

82. "None Like It Anywhere; New-York's New Cancer Hospital for Women," *New York Times*, November 24, 1887.

83. "The Astor Pavilion Opened; The Good Work of the Cancer Hospital Ready to Begin," *New York Times*, December 7, 1887.

84. *The New York Cancer Hospital Fourth Annual Report* (New York: New York Cancer Hospital, 1888).

85. "Society," *New York Times*, October 11, 1896.

86. "Society Events of the Week," *New York Times*, November 22, 1896.

87. "Society," *New York Times*, October 24, 1897.

88. "Loving Cup to Mrs. Speyer; Irene Club, of Which She Was a Founder, Now 35 Years Old," *New York Times*, February 15, 1919.

89. Francelia Butler, "President Cleveland Scoops the Press," in *Cancer Through the Ages*, 73–78.

90. "Cleveland's Health. The President Said to Be in Bad Condition Physically," *Argus-Leader, Sioux Falls*, August 22, 1893.

91. "The President a Very Sick Man—An Operation Performed on Him on Mr. Benedict's Yacht—Part of the Jaw Removed," *Philadelphia Press*, August 29, 1893. As told by Matthew Algeo in *The President Is a Sick Man: Wherein the Supposedly Virtuous Grover Cleveland Survives a Secret Surgery at Sea and Vilifies the Courageous Newspaperman Who Dared Expose the Truth* (Chicago: Chicago Review, 2011), 141–53, the journalist Elisha J. Edwards wrote the 1893 story.

92. "Is Grover Ill? President Cleveland Said to Have Undergone Severe Surgical Treatment," *Buffalo Evening News*, August 30, 1893.

93. William W. Keen, *The Surgical Operations on President Cleveland in 1893* (Philadelphia: G. W. Jacobs, 1917).

94. *The New York Cancer Hospital Fifth Annual Report* (New York: New York Cancer Hospital, 1889).

95. *The New York Cancer Hospital Sixth Annual Report* (New York: New York Cancer Hospital, 1890).

96. "Mrs. C. P. Huntington's Gift; Presents $100,000 to General Memorial Hospital for Treatment of Cancer and Allied Diseases," *New York Times*, May 24, 1902.

97. Donald L. Trump and Edwin A. Mirand, *Rock Paper Scissors: How a Partnership Between a Visionary Surgeon and a Newspaper Publisher Led to the Establishment of the World's First Cancer Center* (Buffalo, NY: Roswell Park Cancer Institute, 2011).

98. "Bequest for Study of Cancer. Mrs. Croft Willed $100,000 to Harvard for This Purpose," *Boston Herald*, January 6, 1900.

2. CANCER'S SPRING (1900–1920)

1.   "Rich Women Begin a War on Cancer; Mrs. Sage, Mrs. F. W. Vanderbilt, and Mrs. Speyer Helping to Plan National Campaign," *New York Times*, April 23, 1913.

2.   Frederick S. Dennis, "The Treatment of Malignant Disease," *JAMA* 37, no. 16 (October 19, 1901): 1013–19, https://doi.org/10.1001/jama.1901.62470420001001.

3.   Samuel H. Adams, "The Great American Fraud: A Series of Articles on the Patent Medicine Evil," *Collier's Weekly*, 1905–1906.

4.   James T. Patterson, "The Rise of the Doctors," in *The Dread Disease: Cancer and Modern American Culture* (Cambridge, MA: Harvard University Press, 1987), 36–55.

5.   "The Beard Treatment of Cancer," *JAMA* 49, no. 21 (November 23, 1907): 1779, https://doi .org/10.1001/jama.1907.02530210051009.

6.   William. B. Coley, "The Treatment of Inoperable Sarcoma by Bacterial Toxins," *Proceedings of the Royal Society of Medicine* 3, Surgical Section (1910): 1–48.

7.   Eric Faure, "Puzzling and Ambivalent Roles of Malarial Infections in Cancer Development and Progression," *Parasitology* 143, no. 14 (September 13, 2016): 1811–23, https://doi .org/10.1017/S0031182016001591.

8.   "Frogs Fail to Cure Cancer; Animals Were Applied to Patient's Neck, but He Is Dead Now," *New York Times*, July 19, 1908.

9.   Roswell Park, "The Recent Buffalo Investigations Regarding the Nature of Cancer," *Medical Record* 59, no. 20 (May 18, 1901): 761–67.

10. Leo Loeb, "Etiology of Cancer of the Skin," *JAMA* 55, no. 19 (November 5, 1910): 1607–11, https://doi.org/10.1001/jama.1910.04330190003002.

11. Snow, Herbert, "Cancer Facts and Cancer Falacies," *Lancet* 164 (September 17, 1904), 822 - 824, https://doi.org/10.1016/S0140-6736(01)31881-0.

12. Steven I. Hajdu, "A Note from History: Landmarks in History of Cancer, Part 4," *Cancer* 118, no. 20 (October 15, 2012): 4914–28, https://doi.org/10.1002/cncr.27509.

13. "Divine Healer Depends Upon Faith to Cure," *Sunday Oregonian*, September 13, 1903.

14. " 'Not Hypnotism but, Rebuke to Devil, Is Cure': Woman Testifies Faith Is Secret of Success," *Boston Journal*, August 29, 1913.

15. "Cure for Cancer Sought Through Study of Fish; President Taft Urges Congress to Make Appropriation for a Laboratory to Investigate the 'Incurable' Disease," *New York Times Magazine*, April 17, 1910.

16. *Hearings Before the Committee on Interstate and Foreign Commerce of the House of Representatives on Bills Relating to Health Activities of the General Government*, 61st Cong., 2nd Sess. 4–6 (1910).

17. James T. Patterson, "The Alliance Against Cancer," in *The Dread Disease: Cancer and Modern American Culture* (Cambridge, MA: Harvard University Press, 1987), 56–87.

18. "Laboratory Report Shows Germs Cause Fish Cancer," *New York Times Magazine*, January 25, 1914.

19. James T. Patterson, *The Dread Disease: Cancer and Modern American Culture* (Cambridge, MA: Harvard University Press, 1987), 59–60.

20. Edmund Andrews, "Supposed Increase of Cancer: A Statistic Error," *JAMA* 32, no. 25 (June 24, 1899): 1406–9, https://doi.org/10.1001/jama.1899.92450520001002.

21. Lawrence Irwell, "Is Cancer Increasing? Statistician Explains Reasons for Apparent Growth," letter to the editor, *New York Times*, May 7, 1913.

22. Burton J. Hendrick, "What We Know About Cancer," *McClure's Magazine*, July 1909.

23. "Clement Cleveland," in *Harvard College (1780–). Class of 1867, Secretary's Report: no. 14* (Boston: Geo. H. Ellis, 1918), 37–38.

24. Ella Hoffman Rigney, *The Story of Cancer Education and the Role Played by Elsie Cleveland Mead, 1913–1938* (New York, 1939). Dr. John C. A. Gerster, a surgeon and president of the New York City Cancer Committee, and Susan M. Wood contributed as editors or co-authors of this short book.

25. "Meade—Cleveland," *New York Times*, November 10, 1898.

26. Donald Francis Shaughnessy, "The Story of the American Cancer Society" (PhD diss., Columbia University, 1957), Elsie Mead's role, 33, 43–44, 53–55.

27. Barbara Seaman and Susan F. Wood, "Role of Advocacy Groups in Research on Women's Health," in *Women and Health*, ed. Marlene B. Goldman and Maureen C. Hatch (San Diego: Academic, 2000), 27–36.

28. "Clement Cleveland, A.M., M.D.," in *New York Journal of Gynaecology and Obstetrics* 3: 307–8.

29. "Cleveland, Clement," in *The National Cyclopaedia of American Biography: Being the History of the United States as Illustrated in the Lives of the Founders, Builders, and Defenders of the Republic, and of the Men and Women Who Are Doing the Work and Moulding the Thought of the Present Time*, vol. 14, ed. James Terry White (New York: James T. White, 1910), 426–27.

30. Clement Cleveland, "The Palliative Treatment of Incurable Carcinoma Uteri. Based Upon Observations at the New York Cancer Hospital," in Transactions of the American Gynecological Society Volume 14 for the Year 1889 (Boston: Massachusetts Institute of Technology and American Gynecological Society, 1889), 462–67.

31. "Medical Notes: 'Anti-Cancer Association,'" *Boston Medical and Surgical Journal* 168, no. 23 (June 5, 1913): 856, https://doi.org/10.1056/nejm191306051682310.

32. "To Extend Fight on Cancer; Laymen and Physicians Form a Nation-Wide Organization," *New York Times*, May 23, 1913.

33. Judith Robinson, *Tom Cullen of Baltimore* (Toronto, ON: Oxford University Press, 1949), 245–50.

34. Thomas S. Cullen, "The Radical Operation for Cancer of the Uterus," in *Transactions of the American Gynecological Society Volume 37 for the Year 1912* (Philadelphia: American Gynecological Society, 1912), 329–44.

35. *Transactions of the American Gynecological Society Volume 37 for the Year 1912* (Philadelphia: American Gynecological Society, 1912). The 1912 annual meeting of the American Gynecological Society took place in Baltimore from May 28 to May 30.

36. J. Craig Neel, "Results After the Wertheim Operation for Carcinoma of the Cervix of the Uterus," in *Transactions of the American Gynecological Society Volume 37 for the Year 1912* (Philadelphia: American Gynecological Society, 1912), 345–75. Drs. Seth Gordon, Fred Taussig, Thomas Cullen, and others comment in published discussion of Dr. Neel's paper.

37. Joseph C. Bloodgood, "The Great Danger of Incomplete Operations for Cancer in the Early Stage of the Disease," *Medical Herald* 32, no. 11 (November 1913).

38. Joseph Colt Bloodgood, "Control of Cancer," *JAMA* 61, no. 26 (December 27, 1913): 2283–86, https://doi.org/10.1001/jama.1913.04350270001001.

39. Samuel V. Kennedy, *Samuel Hopkins Adams and the Business of Writing* (Syracuse, NY: Syracuse University Press, 1999).

40. Samuel Hopkins Adams, "What Can We Do About Cancer?," *Ladies' Home Journal*, May 1913, 21–22.

41. Samuel Hopkins Adams, "Saving Hope in Cancer: Which Will You Believe In?—Science?—or Quackery?," *Collier's Weekly*, April 26, 1913.

42. Samuel Hopkins Adams, "The New Hope in Cancer," *McClure's Magazine*, May 1913.

43. Thomas S. Cullen, "The Cancer Problem: Anniversary Discourse Before the Academy of Medicine of Northern New Jersey, March 18, 1914," *Journal of the Medical Society of New Jersey* 11, no. 4 (April 1914): 163–69.

44. "Abstract of Discussion" [following] Emil Ries, "Theoretical and Practical Foundations of a Radical Operation for Carcinoma of the Cervix Uteri," *JAMA* 61, no. 14 (October 4, 1913): 1266–70, https://doi.org/10.1001/jama.1913.04350150022008. See also, "The Minneapolis Session: American Medical Association Sixty-Fourth Annual Session, Minneapolis, June 17–20, 1913," *JAMA* 60, no. 19 (May 10, 1913): 1431–59, https://doi.org/10.1001/jama.1913.04340190025012.

45. "J. Henry Carstens, MD," *Wayne State University School of Medicine Physician Biography Records*, Walter P. Reuther Library, Wayne State University School of Medicine, Detroit, https://reuther.wayne.edu/files/WSP000126.pdf.

46. "Fight Against Spread of Cancer in Pittsburgh Now in Full Blast," *Pittsburgh Post*, February 4, 1914.

47. "Cancer to Be Discussed," *New York Tribune*, March 16, 1914.

48. "Experts Disagree on Treating Cancer; Dr. Ewing Upholds Radium as a Cure, but Thinks an Overdose Killed Bremner," *New York Times*, March 24, 1914.

49. "Phipps to Give $15,000,000 for Radium Supply. Pittsburgh Millionaire Plans to Equip Institutes to Treat Cancer," *Philadelphia Inquirer*, January 22, 1914.

50. Ben F. Allen, "Phipps Will Equip Radium Hospitals Pittsburg–New York Millionaire Backs $15,000,000 Fight Against Cancer," Cleveland *Plain Dealer*, January 22, 1914.

2. CANCER'S SPRING (1900–1920)   271

51. Notes, April–June 1913; May 1914, in "American Society for the Control of Cancer, 1913–1917," box 68, no. 606, Personal Giving, Subseries 1: Institutions, Russell Sage Foundation Records, Rockefeller Archive Center. The *New York Times* headlined Sage's participation in this meeting. (See note 1 for this chapter.) However, review of Olivia Sage's letters indicates that she declined Cleveland's invitation and, upon his request for her to reconsider, held firm; she was not interested in supporting the anticancer cause.

52. "Mrs. Russell Sage Dies at Her Home," *New York Times*, November 4, 1918.

53. Ruth Crocker, *Mrs. Russell Sage: Women's Activism and Philanthropy in Gilded Age and Progressive Era America* (Bloomington: Indiana University Press, 2008). Sage and the cancer society, 277–79; her will, 306–11.

54. Hoffman's 1892 "Vital Statistics of the Negro" (*Arena* 29 April 1892: 556–67) landed him his job with Prudential Insurance in Newark, after which his actuarial career took off. Hoffman's flawed analysis, attributing lower longevity among Black people to physical "inferiority" rather than to lesser circumstances including poverty, along with an expanded 1896 volume, "Race Traits and Tendencies of the American Negro" (published by the American Economic Association), "justified" denial of insurance policies to Black Americans. Hoffman's racist ideas drew contemporary rebukes such as that by W. E. B. Du Bois in 1896: "Review of 'Race Traits and Tendencies of the American Negro,'" *Annals of the American Academy of Political and Social Science* 9: 127–33.

 Hoffman's work on cancer is widely cited. He received many honors. Before World War I, Hoffman was president of the American Statistical Association. He received an honorary LLD from Tulane University and honorary AMA membership.

 Critical modern scholarship on Hoffman is limited and includes publications by Francis J. Rigney Jr. (Hoffman's grandson), *Frederick L. Hoffman: His Life and Works*, ed. F. J. Sypher (Philadelphia: Xlibris, 2002); and by Beatrix Hoffman (unrelated), "Scientific Racism, Insurance, and Opposition to the Welfare State: Frederick L. Hoffman's Transatlantic Journey," *Journal of the Gilded Age and Progressive Era* 2, no. 2 (2003): 150–90, http://www.jstor.org/stable/25144326; Megan J. Wolff, "The Myth of the Actuary: Life Insurance and Frederick L. Hoffman's 'Race Traits and Tendencies of the American Negro,'" *Public Health Reports* 121, no. 1 (2006): 84–91.

55. "The Sixth Annual Meeting of the Eugenics Research Association," July 21, 1918, *Eugenical News* 3 (Cold Spring Harbor, NY: Eugenics Record Office, 1918), image id 1875, accessed May 22, 2022, http://www.eugenicsarchive.org/eugenics/image_header.pl?id=1875. With attendance "depleted" by war, "Dr." Frederick L. Hoffman was invited to preside over the June 1918 meeting of the Eugenics Research Association and elected to the executive council.

56. "Joint Session of The Eugenics Research Association and The American Eugenics Society: American Museum of Natural History" June 2, 1928, historical image published by the Dolan DNA Learning Center, Cold Spring Harbor Laboratory, New York, accessed May 7, 2022, http://www.eugenicsarchive.org/eugenics/image_header.pl?id=252.

57. Beatrix Hoffman, "Scientific Racism, Insurance, and Opposition to the Welfare State: Frederick L. Hoffman's Transatlantic Journey," *Journal of the Gilded Age and Progressive Era* 2, no. 2 (April 2003): 150–90.

58. Joseph C. Bloodgood, *What Every One Should Know About Cancer* (Chicago: Council on Health and Public Instruction of the American Medical Association, 1914).

59.   "Lecture Notes," *ASCC Campaign Notes* 1, no. 3 (March 15, 1918).

60.   "Lecture Notes," *ASCC Campaign Notes* 1, no. 4 (April 15, 1918).

61.   "A War Department Lecture on Cancer," *ASCC Campaign Notes* 1, no. 6 (September 1, 1918).

62.   "Lecture Notes," *ASCC Campaign Notes* 1, no. 5 (May 1, 1918).

63.   "6,000,000 Workmen Read Warning Signs of Cancer," *ASCC Campaign Notes* 1, no. 4 (April 15, 1918).

64.   "Advice for Preventing Unnecessary Sickness in Texas," *ASCC Campaign Notes* 1, no. 3 (March 15, 1918).

65.   "Personal Notes," *ASCC Campaign Notes*1, no. 6 (September 1, 1918).

66.   "Cleveland Compares Cancer to the Germans," *ASCC Campaign Notes* 1, no. 7 (October 1, 1918).

67.   "Meetings in Atlanta," *ASCC Campaign Notes* 1, no. 13 (May 1, 1919).

68.   "Cancer Literature Now Available," *ASCC Campaign Notes*, 1, no. 18 (October 1, 1919).

3. EDUCATIONAL CAMPAIGNS (1920–1930)

1.   "Mme. Curie Plans to End All Cancers," *New York Times*, May 12, 1921.

2.   Ann M. Lewicki, "Marie Sklodowska Curie in America, 1921," *Radiology* 223, no. 2 (May 1, 2002): 299–303, https://doi.org/10.1148/radiol.2232011319.

3.   Mrs. William Brown Meloney, "That Millions Shall Not Die!" *Delineator*, April 1921, 1.

4.   "New York Women Arrange Welcome for Mme. Curie," *New York Herald*, May 1, 1921.

5.   "Gramme of Radium Gift to Mme. Curie," *New York Herald*, February 8, 1921.

6.   Mrs. William Brown Meloney, "The Greatest Woman in the World," *Delineator*, April 1921, 15–17.

7.   "Notes and Correspondence: Madame Curie Receives Gram of Radium and Many Honors," *Journal of Industrial and Engineering Chemistry* 13, no. 6 (June 1921): 573, https://doi.org/10.1021/ie50138a039.

8.   "Praise Mme. Curie at Luncheon Here," *New York Evening World*, May 17, 1921.

9.   "Radium Presented to Madame Curie," *New York Times*, May 21, 1921.

10.   "Madame Curie Pays Visit to Canonsburg Radium Plant," *Pittsburgh Post*, May 28, 1921.

11.   "Spirit of West and Scenery at Grand Canyon Bring High Praise from Madame Curie," *Bisbee Daily Review* (Bisbee, AZ) June 14, 1921.

12.   "Mme. Curie Ill in East; May Cancel Trip Plans," *Los Angeles Times*, May 27, 1921.

13.   "Mme. Curie Cancels Trip to Pacific Coast," *Baltimore Sun*, May 29, 1921.

14.   "Mme. Curie Taken Ill on Arrival Here from Falls," *Buffalo Morning Express*, June 17, 1921.

15.   "Memorial Hospital Greets Mme. Curie," *New York Times*, May 29, 1921.

16.   "Box with One Gram of Radium Presented to Madame Curie," *Popular Mechanics*, September 1921, 371.

17.   Warren G. Harding, *Remarks of the President in Presenting to Madam Curie a Gift of Radium from the American People: 3 p.m., May 20, 1921* (Washington, DC: Government Printing Office, 1921), https://www.loc.gov/item/21026534/.

18.   *What Everyone Should Know About Cancer* (New York: ASCC, 1922). The ASCC distributed later versions of this pamphlet, including 1924, 1927, and 1930 editions.

19. ASCC, *Bulletin*, vols. 1–5 (New York: ASCC, 1920–1923).

20. "Notice to Members," *ASCC Campaign Notes* 2, no. 2 (February 1920).

21. "Wanted: 3,000 Members by December 31, 1920," *ASCC Campaign Notes* 2, no. 8 (August 1920).

22. "Report of the Annual Meetings," *ASCC Campaign Notes* 5, no. 3 (March 1923).

23. George A. Soper, "Flood of Cancer 'Cures' Sweeps Over Country; Public Warned Against Quacks Who Say They Can Eradicate Disease with Medicine or Serum—Secrecy About Cancer Deplored," *New York Times*, July 27, 1924, https://www.nytimes.com/1924/07/27/archives/flood-of-cancer-cures-sweeps-over-country-public-warned-against.html.

24. "Minnesota," *ASCC Campaign Notes*, no. 4 (April 1922).

25. "Scranton's 'Cancer Day,'" *ASCC Campaign Notes* 2, no. 6 (June 1920).

26. "More Cancer Days in Pennsylvania," *ASCC Campaign* 3, no. 6 (June 1921).

27. "Colorado Area Organized," *ASCC Campaign Notes* 2, no. 11 (November 1920).

28. "Denver's Cancer Campaign," *ASCC Campaign Notes* 2, no. 12 (December 1920).

29. "Dr. Charles A. Powers Drops Dead in Club; President of American Society for Control of Cancer Served in France with Rank of Major," *New York Times*, December 24, 1922.

30. Frank J. Osborne, "Good News of a Bad Subject," *Delineator* 96 (April 1920). This article appeared with an introduction by Carolyn Conant Van Blarcom, health editor of the *Delineator*.

31. Frank J. Osborne, "Good News of a Bad Subject," *ASCC Campaign Notes* 2, no. 8 (August 1920).

32. "Lantern Slides on Cancer," *ASCC Campaign Notes* 1, no. 14 (June 1919).

33. "United States Public Health Service Stereopticon Loan Library," *ASCC Campaign Notes* 2, no. 1 (January 1920).

34. "'Merchant of Venice' to Be Staged as Benefit: Performances to Be Given in Aid of American Society for Control of Cancer," *New-York Tribune*, June 6, 1920.

35. "Theatrical Production," *ASCC Campaign Notes* 3, no. 2 (February 1921).

36. "Lectures in Cooperation with the Young Men's Christian Association," *ASCC Campaign Notes* 2, no. 7 (July 1920).

37. "Cancer Exhibit at the Museum of Natural History," *ASCC Campaign Notes* 2, no. 7 (July 1920).

38. David Cantor, "A Rediscovered Cancer Film of the Silent Era," Medicine On Screen, August 2, 2013, accessed May 7, 2022, https://www.nlm.nih.gov/hmd/collections/films/medicalmoviesontheweb/rewardofcourageessay.html.

39. "American Cancer Society—General Correspondence, 1913, 1915–1929," box 6, no. 42, Office of the Messrs. Rockefeller Records, Rockefeller Archive Center, Sleepy Hollow, NY.

40. "The Rockefeller Gift," *ASCC Campaign Notes* 3, no. 5 (May 1921).

41. "Letter from President Harding," *ASCC Campaign Notes* 3, no. 11 (November 1921).

42. *The Reward of Courage* (Providence, RI: Eastern Film Corporation and the American Society for the Control of Cancer, 1921), http://resource.nlm.nih.gov/101570969.

43. "Gleanings from Cancer Week," *ASCC Campaign Notes* 3, no. 12 (December 1921).

44. "'The Reward of Courage,'" *ASCC Campaign* Notes 4, no. 2 (February 1922).

45. "Three Outstanding Events—B. Cancer Film," *ASCC Campaign Notes* 4, no. 3 (March 1922).

46.   "Further Reports on Cancer Week," table: Film (Showings), *ASCC Campaign Notes* 4, no. 4 (April 1922).

47.   David Cantor, "Uncertain Enthusiasm: The American Cancer Society, Public Education, and the Problems of the Movie, 1921–1960," *Bulletin of the History of Medicine* 81, no. 1 (Spring 2007): 39–69, https://doi.org/10.1353/bhm.2007.0002.

48.   "Methods Developed During Cancer Week," *ASCC Campaign Notes* 3, no. 11 (November 1921).

49.   "Further Reports on Cancer Week: Nebraska," *ASCC Campaign Notes* 4, no. 1 (January 1922).

50.   "Further Reports on Cancer Week: St. Louis," *ASCC Campaign Notes* 4, no. 1 (January 1922).

51.   "Letter from Archbishop Hayes to All Priests in the New York Diocese. Read in Churches Sunday, Oct. 30, 1921," *ASCC Campaign Notes* 4, no. 4 (April 1922).

52.   "Gleanings from Cancer Week: Georgia," *ASCC Campaign Notes* 3, no. 12 (December 1921).

53.   "Maryland Committee Letter," *ASCC Campaign Notes* 3, no. 12 (December 1921).

54.   "Miscellany: Cancer Decalogue Prepared by the Standing Committee on the Control of Cancer of the Massachusetts Medical Society," *Boston Medical and Surgical Journal* 177, no. 2 (July 12, 1917): 62.

55.   "Arkansas Medical Society: Cancer Decalogue," *ASCC Campaign Notes* 1, no. 8 (November–December 1918).

56.   "Dr. Martin's Commandments," *ASCC Campaign Notes* 3, no. 9 (September 1921).

57.   Franklin H. Martin, "Ten Commandments of Cancer," *ASCC Campaign Notes* 3, no. 9 (September 1921).

58.   Lasker Memorial in *ASCC Campaign Notes* 4, no. 3 (March 1922); 4, no. 9 (September 1922); 4, no. 12 (December 1922).

59.   "Gleanings from Cancer Week: Delaware," *ASCC Campaign Notes* 3, no. 12 (December 1921).

60.   "Four Notable Contributions to National Cancer Week: Metropolitan Life Insurance Company," *ASCC Campaign Notes* 4, no. 1 (January 1922).

61.   Frederick L. Hoffman, *Some Cancer Facts and Fallacies: An Address Delivered, in Substance, Before the Mayo Foundation* (Newark, NJ: Prudential Insurance, 1925).

62.   "Cancer Week," *JAMA* 77, no. 18 (October 29, 1921): 1426, https://doi.org/10.1001/jama.1921.02630440046021.

63.   "Cancer Phobia," *JAMA* 77, no. 18 (October 29, 1921): 1427, https://doi.org/10.1001/jama.1921.02630440046021.

64.   Byron B. Davis, "Carcinoma of the Breast with a Consideration of Precancerous Conditions," *JAMA* 78, no. 11 (March 18, 1922): 779–84, https://doi.org/10.1001/jama.1922.02640640007002.

65.   "One of the Letters Prepared by Dr. J. Shelton Horsley, Chairman of the Publicity Committee, for Virginia Newspapers," *ASCC Campaign Notes* 4, no. 2 (February 1922).

66.   "The Propaganda for Reform," *JAMA* 86, no. 1 (January 2, 1926): 55–57, https://doi.org/10.1001/jama.1926.02670270059027.

67.   David Cantor, "Cancer, Quackery and the Vernacular Meanings of Hope in 1950s America," *Journal of the History of Medicine and Allied Sciences* 61, no. 3 (July 1, 2006): 324–68, https://doi.org/10.1093/jhmas/jrj048.

68.   Morris Fishbein, "History of Cancer Quackery," *Perspectives in Biology and Medicine* 8, no. 2 (Winter 1965): 139–66, https://doi.org/10.1353/pbm.1965.0022.

69.   James Harvey Young, "The Most Heartless," in *The Medical Messiahs: A Social History of Medical Quackery in 20th Century America* (Princeton, NJ: Princeton University Press, 1967): 360–89.

70.   "Hoxsey, Harry M. (1909–1990)," boxes 370, S01, Health Fraud Collection, Department of Investigation, AMA, Chicago, IL.

71.   Kirsten E. Gardner, *Early Detection: Women, Cancer, and Awareness Campaigns in the Twentieth-Century United States* (Chapel Hill: University of North Carolina Press, 2006), "Cancer education targeted a white and middle-class audience," 14.

72.   Keith Wailoo, "White Plague," in *How Cancer Crossed the Color Line* (New York: Oxford University Press, 2011), 13–37.

73.   Keith Wailoo, "Primitive's Progress," in *How Cancer Crossed the Color Line* (New York: Oxford University Press, 2011), 40–63.

74.   "Campaigns and Cancer Weeks," in *The American Society for the Control of Cancer: Its Objects and Methods and Some of the Visible Results of Its Work* (New York: ASCC, 1925), 17–19.

75.   "Bulkley, Lucius," folders in box 104 boxes 104, 105, Health Fraud Collection, Department of Investigation, AMA, Chicago IL.

76.   Albert G. Hulett, "L. Duncan Bulkley and 'Cancer,'" letter to the editor, *JAMA* 82, no. 16 (April 19, 1924): 1285, https://doi.org/10.1001/jama.1924.02650420049031.

77.   *Cancer Control: Report of an International Symposium Held Under the Auspices of the American Society for the Control of Cancer, Lake Mohonk, New York, U.S.A., September 20–24, 1926* (Chicago: Surgical Publishing, 1927).

78.   "Experts Outline Data Known in Fight Against Dreaded Cancer," *Orlando Sentinel*, October 3, 1926.

79.   "Cancer Control Facts Disclosed," *Evening Star* (Washington, DC), September 25, 1926.

80.   Welch encouraged and defended medical research in humans to a degree considered unethical by some of his contemporaries and modern scholars. See Susan E. Lederer, *Subjected to Science: Human Experimentation in America Before the Second World War* (Baltimore, MD: Johns Hopkins University Press, 1995), 56–58; 65–68; 82.

81.   William H. Welch, "Greeting of the Foreign Guests on Behalf of the American Medical Profession," in *Cancer Control: Report of an International Symposium Held Under the Auspices of the American Society for the Control of Cancer, Lake Mohonk, New York, U.S.A., September 20–24, 1926*, ed. ASCC (Chicago: Surgical Publishing, 1927), 11–14.

82.   "Assails Overeating as Cause of Cancer," *New York Times*, September 23, 1926.

83.   Harry C. Saltzstein, "Newspaper Publicity in the Control of Cancer," in *Cancer Control: Report of an International Symposium Held Under the Auspices of the American Society for the Control of Cancer, Lake Mohonk, New York, U.S.A., September 20–24, 1926* (Chicago: Surgical Publishing, 1927), 299–307.

84.   "Peacock Point Fete Attracts Throngs; Society Attends Circus on Mrs. Davison's Estate to Aid Fight on Cancer," *New York Times*, September 13, 1927.

85.   *Cancer as a Subject for Popular Entertainment* (New York: ASCC, 1926).

86.   John C. A. Gerster and Susan M. Wood, "Cancer Education in New York City," *American Journal of Cancer* 15, no. 1 (January 1931): 286–98.

87.   Francis J. Rigney's wife, Ella Hoffman Rigney, was the daughter of statistician Frederick Hoffman and future curator of NYC Cancer Committee exhibits.

88.   George H. Bigelow and Herbert L. Lombard, *Cancer and Other Chronic Diseases in Massachusetts* (Boston: Houghton Mifflin, 1933).

89.   Robert B. Greenough, "The Service of the Pondville Hospital at Norfolk," *Boston Medical and Surgical Journal* 197, no. 14 (October 6, 1927): 560–61, https://doi.org/10.1056/nejm192710061971408.

90.   George L. Parker, "The Pondville State Cancer Hospital, 1927–1947," *New England Journal of Medicine (NEJM)* 238, no. 23 (June 3, 1948): 800–804, https://doi.org/10.1056/NEJM194806032382303.

91.   *Report for the Year Ended March 31, 1928* (New York: ASCC, 1928).

92.   James T. Patterson, *The Dread Disease: Cancer and Modern American Culture* (Cambridge, MA: Harvard University Press, 1987), 88–90.

4. FIGHTING WORDS (1930–1945)

1.   Mrs. Carl W. (Marjorie) Illig, Letter to GFWC Health Chairmen, October 16, 1934, Archives, Division of Public Health, Women's History and Resource Center, General Federation of Women's Clubs, Washington, DC.

2.   Kristin Kate White, "Training a Nation: The General Federation of Women's Clubs' Rhetorical Education and American Citizenship, 1890–1930" (PhD diss., Ohio State University, 2010), 71, http://rave.ohiolink.edu/etdc/view?acc_num=osu1279827080. White estimates there had been "close to two million" GFWC members in the early 1920s, citing "Program records, 1922–1924."

3.   Mrs. Carl W. (Marjorie) Illig, Jr. "Annual Report of the Division of Public Health," General Federation of Women's Clubs 1933–1934, Archives, Division of Public Health, Women's History and Resource Center, General Federation of Women's Clubs, Washington, DC.

4.   "Progress of the Women's Field Army," *Bulletin of the American Society for the Control of Cancer (ASCC Bulletin)* 18, no. 7 (July 1936): 10–12.

5.   Walter E. Heston, "Clarence Cook Little," *Cancer Research* 32, no. 6 (June 1972): 1354–56.

6.   George D. Snell, "Clarence Cook Little 1888–1971: A Biographical Memoir," in *Biographical Memoirs* (Washington, DC: National Academy of Sciences, 1975), 239–63.

7.   Rachel A. Snell, "C. C. Little: A Complicated Legacy," Khronikos (blog), June 21, 2013, https://khronikosum.wordpress.com/2013/06/21/c-c-little-a-complicated-legacy/.

8.   Kirsten E. Gardner, *Early Detection: Women, Cancer, and Awareness Campaigns in the Twentieth-Century United States* (Chapel Hill: University of North Carolina Press, 2006). C. C. Little's meeting with GFWC leadership, 70–74.

9.   Marjorie B. Illig, "Health Programs of National Women's Organizations" *Journal of Social Hygiene* 22, no. 7 (October 1, 1936): 310–11.

10.   "Cancer Education Program," in *Report of the Division of Public Health, General Federation of Women's Clubs 1932–1935* (Washington, DC: General Federation of Women's Clubs, 1935).

11.   "Cancer Education Program" flyer (Washington, DC: General Federation of Women's Clubs, 1935).

12. Irvin D. Fleming, Harmon J. Eyre, and Jan Pogue, *The American Cancer Society: A History of Saving Lives* (Atlanta: American Cancer Society, 2010), 23–26.
13. "The Propaganda for Reform," *JAMA* 86, no. 1 (January 2, 1926): 55–57, https://doi.org/10.1001/jama.1926.02670270059027.
14. Oliver Field, "The Nature of the American Medical Association Fight Against Quackery in Medicine," *Food, Drug, Cosmetic Law Journal* 9, no. 4 (April 1954): 213–21.
15. Terra Ziporyn, "AMA's Bureau of Investigation Exposed Fraud," *JAMA* 254, no. 15 (October 18, 1985): 2043–46, https://doi.org/10.1001/jama.1985.03360150017002.
16. James T. Patterson, "Hymns to Science and Prayers to God," in *The Dread Disease: Cancer and Modern American Culture* (Cambridge, MA: Harvard University Press, 1987), 137–70.
17. Robert B. Greenough, "The Service of the Pondville Hospital at Norfolk," *Boston Medical and Surgical Journal* 197, no. 14 (October 6, 1927): 560–61, https://doi.org/10.1056/nejm192710061971408.
18. George H. Bigelow and Herbert L. Lombard, "Economics of the Massachusetts Cancer Program," *NEJM* 207, no. 22 (December 1, 1932): 972–74, https://doi.org/10.1056/nejm193212012072202.
19. George H. Bigelow and Herbert L. Lombard, *Cancer and Other Chronic Diseases in Massachusetts* (Boston: Houghton Mifflin, 1933).
20. Albert Soiland, "Some Economic Aspects of the Cancer Problem," *Radiology* 14, no. 3 (March 1, 1930): 240–53, https://doi.org/10.1148/14.3.240.
21. "Norman Baker Versus the American Medical Association," *JAMA* 98, no. 11 (March 12, 1932): 890, https://doi.org/10.1001/jama.1932.02730370030014.
22. Warren B. Smith, "Norman Baker—King of the Quacks," *Iowan* 7 (December 1958–January 1959).
23. Morris Fishbein, "History of Cancer Quackery," *Perspectives in Biology and Medicine* 8, no. 2 (Winter 1965): 139–66, https://doi.org/10.1353/pbm.1965.0022.
24. "Hoxsey, Harry M. (1909–1990)," boxes 365, 370–72, S01, Health Fraud Collection, Department of Investigation, AMA, Chicago, IL.
25. James Harvey Young, "The Most Heartless," in *The Medical Messiahs: A Social History of Medical Quackery in 20th Century America* (Princeton, NJ: Princeton University Press, 1967): 360–89.
26. *The Castle in the Air Atop the Ozarks Where Sick Folks Get Well Without Operation, Radium or X-Ray* (Eureka Springs, AR: Norman Baker, Inc., 1939), Hayes Martin Papers, box 6, folder 91, Memorial Sloan Kettering Cancer Center Archives, Rockefeller Archive Center, Sleepy Hollow, NY.
27. Rife ray machines for treating cancer were sold at least through the 1990s. Videos and other propaganda supporting their use remain on the internet.
28. "Electrotherapy, Rife, Royal Raymond," box 233, Health Fraud Collection, Department of Investigation, AMA, Chicago, IL.
29. H. H. Dunn, "Movie: New Eye of Microscope in War on Germs," *Popular Science* (June 1931).
30. "New Cancer Foe Hailed: Powerful Ray Credited with Killing Germs, Homeopathic Group Told," *Los Angeles Times*, May 18, 1940.
31. "Mrs. Starling W. Childs," *New York Times*, October 22, 1936.

32. "Jane C. Childs Left a $4,783,181 Estate," *New York Times*, February 1, 1938.
33. "History," Jane Coffin Childs Memorial Fund for Medical Research, accessed May 9, 2022, https://www.jccfund.org/about-fund/history/.
34. Jane inherited a fortune from her father, Charles A. Coffin, who led General Electric.
35. "$210,000 Given to U. of P. for War on Cancer," *Philadelphia Inquirer*, January 26, 1930.
36. "More Time Is Granted for Cancer Seal Contest," *Chicago Tribune*, March 6, 1930.
37. "$100,000 Given for Clinic at U.C. Hospital," *Oakland Tribune*, June 10, 1930.
38. "Contributes to Cancer Clinic," *Hammond Indiana Times*, August 3, 1937.
39. "Funds for Cancer Research and Treatment," *ASCC Bulletin* 20, no. 2 (February 1938): 9.
40. "Announcement," *American Journal of Cancer* 15, no. 1 (January 1931): 1–3.
41. *ASCC Bulletin* 13, no. 1 (January, 1931): 7.
42. New York City Cancer Committee, *Cancer: Then and Now* (New York: Chemical Foundation, 1932).
43. "The Coffey–Humber Cancer Treatment," *Radiology* 14, no. 6 (June 1, 1930), 607, https://doi.org/10.1148/14.6.607a.
44. "Coffey–Humber Treatment for Cancer," *JAMA* 95, no. 18 (November 1, 1930): 1349–50, http://dx.doi.org/10.1001/jama.1920.02720180043016.
45. "Hope Abandoned for Woman Making Air Trip to Hospital to Try New Cure for Cancer," *Montana Standard*, February 16, 1930.
46. W. B. Coffey and J. D. Humber, "The Coffey–Humber Treatment," letter, *JAMA* 94, no. 9 (March 1, 1930): 652, https://doi.org/10.1001/jama.1930.02710350052023.
47. "California v. New York," *Time*, May 25, 1931, 31–32.
48. William J. Mayo, "Again the Cancer Problem," *ASCC Bulletin* 12, no. 9 (September 1930): 1–2.
49. Rowland H. Harris, "The Coffey–Humber Extract of Suprarenal Cortex Substance: A Clinical Study of Four Hundred and Fifteen Patients with Malignant Tumors Who Received Experimental Injections," *JAMA* 97, no. 20 (November 14, 1931): 1457–63, https://doi.org/10.1001/jama.1931.02730200033008.
50. "Coast Cancer 'Cure' Held of Little Use," *New York Times*, November 21, 1931.
51. "Cause and Effect in Cancer Research," *ASCC Bulletin* 15, no. 6 (June 1933): 9–10.
52. Louis I. Dublin, "Statistics on Morbidity and Mortality from Cancer in the United States," *American Journal of Cancer* 29, no. 4 (April 1937): 736–42.
53. "With the Women's Field Army," *ASCC Bulletin* 19, no. 4 (April 1937): 10–12.
54. "Cancer and the Press," editorial, *ASCC Bulletin* 15, no. 3 (March 1933): 9.
55. "Press and Cancer Control" (initialed by Clarence C. Little) and "For the Future," *National Bulletin of the American Society for the Control of Cancer* 21, no. 3 (March 1939): 2, 7–9.
56. "The Science Writers' Questions," *National Bulletin of the American Society for the Control of Cancer* 22, no. 4 (April 1940): 6–9.
57. William A. O'Brien, "The Use of the Radio in Cancer Education," *ASCC Bulletin* 18, no. 5 (May 1936): 7–9.
58. "The Radio as a Pioneer in Cancer Education," *ASCC Bulletin* 18, no. 4 (April 1936): 9–10.
59. "With the Women's Field Army," *ASCC Bulletin* 19, no. 1 (January 1937): 9–12.

60. C. C. Little, "Publicity and Cancer," *National Bulletin of the American Society for the Control of Cancer* 21, no. 8 (August 1939): 2–3.

61. "Cancer Army," *Time*, March 22, 1937.

62. "U.S. Science Wars Against an Unknown Enemy: Cancer," *Life*, March 1, 1937.

63. Editors of "Fortune," *Cancer: The Great Darkness* (Garden City, NY: Doubleday, Doran, 1937). Discussion of cancer research funding, 5–10.

64. "Movie Wins Medal of Cancer Group Here; March of Time Honored for War on Disease," *New York Times*, October 28, 1937.

65. "An Extraordinary Year in the History of Cancer," *ASCC Bulletin* 19, no. 12 (December 1937): 10–11.

66. "Signs Cancer Study Bill; Roosevelt Acts on Measure to Set Up National Institute," *New York Times*, August 6, 1937.

67. Christine Sadler, "'Conquer Cancer' Adapted as Battle Cry of the Public Health Service," *Washington Post*, August 8, 1937.

68. Devra M. Breslow, "The National Cancer Institute Act of 1937," in *A History of Cancer Control in the United States, 1946–1971: Book Two: A History of Programmatic Developments in Cancer Control*, ed. Lester Breslow and the History of Cancer Control Project (Washington, DC: U.S. National Cancer Institute, Division of Cancer Control and Rehabilitation, 1979): 507–14.

69. James T. Patterson, "Government Joins the Fight," in *The Dread Disease: Cancer and Modern American Culture* (Cambridge, MA: Harvard University Press, 1987), 114–36.

70. William A. Yaremchuk, "The Origins of the National Cancer Institute," *Journal of the National Cancer Institute* 59, no. S2 (August 1977): 551–58.

71. Michael B. Shimkin, "As Memory Serves—An Informal History of the National Cancer Institute, 1937–57," *Journal of the National Cancer Institute* 59, no. S2 (August 1977): 559–600.

72. Clifton R. Read, "April: Cancer Control Month," *ASCC Bulletin* 20, no. 4 (April 1938): 9.

73. "Report on the Activities of the American Society for the Control of Cancer: 1937–38; 1938–39," *National Bulletin of the American Society for the Control of Cancer* 21, no. 10 (October 1939): 2–12.

74. Marjorie B. Illig, "With the Women's Field Army," *National Bulletin of the American Society for the Control of Cancer* 21, no. 4. (April 1939): 10–12.

75. Howard M. Clute, "Talk on Cancer," *ASCC Bulletin* 19, no. 9 (September 1937): 1–3.

76. Mary Hastings Bradley, "Pattern for Three," *Redbook*, March 1936.

77. Mary Hastings Bradley, *Pattern of Three* (New York: D. Appleton-Century, 1937).

78. "Remarks by Representative Edith Nourse Rogers of Massachusetts and Mrs. Marjorie B. Illig, National Commander of the Women's Field Army of the American Society for the Control of Cancer, Made Over a National Broadcasting Company Network on Wednesday, February 9th," Press release, February 10, 1938, National Broadcasting Company, February 10, 1938. Archives, Women's History and Resource Center, GFWC Headquarters, Washington DC.

79. Howard W. Blakeslee, "Deaths from Cancer Can Be Cut by 50 Per Cent, Society Is Told," *Chattanooga Daily Times*, March 26, 1938.

80. "Twenty-Fifth Anniversary Celebration," *ASCC Bulletin* 20, no. 3 (March 1938): 10.

81. James Ewing, "The Public and the Cancer Problem," *Science* 87, no. 2262 (May 6, 1938): 399–407, https://doi.org/10.1126/science.87.2262.399.

82. James B. Murphy, "James Ewing 1866–1943: A Biographical Memoir," in *Biographical Memoirs* (Washington, DC: National Academy of Sciences, 1951), 44–60.

83. LaSalle D. Leffall Jr., "James Ewing, MD: Contemporary Oncologist Exemplar: The James Ewing Lecture," *Archives of Surgery* 122, no. 11 (November 1987): 1240–43, https://doi .org/10.1001/archsurg.1987.01400230026003.

84. "Hospitals—Memorial Hospital, 1931–1940," OMR box 24, folder 190, Medical Interests, Office of the Messrs. Rockefeller Records, Rockefeller Archive Center, Sleepy Hollow, NY.

85. "Rockefeller Provides $3,000,000 to Build Cancer Hospital Here," *New York Times*, April 28, 1936.

86. "'Cancer Club' Asks 25,000 to Join; That Number Is Said to Have Been Successfully Treated," *New York Times*, March 25, 1938.

87. Clifton R. Read, "Progress in Lay Cancer Education: Pioneers in the Educational War Against Cancer," *ASCC Bulletin* 20, no. 5 (May 1938): 7.

88. "Cured Cancer Patients Will Organize Club," *Tampa Tribune*, April 28, 1938.

89. *CBS Radio Program Book* (New York: Columbia Broadcasting System, 1939). *Highways to Health* was broadcast on Tuesdays from 4:00 to 4:15 p.m. The April 25, 1939, program featured the Cured Cancer Club.

90. James P. Roe, Anna C. Palmer, and Frank E. Adair, "Cancer Can Be Cured," *National Bulletin of the American Society for the Control of Cancer* 21, no. 7 (July 1939): 8–11.

91. Bowman C. Crowell, "The Women's Field Army Against Cancer," *National Bulletin of the American Society for the Control of Cancer* 21, no. 4 (April 1939): 3–5.

92. George Gallup, "Survey Reveals Need of Cancer Education," *National Bulletin of the American Society for the Control of Cancer* 21 (June 1939): 7–8.

93. George Gallup, "Public Mistaken on Cancer, Poll by Gallup Shows: Many Believe It Contagious or Incurable, but Majority Know Disease Can Be Beaten at Start," *Atlanta Constitution*, April 16, 1939.

94. George Gallup, "Mistaken Ideas About Cancer Widespread, Poll Shows," *Lincoln Star*, April 16, 1939.

95. "Modley's Little Men," *New Yorker*, February 19, 1938, 16–17.

96. Marjorie B. Illig, "With the Women's Field Army," *National Bulletin of the American Society for the Control of Cancer* 21, no. 1 (January 1939): 10–12.

97. Marjorie B. Illig, "With the Women's Field Army," *National Bulletin of the American Society for the Control of Cancer*, 23, no. 3 (March 1939): 10–12.

98. Ella Hoffman Rigney, "An Exhibit on Cancer," *Quarterly Review, New York City Cancer Committee*, 3, no. 4 (January 1939): 81–93.

99. Ella Hoffman Rigney, "Is a Cancer Exhibit Worth While?," *Quarterly Review, New York City Cancer Committee*, 4, no. 2–3 (July–October 1939): 59–63.

100. Clifton R. Read, "V. National Publicity: Report of Publicity Director," *National Bulletin of the American Society for the Control of Cancer* 21, no. 10 (October 1939): 11–12.

101. Frank E. Adair, "Is There Evidence That the Education of the Public on the Early Signs of Cancer Is Accomplishing the Aims of the American Society for the Control of Cancer?," *National Bulletin of the American Society for the Control of Cancer*, 21 no. 4 (April 1939): 6–7.

102. *Dark Victory*, directed by Edmund Goulding (Burbank, CA: Warner Bros., 1939), 104 min.

103. George E. Brewer Jr., *In Time's Course* (Ipswich, MA: George E. Brewer Jr., 1932).

104. Frank S. Nugent, "Bette Davis Scores New Honors in 'Dark Victory,'" *New York Times*, April 21, 1939.

105. Susan E. Lederer, "Dark Victory: Cancer and Popular Hollywood Film," *Bulletin of the History of Medicine* 81, no. 1 (Spring 2007): 94–115.

106. Daphne Du Maurier, *Rebecca* (New York: P.F. Collier, 1938).

107. *Rebecca*, directed by Alfred Hitchcock (Beverly Hills, CA: United Artists, 1940), 130 min.

108. "An Appeal to Writers," *National Bulletin of the American Society for the Control of Cancer* 22, no. 6 (June 1940): 9.

109. Marjorie B. Illig, "With the Women's Field Army," *National Bulletin of the American Society for the Control of Cancer* 22, no. 5 (May 1940): 10–12.

110. Marjorie B. Illig, "With the Women's Field Army," *ASCC Bulletin* 23, no. 6 (June 1941): 7–11.

111. Marjorie B. Illig, "April Is Our Battle Month," *ASCC Bulletin* 23, no. 3 (March 1941): 2.

112. "War Cancels National Assembly," *ASCC Bulletin* 24, no. 1 (January 1942): 11.

113. Mrs. H. W. Peterson, "Montana Training School," *ASCC Bulletin* 25, no. 12 (December 1943): 139-40.

114. Donald Francis Shaughnessy, "The Story of the American Cancer Society" (PhD diss., Columbia University, 1957), 204–6.

115. C. C. Little, "Campaign—1943," *ASCC Bulletin* 25, no. 3 (March 1943): 26.

5. A CELEBRITY CAUSE (1945–1960)

1. Rebecca Skloot, *The Immortal Life of Henrietta Lacks* (New York: Crown, 2010). Lacks's diagnosis and treatment are detailed in Part 1, 13–86.

2. Vincent T. DeVita Jr. and Edward Chu, "A History of Cancer Chemotherapy," *Cancer Research* 68, no. 21 (November 1, 2008): 8643–53, https://doi.org/10.1158/0008-5472.CAN-07-6611.

3. Steven I. Hajdu and Manjunath Vadmal, "A Note from History: Landmarks in History of Cancer, Part 6," *Cancer*, 119 no. 23 (December 1, 2013): 4058–82, https://doi.org/10.1002/cncr.28319.

4. Siddhartha Mukherjee, "Poisoning the Atmosphere," in *The Emperor of All Maladies: A Biography of Cancer* (New York: Scribner, 2010), 89–92.

5. Vincent T. DeVita Jr. and Elizabeth DeVita-Raeburn, "The Chemotherapists," in *The Death of Cancer: After Fifty Years on the Front Lines of Medicine, a Pioneering Oncologist Reveals Why the War on Cancer Is Winnable—and How We Can Get There* (New York: Sarah Crichton, 2015) 33–60.

6. Louis S. Goodman, Maxwell M. Wintrobe, William Dameshek, Morton J. Goodman, Alfred Gilman, and Margaret T. McLennan, "Nitrogen Mustard Therapy: Use of Methyl-Bis(Beta-Chloroethyl)amine Hydrochloride and Tris(Beta-Chloroethyl)amine Hydrochloride for Hodgkin's Disease, Lymphosarcoma, Leukemia and Certain Allied and Miscellaneous Disorders," *JAMA* 132, no. 3 (September 21, 1946): 126–32, https://jamanetwork.com/journals/jama/fullarticle/288442.

7.   Susan L. Smith, "War! What Is It Good For? Mustard Gas Medicine," *Canadian Medical Association Journal* 189, no. 8 (February 27, 2017): E321–22, https://doi.org/10.1503/cmaj.161032.

8.   William James Maloney and Mea A. Weinberg, "A Comprehensive Analysis of Babe Ruth's Head and Neck Cancer," *Journal of the American Dental Association* 139, no. 7 (July 2008): 926–32, https://doi.org/10.14219/jada.archive.2008.0279.

9.   David P. Steensma, Marc A. Shampo, and Robert A. Kyle, "George Herman 'Babe' Ruth Jr: Baseball Star and Early Participant in a Cancer Clinical Trial," *Mayo Clinic Proceedings* 83, no. 11 (November 1, 2008): 1262, https://dx.doi.org/10.4065/83.11.1262.

10. Nadim B. Bikhazi, Alan M. Kramer, Jeffrey H. Spiegel, and Mark I. Singer, "'Babe' Ruth's Illness and Its Impact on Medical History," *Laryngoscope* 109, no. 1 (January 1999): 1–2, https://doi.org/10.1097/00005537-199901000-00001.

11. Lawrence K. Altman, "The Doctor's World; The Babe's Other Record: Cancer Pioneer," *New York Times*, December 29, 1998.

12. Babe Ruth and Bob Considine, *The Babe Ruth Story* (New York: Dutton, 1948; New York: Signet, 1992), 243–44. Citations refer to the Signet edition.

13. "Cure for Cancer? New Synthetic Drugs Appear to Halt Growth of Malignant Tumors," *Wall Street Journal*, September 11, 1947.

14. "Teropterin and Babe Ruth," *New York Times*, August 19, 1948.

15. Otis L. Guernsey Jr., "On the Screen: The Babe's Worst Inning," *New York Herald Tribune*, July 27, 1948.

16. "Ruth Sees Premiere of Film on His Life," *New York Times*, July 27, 1948.

17. John McCarten, "The Current Cinema: Wet Grounds," *New Yorker*, August 7, 1948.

18. "'Babe Ruth,' June 1948–Aug 1948," Public Affairs, series 4.3: "Scrapbooks," reel 2 (microfilm), Memorial Sloan Kettering Cancer Center Archives, Rockefeller Archive Center, Sleepy Hollow, NY.

19. "Original Jimmy Fund Radio Fund Broadcast," *Truth or Consequences*, radio broadcast, NBC, New York, NY, May 22, 1948. Available at https://youtu.be/eXeYrG-L9L8.

20. Gretchen Marie Krueger, "'For Jimmy and the Boys and Girls of America': Publicizing Childhood Cancers in Twentieth-Century America," *Bulletin of the History of Medicine* 81, no. 1 (Spring 2007): 70–93. http://www.jstor.org/stable/44451739.

21. Siddhartha Mukherjee, "The Goodness of Show Business" and "The House That Jimmy Built," in *The Emperor of All Maladies: A Biography of Cancer* in *The Emperor of All Maladies: A Biography of Cancer* (New York: Scribner, 2010), 93–100, 101–4.

22. "History of Dana-Farber Cancer Institute," Dana-Farber Cancer Institute, accessed May 3, 2022, https://www.dana-farber.org/about-us/history-and-milestones/.

23. "Dana Laboratories Are Dedicated at Jimmy Fund Bldg.," *Boston Globe*, December 1, 1962.

24. Herbert Black, "Cancer Center for Adults Fruition of Dr. Farber Dream," *Boston Globe*, June 28, 1976.

25. "About Us," Pan-Mass Challenge, accessed May 3, 2022, https://www.pmc.org/about.

26. "Billy Starr," *Boston Globe*, March 8, 1982.

27. Stan Grossfeld, "Spokesman for Cause: Founder Starr Is Pan-Mass Challenge's Biggest Wheel," *Boston Globe*, July 29, 2009.

28. Margo Miller, "People and Places," *Boston Globe*, November 29, 1982.

29. Dan Shaughnessy, "Jimmy Fund Gets 50th Anniversary Gift: 'Jimmy,'" *Boston Globe*, May 17, 1998.

30. Pamela Ferdinand, "'This Is Jimmy. Heard You Were Lookin' for Me': Famed Cancer Patient Turns Up After 40 Years," *Washington Post*, May 22, 1998.

31. Alec Foege, "Jimmy Found," *People*, June 8, 1998.

32. Douglas Martin, "Einar Gustafson, 65, 'Jimmy' of Child Cancer Fund, Dies," *New York Times*, January 24, 2001.

33. Walter Sanford Ross, *Crusade: The Official History of the American Cancer Society* (New York: Arbor House, 1987), 33–40.

34. James T. Patterson, "The Research Explosion," in *The Dread Disease: Cancer and Modern American Culture* (Cambridge, MA: Harvard University Press, 1987), 171–200; the Laskers' ACS overhaul 172–74.

35. Siddhartha Mukherjee, "They Form a Society," in *The Emperor of All Maladies: A Biography of Cancer* (New York: Scribner, 2010), 107–15.

36. "Biographical Overview," Mary Lasker, National Library of Medicine Profiles in Science, accessed May 3, 2022, https://profiles.nlm.nih.gov/spotlight/tl/feature/biographical -overview.

37. Donald Francis Shaughnessy, "The Story of the American Cancer Society" (PhD diss., Columbia University, 1957), Mary Lasker, Louis Mattox Miller, and the *Reader's Digest* stories, 226–27.

38. Eric Pace, "Mary W. Lasker, Philanthropist for Medical Research, Dies at 93," *New York Times*, February 23, 1994.

39. Jeffrey L. Cruikshank and Arthur W. Schultz, *The Man Who Sold America: The Amazing (but True!) Story of Albert D. Lasker and the Creation of the Advertising Century* (Boston: Harvard Business School, 2010), "Reach for a Lucky Instead" campaign, 254.

40. "Reminiscences of Mary Lasker," part 1, Session 16 (transcript), *Notable New Yorkers*, interviewed by John T. Mason Jr., June 12, 1963 (New York: Oral History Research Office, Columbia University Libraries), 471–506.

41. "Reminiscences of Mary Lasker," part 1, Session 4 (transcript), *Notable New Yorkers*, interviewed by John T. Mason Jr., November 5, 1962 (New York: Oral History Research Office, Columbia University Libraries), 105–6.

42. "Sloan, Kettering to Combat Cancer; Studying Sketch of Proposed Cancer Research Institute," *New York Times*, August 8, 1945.

43. Memorial Hospital, Public Affairs, record group 375, series 3, Box 1, folder 11 (1945), Memorial Sloan Kettering Cancer Center Archives, Rockefeller Archive Center, Sleepy Hollow, NY.

44. Mary F. Czufin, director, Women's Division, New York City Committee of the American Cancer Society, Inc., to Mary Lasker Mary Lasker Papers, 1940–1993, box 94, Columbia University Libraries, Rare Book and Manuscript Library, New York, NY.

45. Memorial Hospital, Public Affairs, record group 375, series 3, Box 1, folder 12 (1946), Public Affairs, Memorial Sloan Kettering Cancer Center Archives, Rockefeller Archive Center, Sleepy Hollow, NY.

46. Mary Lasker Papers, 1940–1993, boxes 94, 95, 121, Columbia University Libraries, Special Collections, New York, NY. These boxes hold documents concerning the relationship

between the ACS and NYC Cancer Committee and their finances in the early postwar period.

47. "$12,000,000 Is Goal in Fight on Cancer," *New York Times*, April 2, 1946.

48. "Use of Atom Against Cancer Demonstrated: Guests at Dinner Opening Drive for 1,072,000 See Progress of Science," *New York Herald Tribune*, April 2, 1946.

49. Devra M. Breslow, "Federal Cancer Control Program 1946–1957," *A History of Cancer Control in the United States, 1946–1971: Book Two: A History of Programmatic Developments in Cancer Control*, ed. Lester Breslow and the History of Cancer Control Project (Washington, DC: U.S. National Cancer Institute, Division of Cancer Control and Rehabilitation, 1979). Breslow notes: "The geographic spread was encouraging: by the early 1950s, centers for clinical oncology were not limited to Memorial Hospital; pockets of competence were emerging throughout the nation," 550.

50. "Medicine: Frontal Attack," *Time*, June 27, 1949.

51. C. Chester Stock, "Obituary: Cornelius Packard Rhoads, 1898–1959," *Cancer Research* 20, no. 3 (April 1960): 409–11.

52. Susan E. Lederer, "'Porto Ricochet': Joking About Germs, Cancer, and Race Extermination in the 1930s," *American Literary History* 14, no. 4 (Winter 2002): 720–46, http://www .jstor.org/stable/3568022.

53. Douglas Starr, "Revisiting a 1930s Scandal, AACR to Rename a Prize," *Science* 300, no. 5619 (April 25, 2003): 573–74, https://doi.org/10.1126/science.300.5619.573.

54. "Postal Truck Posters," *American Cancer Society 1946 Campaign Progress Bulletin*, no. 11 (March 20, 1946): 3.

55. "Our Founding," Damon Runyon Cancer Research Foundation, accessed May 11, 2022, https://www.damonrunyon.org/our-strategy/our-history.

56. "Milton's Marathon," *Life*, April 25, 1949, 112–16.

57. Olivia B. Waxman, "This Is How Telethons Became a Fundraising Tradition," *Time*, September 12, 2017.

58. "Our History: Hope Rises from Loss," Leukemia & Lymphoma Society, accessed May 3, 2022, https://www.lls.org/our-history.

59. "Award to Be Given," *Times Dispatch* (Richmond, VA), March 24, 1950.

60. Shawn G. Kennedy, "Leukemia Society Offers Patients a Variety of Aid," *New York Times*, November 25, 1982.

61. "CRI History," Cancer Research Institute, accessed May 3, 2022, https://www.cancer research.org/about-cri/cri-history.

62. Eric Nagourney, "Helen C. Nauts, 93, Champion of Her Father's Cancer Work," *New York Times*, January 9, 2001.

63. "'Cured Cancer Club' of 100 Shows Value of Fund Drive," *Globe and Mail*, April 3, 1946.

64. "Massachusetts Medical Society, Deaths," *NEJM* 230, no. 11 (March 16, 1944): 336, https:// doi.org/10.1056/nejm194403162301108.

65. "Cured Cancer Club Adding 2 Chapters," *Washington Post*, August 27, 1953.

66. "'Cured Cancer Club' Organized Here by 50 Lansing Residents," *Lansing State Journal* (Lansing, MI), November 2, 1939.

67. "Early American Styles Will Vie with Modern," *Washington Post*, May 14, 1950.

68. "Overcoming Fear" *Washington Post*, September 9, 1953 June 10, 1952.

69. Frank Carey, "Patients Cured of Cancer Stage Capital Club Dinner," *Hartford Courant*, July 25, 1954.

70. "Cured Patient to Address Cancer Society," *Courier-Journal* (Louisville, KY), November 4, 1954.

71. "Cured Victim of Cancer to Launch Appeal Here," *Los Angeles Times*, March 30, 1955.

72. Edward F. Reid, "Another Couple Tell of Recovery from Cancer," *Tipton Daily Tribune* (Tipton, IN), April 9, 1958.

73. "Bush Proposes Creation of 'Cured Cancer Club,'" *Hartford Courant*, March 29, 1956. As reported, "a 'cured cancer club' . . . would operate in somewhat the same manner to aid cancer victims as Alcoholics Anonymous works."

74. Our Medical Correspondent, "Link Between Smoking and Cancer: Tobacco Firms' Research Offer," *Manchester Guardian*, February 13, 1954.

75. "Rejoinder by Companies: 'No Proof,'" *Manchester Guardian*, February 13, 1954.

76. Russell W. Baker, "Sure Smoking–Lung Cancer Link Reported in Britain," *Baltimore Sun*, February 13, 1954.

77. "Smoker-Grandma Dies at Age of 101," *Baltimore Sun*, February 13, 1954.

78. "British Medics Link Smoking with Cancer," *Los Angeles Times*, February 13, 1954.

79. "Tobaccos Issues Decline in London; Remarks on Cancer, Smoking by Health Minister Cause Sharp Price Reaction," *New York Times*, February 13, 1954.

80. "Is There Proof That Smoking Causes Cancer?, Interview with E. Cuyler Hammond, Director of Statistical Research, American Cancer Society," *U.S. News* 36 (February 26, 1954): 62–71.

81. E. Cuyler Hammond and Daniel Horn, "The Relationship Between Human Smoking Habits and Death Rates: A Follow-Up Study of 187,766 Men," *JAMA* 155, no. 15 (August 7, 1954): 1316–28, https://doi.org/10.1001/jama.1954.03690330020006.

82. James T. Patterson, "Smoking and Cancer," in *The Dread Disease: Cancer and Modern American Culture* (Cambridge, MA: Harvard University Press, 1987), 201–30.

83. "Doctor Lauds Smoking," *New York Times*, September 22, 1954.

84. Naomi Oreskes and Erik M. Conway, "Doubt Is Our Product," in *Merchants of Doubt: How a Handful of Scientists Obscured the Truth on Issues from Tobacco Smoke to Global Warming* (New York: Bloomsbury, 2010), 10–35. An essential account of how the tobacco industry conspired to question, discredit, and dilute evidence of smoking's harms.

85. Robert K. Plumb, "Study on Smoking and Cancer Is Set," *New York Times*, October 20, 1954.

86. Bill Fay, "Cancer Quacks," *Collier's*, May 26, 1951.

87. *Cold Cancer Facts* (Denver, CO: Spears Chiropractic Sanitarium and Hospital, circa 1946), Ebling Library for the Health Sciences, Rare Books and Special Collections, University of Wisconsin–Madison.

88. Eugene F. Jannuzi, "Cancer Treatment Is Revealed as Hoax," *Pittsburgh Post-Gazette*, October 4, 1948.

89. "Unproven Methods of Cancer Treatment," *CA: A Cancer Journal for Clinicians* 11, no. 1 (January/February 1961): 17–18, https://doi.org/10.3322/canjclin.11.1.17.

90. Lorna Doone Burks, *I Die Daily: The Story of a Woman Whose Love Will Live Forever* (New York: Rockport, 1946)."My experience might teach someone else," 14; "She had been

operated on in San Francisco," 15; an "account" with "the Father," 16; "pride was the cause," 55; "a shameful thing," 55; It *is* unclean, this cancer," 55; expenses "more than twice my husband's entire salary," 16; "It would be better for all concerned," 16; see also 111–13 (caregiver covers bills, car has been sold); "None wanted me, when told that I was dying of cancer," 47; "No busy doctor in wartime," 47; "hophead" episode, denied morphine, 69–76.

91.   J. F., "Scourge and Remedy: I Die Daily," *New York Times*, April 27, 1947.

92.   Barbara Bush, *Barbara Bush: A Memoir* (New York: Scribner 2015), 39–49.

93.   Hagop M. Kantarjian and Robert A. Wolff, "A Brief History of MD Anderson Cancer Center," in *The MD Anderson Manual of Medical Oncology*, 3rd ed. (New York: McGraw-Hill, 2016).

94.   "Who Was MD Anderson?," University of Texas MD Anderson Cancer Center, accessed May 3, 2022, https://www.mdanderson.org/about-md-anderson/facts-history/who-was-md-anderson.html.

95.   United Press, "Star's Operation Set; Specialist to Perform Surgery on Mrs. Zaharias Friday," *New York Times*, April 14, 1953.

96.   Babe Didrikson Zaharias and Harry T. Paxton, *This Life I've Led: My Autobiography* (New York: A. S. Barnes, 1955), 5, 228.

97.   "Babe Zaharias Dies; Athlete Had Cancer," *New York Times*, September 28, 1956.

98.   "President Opens Cancer Crusade," *New York Herald Tribune*, April 2, 1954.

99.   "Ike and Babe Open Campaign, Then Talk Golf," *Chicago Daily Tribune*, April 2, 1954.

100. Irvin D. Fleming, Harmon J. Eyre, and Jan Pogue, *The American Cancer Society: A History of Saving Lives* (Atlanta: American Cancer Society, 2010), 58–59.

101. Rob Roy, "Find Sepia Artists Major Participants in Nation's Drive for Funds to Fight Cancer," *Chicago Defender*, April 17, 1954.

102. Audrey Hepburn and Mel Ferrer, "Public Service Announcement for the American Cancer Society," backstage, Broadway production of *Ondine*, February 28, 1954.

103. "Church Bells Throughout Nation Signal Start of 1955 Crusade," *ACS Bulletin* 4, no. 15 (April 1955) 1.

104. "Church Bells Will Toll—Cancer Fund Campaign to Be Launched Friday," *Shreveport Journal* (Shreveport, LA), March 31, 1955.

105. "Tolling of Church Bells to Launch Cancer Crusade," *Montana Standard*, March 31, 1955.

106. "Pealing Bells to Launch Cancer Drive Tomorrow," *Valley Times* (North Hollywood, CA), March 31, 1955.

107. "Whole Village to Go on Trip to New York," *St. Cloud Times* (St. Cloud, MN), April 29, 1953.

108. John G. Rogers, "Cancer Group Brings a Whole Village Here," *New York Herald Tribune*, May 7, 1953.

109. "Funkley, Minn., to See Ike Today, Tour Capitol Hill," *Minneapolis Tribune*, May 12, 1953.

110. "Little Village—Big Award," *Cancer News*, July 1953, 16-17.

111. "Tiny Funkley Takes a Trip," *Life*, May 25, 1953.

112. *Breast Self-Examination* (New York: American Cancer Society, National Cancer Institute, and U.S. Public Health Service, 1950), 15 min.

113. "The Biennial," *American Journal of Nursing* 50, no. 7 (July 1950): 387–403, https://doi.org/10.2307/3467570.

114. Raymond F. Kaiser, "A Special Purpose Health Education Program: Breast Self-Examination," *Public Health Reports* 70, no. 4 (April 1955): 428–32, https://doi.org/10.2307/4589090.

115. *No Sad Songs for Me*, directed by Rudolph Maté (Culver City, CA: Columbia Pictures, 1950), 188 min.

116. Bosley Crowther, "The Screen in Review: Margaret Sullavan Returns in 'No Sad Songs for Me,'" *New York Times*, April 28, 1950.

117. William Saroyan, *Don't Go Away Mad and Two Other Plays* (New York: Harcourt, Brace, 1949).

118. Fanny Butcher, "Thoughts of Dying Men in a Saroyan Play," *Chicago Tribune*, December 11, 1949.

119. Thomas Quinn Curtiss, "Saroyan in Search of a Moral; Don't Go Away Mad! and Two Other Plays," *New York Times*, November 20, 1949.

120. "Dialogue of New Saroyan Play Is Strong Point," *Indianapolis News*, December 2, 1949.

121. Theresa Loeb Cone, "Drama Group Presents New Saroyan Play," *Oakland Tribune*, July 8, 1952.

122. John Gunther, *Death Be Not Proud* (New York: Harper & Row, 1949).

123. Mark Harris, *Bang the Drum Slowly* (New York: Knopf, 1956).

124. *Bang the Drum Slowly (United States Steel Hour)*, directed by Daniel Petrie (New York: CBS), September 26, 1956, 52 min.

125. Tennessee Williams, *Cat on a Hot Tin Roof* (New York: Signet, 1955).

126. *Cat on a Hot Tin Roof*, written by Tennessee Williams, directed by Elia Kazan, Morosco Theatre, New York, NY, March 24, 1955–November 17, 1956.

127. *Cat on a Hot Tin Roof*, directed by Richard Brooks (Beverly Hills, CA: MGM, 1958), 108 min.

128. "The Living Proof," 1956, series 6 (radio/TV programs), box 1, folder 13, Public Affairs, Memorial Hospital, Memorial Sloan Kettering Cancer Center Archives, Rockefeller Archive Center, Sleepy Hollow, NY.

129. "35,000 Ring Doorbells for Cancer Appeal," *Los Angeles Times*, April 23, 1958.

130. Richard Carter, "Three Women, One Nuisance," and "The Cancer Crusade" in *The Gentle Legions* (Garden City, NY: Doubleday, 1961), 15–23, 139–72; "forever educating itself to educate others," 170. Citations refer to revised edition (New Brunswick, NJ: Transaction Publishers, 1992).

6. OUR BODIES, OUR DECISIONS (1960–1980)

1. Rachel Carson, *Silent Spring* (Cambridge, MA: Houghton Mifflin, 1962).

2. Rachel Carson, "Silent Spring—I," *New Yorker*, June 16, 1962.

3. Rachel Carson, "Silent Spring—II," *New Yorker*, June 23, 1962.

4. Rachel Carson, "Silent Spring—III," *New Yorker*, June 30, 1962.

5. John M. Lee, "'Silent Spring' Is Now Noisy Summer; Pesticides Industry Up in Arms Over a New Book," *New York Times*, July 22, 1962.

6. Lorus Milne and Margery Milne, "There's Poison All Around Us Now," *New York Times*, September 23, 1962.

7. "Rachel Carson Book Is Called One-Sided," *New York Times*, September 14, 1962.

8.   "Pesticides: The Price for Progress," *Time*, September 28, 1962.

9.   William Darby, "Silence, Miss Carson!," *Chemical and Engineering News* 40 (October 1, 1962): 60–63.

10. Bruce N. Ames, "Identifying Environmental Chemicals Causing Mutations and Cancer," *Science* 204, no. 4393 (May 11, 1979): 587–93, https://doi.org/10.1126/science.373122.

11. Bruce N. Ames and Lois S. Gold, "The Causes and Prevention of Cancer: Gaining Perspective," *Environmental Health Perspectives* 105, no. S4 (June 1, 1997): 865–73, https://doi .org/10.1289/ehp.97105s4865.

12. Michael B. Smith, "'Silence, Miss Carson!' Science, Gender, and the Reception of Silent Spring," *Feminist Studies* 27, no. 3 (Autumn 2001): 733–52, https://doi.org/10.2307/3178817.

13. James Delingpole, "Google Celebrates the 20th Century's Greatest Female Mass Murderer, Rachel Carson," *Breitbart News*, May 27, 2014, https://www.breitbart.com/europe/2014/05/27 /google-celebrates-the-20th-century-s-greatest-female-mass-murderer-rachel-carson/.

14. Charles C. Mann, "'Silent Spring & Other Writings' Review: The Right and Wrong of Rachel Carson," *Wall Street Journal*, April 26, 2018.

15. Linda Lear, *Rachel Carson: Witness for Nature* (New York: Henry Holt, 1997).

16. William Souder, *On a Farther Shore* (New York: Random House, 2012).

17. Jill Lepore, "The Right Way to Remember Rachel Carson," *New Yorker*, March 19, 2018.

18. Douglas Brinkley, "Rachel Carson and JFK, an Environmental Tag Team," *Audubon*, May–June 2012.

19. Jay L. McMullen, "The Silent Spring of Rachel Carson," *CBS Reports*, television broadcast, CBS, April 3, 1963.

20. Ellen Leopold, "A Little Private Hell: The Letters of Rachel Carson and Dr. George Crile, Jr., 1960–64," in *A Darker Ribbon* (Boston: Beacon, 1999), 111–50. Leopold provides a rich chapter on Carson's experience with breast cancer and correspondence with Crile.

21. Souder, *On a Farther Shore*, at a dinner for trustees of the National Parks Association, Carson overheard the comment about Sen. Neuberger, 322–23.

22. Linda Lear, *Rachel Carson: Witness for Nature* (New York: Houghton Mifflin Harcourt, 1997), final trip to Cleveland Clinic for hypophysectomy and injection of Yttrium-90, 478–79.

23. Boston Women's Health Collective, *Women and Their Bodies: A Course* (Boston: Boston Women's Health Collective and New England Free Press, 1970).

24. Boston Women's Health Collective, *Our Bodies, Ourselves: A Book by and for Women* (Boston: Boston Women's Health Collective and New England Free Press, 1971).

25. Walter Selove and Mortimer M. Elkind, "Radiation and Man," *Bulletin of the Atomic Scientists* 14, no. 1 (January 1958): 7–8, https://doi.org/10.1080/00963402.1958.11453782.

26. "The AEC's Unsafe Image," editorial, *St. Louis Post-Dispatch*, December 14, 1971.

27. Lowell P. Weicker Jr., "Our Environment: Commitment or Complacency? Keynote Address Delivered Before the Southwestern Connecticut Girl Scout Council Conference on Natural Resources at Hartford, Connecticut, on August 11, 1969," *Vital Speeches of the Day* 35, no. 23 (September 15, 1969): 732–35.

28. David Cantor, "The Frustrations of Families: Henry Lynch, Heredity, and Cancer Control, 1962–1975," *Medical History* 50, no. 3 (July 2006): 279–302, https://doi.org/10.1017 /S0025727300009996.

29. Edwin Silverberg and Arthur I. Holleb, "Cancer Statistics 1972," *CA: A Cancer Journal for Clinicians* 22, no. 1 (January/February 1972): 2–20, https://doi.org/10.3322/canjclin.22.1.2.

30. Advisory Committee to the Surgeon General of the Public Health Service, *Smoking and Health* (Washington, DC: U.S. Department of Health, Education, and Welfare, 1964).

31. National Center for Chronic Disease Prevention and Health Promotion (U.S.) Office on Smoking and Health, "Fifty Years of Change 1964–2014," in *The Health Consequences of Smoking—50 Years of Progress: A Report of the Surgeon General* (Atlanta: Centers for Disease Control and Prevention, 2014).

32. Roy Norr, "Cancer by the Carton," *Reader's Digest*, December 1952. This is an abridged version of the original article published in the *Christian Herald*.

33. Anthony Burgess, *A Clockwork Orange* (New York: Norton, 1962). A glossary of the fictional "Nadsat" language at this novel's end equates "cancer" with "cigarette."

34. "U.S. Panel Says Cigarettes Are Major Cause of Deadly Diseases," *St. Louis Post-Dispatch*, January 11, 1964.

35. "The Smoking Report," editorial, *New York Times*, January 12, 1964.

36. "Cigarette Smoking Branded a Major Health Hazard," *Baltimore Sun*, January 12, 1964.

37. R. T. Ravenholt, "Tobacco's Global Death March," *Population and Development Review* 16, no. 2 (June 1990): 213–40, https://doi.org/10.2307/1971589.

38. Jeffrey L. Cruikshank and Arthur W. Schultz, *The Man Who Sold America: The Amazing (but True!) Story of Albert D. Lasker and the Creation of the Advertising Century* (Boston: Harvard Business School, 2010). "Reach for a Lucky instead," 254.

39. K. L. Lum, J. R. Polansky, R. K. Jackler, and S. A. Glantz, "Signed, Sealed and Delivered: 'Big Tobacco' in Hollywood, 1927–1951," *Tobacco Control* 17, no. 5 (September 25, 2008): 313–23, https://dx.doi.org/10.1136/tc.2008.025445.

40. Howard C. Taylor, "Physicians and Cigarette Smoking," *JAMA* 181, no. 9 (September 1, 1962): 777–78, https://doi.org/10.1001/jama.1962.03050350039009.

41. Bernard DeVoto, "Doctors Along the Boardwalk," *Harper's Magazine*, September 1947, 215–24.

42. Martha N. Gardner and Allan M. Brandt, "'The Doctors' Choice Is America's Choice': The Physician in U.S. Cigarette Advertisements, 1930–1953," *American Journal of Public Health* 96, no. 2 (February 2006): 222–32, https://doi.org/10.2105/ajph.2005.066654.

43. Herbert L. Lombard and Carl R. Doering, "Cancer Studies in Massachusetts: Habits, Characteristics and Environment of Individuals with and Without Cancer," *NEJM* 198, no. 10 (April 26, 1928): 481–87, https://doi.org/10.1056/nejm192804261981002.

44. Ronald A. Fisher, "Cancer and Smoking," *Nature* 182, no. 4635 (August 30, 1958): 596, https://doi.org/10.1038/182596a0.

45. Clarence Cook Little, *Annual Report of the Scientific Director, The Council for Tobacco Research (formerly the Tobacco Industry Research Committee), 1963–64* (New York: Council for Tobacco Research, 1964), https://www.industrydocuments.ucsf.edu/tobacco/docs/#id=tmbv0035.

46. "Smokers Assured in Industry Study; Report by Tobacco Council Finds No Cigarette Link to Cancer and Heart Disease," *New York Times*, August 17, 1964.

47. Clark W. Heath, "Differences Between Smokers and Nonsmokers," *Archives of Internal Medicine* 101, no. 2 (February 1958): 377–88, https://doi.org/10.1001/archinte.1958.00260140209031.

48.   Carl C. Seltzer, "Masculinity and Smoking," *Science* 130, no. 3390 (December 18, 1959): 1706–7, https://doi.org/10.1126/science.130.3390.1706.

49.   James T. Patterson, "Smoking and Cancer," in *The Dread Disease: Cancer and Modern American Culture* (Cambridge, MA: Harvard University Press, 1987), 201–30.

50.   David M. Cutler, "Are We Finally Winning the War on Cancer?," *Journal of Economic Perspectives* 22, no. 4 (Fall 2008): 3–26, https://doi.org/10.1257/jep.22.4.3.

51.   "John Wayne Tells of Cancer Surgery," *New York Times*, December 31, 1964.

52.   "Playboy Interview: John Wayne," *Playboy*, May 1971.

53.   Paul Weeks, "Nat 'King' Cole Dies of Cancer at 45," *Los Angeles Times*, February 16, 1965.

54.   Keith Wailoo, "How the Other Half Dies," in *How Cancer Crossed the Color Line* (New York: Oxford University Press, 2011), 92–119.

55.   John A. Williams, *The Man Who Cried I Am* (Thunder's Mouth, 1967), "The cancer smell of rot and death," 151.

56.   Keith Wailoo, *How Cancer Crossed the Color Line* (New York: Oxford University Press, 2011), 133.

57.   *The Heart Is a Lonely Hunter*, directed by Robert Ellis Miller (Burbank, CA: Warner Bros.–Seven Arts, 1968), 123 min. In the 1940 novel by Carson McCullers, the doctor's diagnosis is tuberculosis; in the movie, the doctor quietly calls it cancer.

58.   Edwin Silverberg and Arthur I. Holleb, "Major Trends in Cancer: 25 Year Survey," *CA: A Cancer Journal for Clinicians* 25, no. 1 (January/February 1975): 2–7, https://doi.org/10.3322/canjclin.25.1.2.

59.   Michael B. Shimkin, Matthew H. Griswold, and Sidney J. Cutler, "Survival in Untreated and Treated Cancer," *Annals of Internal Medicine* 45, no. 2 (August 1, 1956): 255–67, https://doi.org/10.7326/0003-4819-45-2-255.

60.   Jacqueline Susann, *Valley of the Dolls* (New York: Bernard Geis, 1966).

61.   *Valley of the Dolls*, directed by Mark Robson (Los Angeles: 20th Century Fox, 1967), 123 min.

62.   Amy Fine Collins, "Once Was Never Enough," *Vanity Fair*, January 2000.

63.   Barbara Seaman, "Jacqueline Susann," in *Shalvi/Hyman Encyclopedia of Jewish Women*, Jewish Women's Archive, December 31, 1999, Accessed May 13, 2022, https://jwa.org/encyclopedia/article/susann-jacqueline.

64.   A. Patrick Schneider II, Christine M. Zainer, Christopher Kevin Kubat, Nancy K. Mullen and Amberly K. Windisch, "The Breast Cancer Epidemic: 10 Facts," *Linacre Quarterly* 81, no. 3 (August 1, 2014): 244–77, https://doi.org/10.1179/2050854914Y.0000000027.

65.   Lawrence Garfinkel, Catherine C. Boring, and Clark W. Heath Jr., "Changing Trends: An Overview of Breast Cancer Incidence and Mortality," *Cancer* 74, no. S1 (January 1994): 222–27, https://doi.org/10.1002/cncr.2820741304.

66.   Betty Coe Spicer, "New Weapons Against Breast Cancer," *Ladies' Home Journal*, June 1962.

67.   "A New Test for Early Detection of Breast Cancer," *Good Housekeeping*, May 1963, 159–61.

68.   Terese Lasser and William Kendall Clarke, *Reach to Recovery* (New York: Simon and Schuster, 1972), 158.

69.   Barron H. Lerner, "Breast Cancer Patients in Revolt," in *The Breast Cancer Wars: Hope, Fear, and the Pursuit of a Cure in Twentieth-Century America* (New York: Oxford University Press, 2001), 141–69.

70.   Marge Figel, "Reach to Recovery: Help from One Who Knows," *Essence*, January 1974, 34, 88.

71. Margery Wiesenthal, "Reach-to-Recovery Program of the American Cancer Society," *Cancer* 53, no. S3 (February 1, 1984): 825–27.

72. Oliver Cope, "Breast Cancer: Has the Time Come for a Less Mutilating Treatment?," *Radcliffe Quarterly* 54 (June 1970): 6–11.

73. Oliver Cope, "New Hope for Treatment of Breast Cancer to Avoid the Surgery All Women Fear," *Vogue*, October 15, 1970.

74. Fredelle Maynard, "Breast Cancer: Is There An Alternative to Surgery?," *Woman's Day*, November 1970.

75. Era Bell Thompson, "I Was a Cancer Coward," *Ebony*, September 1971.

76. Rosamond Campion [Babette Rosmond], *The Invisible Worm: A Woman's Right to Choose an Alternate to Radical Surgery* (New York: Macmillan, 1972).

77. "Shorter Reviews: The Invisible Worm," *New York Times*, October 1, 1972.

78. *Love Story*, directed by Arthur Hiller (Hollywood: Paramount, 1970), 100 min.

79. Erich Segal, *Love Story* (New York: Harper & Row, 1970).

80. Jennifer's leukemia diagnosis is stated in the book; movie audiences knew about it.

81. A. H. Weiler, "After 'Love Story,'" *New York Times*, December 6, 1970.

82. Vincent Camby, "Screen: Perfection and a 'Love Story': Erich Segal's Romantic Tale Begins Run," *New York Times*, December 18, 1970.

83. Pauline Kael, "The Current Cinema: Epic and Crumbcrusher," *New Yorker*, December 26, 1970, 52–54.

84. Tim Bannon, "Who Was Brian Piccolo? What You Should Know About the Former Chicago Bears Player," *Chicago Tribune*, April 22, 2019.

85. "Understanding Embryonal Cell Carcinoma," Brian Piccolo Cancer Research Fund, accessed May 20, 2022, https://brianpiccolofund.org/research/understanding-embryonal-cell-carcinoma/.

86. *Brian's Song*, directed by Buzz Kulik (Burbank, CA: ABC, November 30, 1971), 74 min.

87. Gale Sayers with Al Silverman, *I Am Third* (New York: Bantam, 1970).

88. John J. O'Connor, "TV: Love Was Link for Tuesday and Wednesday: ABC's 'Brian's Song' Traces a Friendship," *New York Times*, December 3, 1971.

89. Kate Meyers, "Remembering Brian's Song," *Entertainment Weekly*, November 29, 1991.

90. Barron H. Lerner, "No Stone Unturned: The Fight to Save Brian Piccolo's Life," in *When Illness Goes Public: Celebrity Patients and How We Look at Medicine* (Baltimore, MD: Johns Hopkins University Press, 2006): 100–119.

91. *Bang the Drum Slowly*, directed by John D. Hancock (Hollywood: Paramount, 1973), 96 min.

92. Margalit Fox, "Ann Landers, Advice Giver to the Millions, Is Dead at 83," *New York Times*, June 23, 2002. "Eppie" Lederer was said to be the most influential woman in America. Her "Ann Landers" column was syndicated in over a thousand newspapers. She died from multiple myeloma, a blood cancer, in 2002.

93. Ann Landers, "Ann Landers: 'Save Millions of Lives,'" *Oakland Tribune*, April 20, 1971.

94. Ann Landers, "Ann Landers," *Austin American*, April 20, 1971.

95. Ann Landers, "Bill S-34 Gets a Boost from Ann," *Tampa Tribune*, April 20, 1971.

96. Robert J. Bazell, "Cancer Research Proposals: New Money, Old Conflicts," *Science* 171, no. 3974 (March 5, 1971): 877–79, https://doi.org/doi:10.1126/science.171.3974.877.

97. James T. Patterson, "Popular Fears, Official Dreams," in *The Dread Disease: Cancer and Modern American Culture* (Cambridge, MA: Harvard University Press, 1987), 231–54.

98. Siddhartha Mukherjee, "A Moon Shot for Cancer," in *The Emperor of All Maladies: A Biography of Cancer* (New York: Scribner, 2010), 180–90.

99. Richard Nixon Foundation, "From the Archives: President Nixon Signs the National Cancer Act," December 23, 1971, YouTube video, 9:13, uploaded April 20, 2016, https://youtu.be/lQYfC9kisHw.

100. "Washington: For the Record," *New York Times*, December 11, 1971.

101. "To Adopt the Conference Report On S. 1828," December 10, 1971, GovTrack.us, https://www.govtrack.us/congress/votes/92-1971/s412.

102. Jonathan Spivak, "Cancer Bill, Signed by Nixon, Seen Having Major Impact on Future Medical Research," *Wall Street Journal*, December 24, 1971.

103. Stuart Aeurbach, "U.S. Campaign to Find Cancer Cure Is Launched with Nixon's Signature," *Washington Post*, December 24, 1971.

104. Harold M. Schmeck, Jr. "Nixon Signs Cancer Bill; Cites Commitment to Cure," *New York Times*, December 24, 1971.

105. United Press International, "U.S. Cancer Program Signed by President," *Boston Globe*, December 24, 1971.

106. Lucy Eisenberg, "The Politics of Cancer," *Harper's Magazine*, November 1971, 100-105.

107. "Treasurer's Report" and "Support from the Public," in American Cancer Society Annual Report, 1975 (reviewed by the author in June 2019 at the National Library of Medicine in Bethesda, MD).

108. "Georgia Students March Against Cancer," *Cancer News* 21 (Spring 1967): 10–13.

109. "Partridge Stars Plan a Bike-a-Thon," *Los Angeles Times*, September 5, 1972.

110. "Bicyclists to Ride for Cancer Aid," *Orlando Sentinel*, October 15, 1972.

111. "Partridge Clan to Fight Cancer," *Honolulu Star-Bulletin*, October 15, 1972.

112. "Briefly . . . A Nationwide 'Bike-a-Thon'," *Cancer News* 26 (Winter 1973).

113. "Reports Show Bike-a-Thon Nets $249,254," *Los Angeles Times*, January 5, 1973.

114. "Dance the Weekend Away," *Morning Herald* (Hagerstown, MD), November 13, 1970.

115. "UVM Student Is Arranging Music for MS Dance Marathon," *Burlington Free Press* (Burlington, VT), April 7, 1975.

116. *They Shoot Horses, Don't They?*, directed by Sydney Pollack (Burbank, CA: ABC Pictures, 1969), 125 min. The film is based on the 1935 novel of the same name by Horace McCoy.

117. Paula Becker, "Dance Marathons of the 1920s and 1930s," HistoryLink.org, August 25, 2003, https://www.historylink.org/File/5534.

118. Katie Thornton, "The Grim, Depression-Era Origins of Dance Marathons," *Atlas Obscura*, February 8, 2019, http://www.atlasobscura.com/articles/depression-era-dance-marathons.

119. United Press, "Venice to L.A. Marathon Dancers Forced to Quit by Humane Officers," *Oakland Tribune*, April 22, 1927.

120. Associated Press, "Marathon," *York Daily Record* (York, PA), February 5, 1973.

121. "Expanded History," "THON: Penn State IFC Panhellenic Dance Marathon," data from January 17, 2012 retrieved at *Internet Archive*, https://web.archive.org/web/20120117223431/http://www.thon.org/whatisthon/history/expanded#1973.

122. Elaine Schattner, "Time for THON at Penn State: How the World's Largest Student-Run Charity Helps Kids with Cancer," *Forbes*, January 31, 2017.

123.   T. F. James, "Cancer and Your Emotions," *Cosmopolitan*, April 1960, 39–43.

124.   Howard R. and Martha E. Lewis, "Personality Traits That May Lead to Cancer," *Ladies' Home Journal*, April 1972.

125.   Howard R. Lewis and Martha E. Lewis, *Psychosomatics: How Your Emotions Can Damage Your Health* (New York: Viking, 1972).

126.   David M. Kissen, "The Significance of Personality in Lung Cancer in Men," *Annals of the New York Academy of Sciences* 125, no. 3 (January 1966): 820–6, https://doi.org/10.1111/j.1749-6632.1966.tb45433.x.

127.   David M. Kissen, R. I. F. Brown, and Margaret Kissen, "A Further Report on Personality and Psychosocial Factors in Lung Cancer," *Annals of the New York Academy of Sciences* 164, no. 2 (October 1969): 535–44, https://doi.org/10.1111/j.1749-6632.1969.tb14071.x.

128.   "Obituary Notices: D. M. Kissen, B.Sc., M.D.," *British Medical Journal* 1, no. 5594 (March 23, 1968): 773–74.

129.   Claus Bahne Bahnson, "In Memory of Dr. David M. Kissen: His Work and His Thinking," *Annals of the New York Academy of Sciences* 164, no. 2 (October 1969): 313–18, https://doi.org/10.1111/j.1749-6632.1969.tb14046.x.

130.   Lawrence LeShan, "An Emotional Life-History Pattern Associated with Neoplastic Disease," *Annals of the New York Academy of Sciences* 125, no. 3 (January 1966): 780–93, https://doi.org/10.1111/j.1749-6632.1966.tb45427.x.

131.   Legacy Tobacco Industry Documents, http://legacy.library.ucsf.edu/.

132.   Hardy Shinn to Thomas F. Ahrensfeld, DeBaun Bryant, Frederick P. Haas, Cyril F. Hetsko, Henry C. Roemer, Arthur J. Stevens, and Addison Yeaman, August 15, 1972, https://www.industrydocuments.ucsf.edu/docs/nggb0101. "For some time we have been interested in the work of Dr. Claus Bahnson . . ."

133.   A search for "David Kissen" in the Tobacco Industry Documents archive (https://www.industrydocuments.ucsf.edu/tobacco) yields 1,425 hits. Among those, a "List of Special Projects Funded by the Tobacco Industry Research Committee, the Council for Tobacco Research—USA" includes a two-year grant of $48,650.55 to David M. Kissen at the "Psychosomatic Research Unit, Dept. Psychological Medicine, Southern General Hospital, Glasgow, Scotland" for studies of "Psychosocial Factors, Personality and Lung Cancer in Men Aged 55–64; Steroid Excretion Patterns and Personality in Lung Cancer; Psychosomatic Aspects of Cigarette Smoking and Some Diseases," July 1, 1967–June 30, 1969 ($48,500 in 1968 equates to over $372,000 in 2021 dollars).

134.   Ruth Rosenbaum, "Cancer, Inc.," *New Times*, November 25, 1977.

135.   Robert N. Proctor, *Golden Holocaust: Origins of the Cigarette Catastrophe and the Case for Abolition* (Berkeley: University of California Press, 2011), 300–301.

136.   Daniel S. Greenberg, "A Critical Look at Cancer Coverage," *Columbia Journalism Review* 13, no. 5 (January/February 1975): 40–44.

137.   Daniel S. Greenberg, "Cancer: Now, the Bad News," *Washington Post*, January 19, 1975.

138.   Robert N. Proctor, *Cancer Wars: How Politics Shapes What We Know and Don't Know About Cancer* (New York: Basic Books, 1995), 54–55.

139.   G. Edward Griffin, *World Without Cancer* (Westlake Village, CA: American Media, 1974). Chapter 23, "The Double Standard," presents Griffin's view of the FDA: that it unduly restricts sales of "harmless" vitamins and supplements. Chapters 22 and 24 center on laetrile, which in Griffin's view should be available to patients who want it.

140. Gretchen Marie Krueger, "'For Jimmy and the Boys and Girls of America': Publicizing Childhood Cancers in Twentieth-Century America," *Bulletin of the History of Medicine* 81, no. 1 (Spring 2007): 70–93, http://www.jstor.org/stable/44451739.

141. Hampton Sides, "Childhood Leukemia Was Practically Untreatable Until Dr. Don Pinkel and St. Jude Hospital Found a Cure," *Smithsonian*, July/August 2016.

142. "Fred Hutchinson Has Lung Cancer," *Longview Daily News* (Longview, Washington), January 4, 1964.

143. "Hutchinson Begins 'New' Lung Cancer Treatment," *Cincinnati Enquirer*, January 9, 1964.

144. Tom Groeschen, "Honoring Hutch," *Cincinnati Enquirer*, September 1, 1996.

145. "Cancer Center to Honor Baseball Star," *Daily News* (Port Angeles, WA), September 2, 1975.

146. William G. Bradley, "History of Medical Imaging," *Proceedings of the American Philosophical Society* 152, no. 3 (September 2008): 349–61.

147. Sandra Blakeslee, "Shirley Temple Makes Plea Again," *New York Times*, November 9, 1972.

148. Shirley Temple Black, "Don't Sit Home and Be Afraid," *McCall's*, February 1973.

149. Janet R. Osuch, Kami Silk, Carole Price, Janice Barlow, Karen Miller, Ann Hernick, and Ann Fonfa, "A Historical Perspective on Breast Cancer Activism in the United States: From Education and Support to Partnership in Scientific Research," *Journal of Women's Health* 21, no. 3 (March 2012): 355–62, https://doi.org/10.1089/jwh.2011.2862.

150. "Mrs. Ford to Have Surgery Today for Breast Cancer Test," *Los Angeles Times*, September 28, 1974.

151. Harry Nelson, "Mrs. Ford's Breast Is Removed After Cancer Is Detected," *Los Angeles Times*, September 29, 1974.

152. Stuart Auerbach, "Prognosis Is Called Excellent: Mrs. Ford's Right Breast Removed," *Washington Post*, September 29, 1974.

153. Philip Greer, "Mrs. Rockefeller's Breast Removed: Happy Rockefeller's Left Breast Removed After Cancer Is Found," *Washington Post*, October 18, 1974.

154. William Claiborne, "2d Mastectomy Done On Mrs. Rockefeller," *Washington Post*, November 26, 1974.

155. "Mrs. Rockefeller in Good Condition," *Washington Post*, November 27, 1974.

156. Lillian Barney, "Many More Women Seek Breast Cancer Exams, but Find Few Places to Go," *New York Times*, October 20, 1974.

157. Donald E. Henson and Lynn A. Ries, "Progress in Early Breast Cancer Detection," *Cancer* 65, no. S9 (May 1, 1990): 2155–58, https://doi.org/10.1002/1097-0142(19900501)65:9+<2155::AID-CNCR2820651412>3.0.CO;2-O.

158. Mrs. (Marvella) Birch Bayh, letter to "Ann Landers: Mastectomies . . ." *Washington Post*, June 2, 1974.

159. Barbara Gamarekian, "Marvella Bayh Is Dead of Cancer; Senator's Wife Reassured Others," *New York Times*, April 25, 1979.

160. Betty Rollin, *First, You Cry* (Philadelphia: Lippincott, 1976), "I thought of a newspaper interview with Marvella Bayh, the senator's wife who had had a mastectomy, that I had read a few weeks earlier," 37; visits Terese Lasser, 160–73; pages cited refer to Harper Collins paperback edition.

161. Ellen Leopold, "From the Closet to the Commonplace, 1945–75," in *A Darker Ribbon* (Boston: Beacon, 1999), 215–42.

162.   John Rockwell, "Minnie Riperton, 31; Soul Singer Lectured Nationally on Cancer," *New York Times*, July 13, 1979.

163.   Bob Lucas, "Minnie Riperton," *Ebony*, December 1976.

164.   "Cancer Society's '77 Courage Award to Minnie Riperton," *Philadelphia Tribune*, April 5, 1977.

165.   "Minnie Riperton Cited by President Carter," *New York Amsterdam News*, April 16, 1977.

166.   Keith Wailoo, introduction to *How Cancer Crossed the Color Line* (New York: Oxford University Press, 2011).

167.   Rose Kushner, "Breast Cancer Surgery: The Breast-Cancer Controversy," *Washington Post*, October 6, 1974.

168.   Rose Kushner, *Why Me?* (Philadelphia: W. B. Saunders, 1982).

169.   Ellen Leopold, *A Darker Ribbon* (Boston, MA: Beacon, 1999), Kushner's "intention to transform her personal experience into a public platform," 234; "I put another jacket on it [Kushner's book] so I could read it on the subway," 236.

170.   Barron H. Lerner, "No Shrinking Violet: Rose Kushner and the Maturation of Breast Cancer Activism," in *The Breast Cancer Wars* (New York: Oxford University Press, 2001), 170–95.

171.   Gina Kolata, "Rose Kushner, 60, Leader in Breast Cancer Fight," *New York Times*, January 10, 1990.

172.   Norman G. Rollins, "Cancer Hot Lines: Lifesaving Help by Telephone," *Good Housekeeping*, June 1977, 222–23.

173.   "Protesters Assail Refusal of Saks To Hire Woman After Mastectomy," *New York Times*, March 25, 1977; and Lee Miller, *The Cancer Challenge: Sharing the Experience* (Lincoln, NE: iUniverse, 2007), 1–6.

174.   Susan Sontag, *Illness as Metaphor* (New York: Farrar, Straus and Giroux, 1978) "to de-mythecize" conception of disease, 7; "mythology of cancer," Norman Mailer (comments of), Wilhelm Reich and "bio-energetic shrinking," 22–23; on Auden's Miss Gee, 48–49; "As far as I know, no oncologist convinced of the efficacy of polychemotherapy and immunotherapy," 53; "psychological theories of disease assign to the luckless ill the ultimate responsibility both for falling ill and for getting well," 57; "Reporters covering the 'war on cancer'" and "twin distortions," 66–67.

175.   Susan Sontag, "Illness as Metaphor," *New York Review of Books*, January 26, 1978 (part 1); "Images of Illness," *New York Review of Books*, February 9, 1978 (part 2); "Disease as Political Metaphor," *New York Review of Books*, February 23, 1978 (part 3).

176.   David Rieff, *Swimming in a Sea of Death: A Son's Memoir* (New York: Simon & Schuster, 2008). MDS diagnosis was a " 'death sentence,' as she put it," 45.

177.   Margalit Fox, "Susan Sontag, Social Critic with Verve, Dies at 71," *New York Times*, December 29, 2004.

178.   Chapter 7 in *Illness as Metaphor* concerns cancer and emotions, 50–57. In a footnote, Sontag refers to the work of Drs. Claus and Marjorie Bahnson, who "charted a personality pattern" relating to cancer, about whose Council for Tobacco Research ties she was likely unaware, and to Lawrence LeShan, the psychologist quoted in the *Ladies' Home Journal* on cancer's supposed emotional causes.

7. CANCER IN THE TIME OF AIDS (1980–1990)

1.   *Terms of Endearment*, directed by James L. Brooks (Hollywood: Paramount, 1983), 132 min. The film is based on the 1975 novel of the same name by Larry McMurtry.
2.   Larry McMurtry, *Terms of Endearment* (New York: Simon & Schuster, 1975).
3.   Douglas Brinkley, "After the Hurricane Winds Die Down, Larry McMurtry's Houston Trilogy Lives On," *New York Times*, September 14, 2017.
4.   N. Howlader, A. M. Noone, M. Krapcho, D. Miller, A. Brest, M. Yu, J. Ruhl, et al., *SEER Cancer Statistics Review 1975–2016* (Bethesda, MD: National Cancer Institute, 2019): table 2.8, https://seer.cancer.gov/archive/csr/1975_2016/results_single/sect_02_table.08.pdf.
5.   Shirley M. Bluethmann, Angela B. Mariotto, and Julia H. Rowland, "Anticipating the 'Silver Tsunami': Prevalence Trajectories and Comorbidity Burden Among Older Cancer Survivors in the United States," *Cancer Epidemiology, Biomarkers and Prevention* 25, no. 7 (2016): 1029–36, https://doi.org/10.1158/1055-9965.EPI-16-0133.
6.   Lawrence K. Altman, "Rare Cancer Seen in 41 Homosexuals," *New York Times*, July 3, 1981.
7.   Larry Kramer, "A Personal Appeal," *New York Native*, August 24–September 6, 1981. Reprinted in Larry Kramer, *Reports from the Holocaust: The Making of an AIDS Activist* (New York: St. Martin's, 1989), 8–9.
8.   Susan M. Chambré, "Managing the Madness," in *Fighting for Our Lives: New York's AIDS Community and the Politics of Disease* (New Brunswick, NJ: Rutgers University Press, 2006), GMHC founding and early years, 13–27.
9.   Randy Shilts, *And the Band Played On: Politics, People, and the AIDS Epidemic* (New York: St. Martin's, 1987), meeting in Larry Kramer's apartment, 90-1; Ward 5B 355–57, 394–6.
10. Sally Smith Hughes, "The Kaposi's Sarcoma Clinic at the University of California, San Francisco: An Early Response to the AIDS Epidemic," *Bulletin of the History of Medicine* 71, no. 4 (Winter 1997): 651–88.
11. David France, *How to Survive a Plague: The Inside Story of How Citizens and Science Tamed AIDS* (New York: Alfred A. Knopf, 2016), Denver meeting, "Fighting for Our Lives," 106–110; photo of "Gay Cancer" flyer in Castro Street pharmacy window (between 180–81).
12. "History," APLA Health, accessed May 19, 2022, https://aplahealth.org/about/history/.
13. Michael VerMeulen, "The Gay Plague," *New York Magazine*, May 31, 1982.
14. "Current Trends Update on Acquired Immune Deficiency Syndrome (AIDS)—United States," *Morbidity and Mortality Weekly Report* 31, no. 37 (September 24, 1982): 507–8, 513–14.
15. Katherine Bishop, "Ward 5B: A Model of Care for AIDS," *New York Times*, December 14, 1985.
16. Catherine Lucas, "The San Francisco Model and the Nurses of Ward 5B," *Lancet HIV* 6, no. 12 (August 9, 2019): E819, https://doi.org/10.1016/S2352-3018(19)30267-X.
17. Terry Gross, "First AIDS Ward '5B' Fought to Give Patients Compassionate Care, Dignified Deaths," *Fresh Air*, radio broadcast, NPR, Washington, DC, June 26, 2019, 41 min, https://www.npr.org/sections/health-shots/2019/06/26/736060834/1st-aids-ward-5b-fought-to-give-patients-compassionate-care-dignified-deaths.
18. Lindsey Gruson, "1,500 Attend Central Park Memorial Service for AIDS Victim," *New York Times*, June 14, 1983.

19. United Press International, "Thousands Expected at AIDS Candlelight Vigils," *San Francisco Examiner*, October 8, 1983.

20. Hugh Martin, "Candlelight Vigil Held for AIDS Sufferers," *Tampa Tribune-Times*, October 9, 1983.

21. United Press International, "Vigils Held for AIDS Victims," *New York Times*, October 9, 1983.

22. Audre Lorde, *The Cancer Journals* (San Francisco: Aunt Lute, 1980). Citations refer to 1997 Special Edition (paperback).

23. Lorde, *Cancer Journals*, Lorde learned that her brother-in-law's sister had had a mastectomy for breast cancer, 50–51.

24. Lorde, *Cancer Journals*, "Other one-breasted women hide behind the mask of prosthesis," 14; emphasis on wearing a prosthesis, 49.

25. Lorde, *Cancer Journals*, Reach to Recovery visitor, 57.

26. Lorde, *Cancer Journals*, "Well, women with breast cancer are warriors," 61–62.")

27. Genevieve Richardson, "Why I Refuse to Use Cancer Metaphors About a 'War,' 'Fight,' or 'Battle,'" *Self*, December 7, 2020, https://www.self.com/story/cancer-metaphors.

28. Jonathan M. Marron, Don S. Dizon, Banu Symington, Michael A. Thompson, and Abby R. Rosenberg, "Waging War on War Metaphors in Cancer and COVID-19," *JCO Oncology Practice* 16, no. 10 (October 1, 2020): 624–27, https://doi.org/10.1200/op.20.00542.

29. Alia E. Dastagir, "Characterizing Cancer as a 'War' Assumes It Can be Won. Is That Too Simple?," *USA Today*, October 7, 2021.

30. Lorde, *The Cancer Journals*, "I AM NOT ALONE," 63."

31. "Terry's Story," Terry Fox Foundation, accessed May 15, 2022, https://terryfox.org/terrys-story/.

32. Roy MacGregor, "The Nature of Heroism," *Maclean's*, January 12, 1981.

33. André Picard, "Terry Fox's Latest Contribution to Cancer Care: The Marathon of Hope Cancer Networks," *Globe and Mail*, April 12, 2019.

34. Gary Arnold, "Movie Hero Steve McQueen Dies of Heart Attack at Age of 50," *Washington Post*, November 8, 1980.

35. Barron H. Lerner, "McQueen's Legacy of Laetrile," *New York Times*, November 15, 2005.

36. Barron H. Lerner, "Unconventional Healing: Steve McQueen's Mexican Journey," in *When Illness Goes Public: Celebrity Patients and How We Look at Medicine* (Baltimore, MD: Johns Hopkins University Press, 2006), 139–58.

37. Timothy White, "Bob Marley: 1945–1981—The King of Reggae Finds His Zion," *Rolling Stone*, June 25, 1981.

38. Kat Arney, "Bob Marley, Genomics, and a Rare Form of Melanoma," Cancer Research UK (blog), August 20, 2014, https://scienceblog.cancerresearchuk.org/2014/08/20/bob-marley-genomics-and-a-rare-form-of-melanoma/.

39. Neil Singh, "Decolonising Dermatology: Why Black and Brown Skin Need Better Treatment," *Guardian*, August 13, 2020, https://www.theguardian.com/society/2020/aug/13/decolonising-dermatology-why-black-and-brown-skin-need-better-treatment.

40. Tara Westover, *Educated: A Memoir* (New York: Random House, 2018), 257–58.

41. Sue Smith, "Evangelist Oral Roberts Dedicates City of Faith," *Daily Oklahoman*, November 2, 1981.

42. Russell Chandler (Los Angeles Times Service), "Evangelist Says God Chose Him to Cure Cancer," *Austin American-Statesman*, January 18, 1983.

43. Wayne Biddle and Margo Slade, "Oral Roberts's Word on Cancer," *New York Times*, January 30, 1983.

44. Dan Balz, "Oral Roberts Quotes Plea from God," *Washington Post*, February 2, 1983.

45. "Financial Crisis Grips Oral Roberts's Medical Complex," *Christianity Today*, August 10, 1984, 46.

46. Paul Taylor, "Evangelist's Hospital Finds Debt in Empty Beds," *Washington Post*, July 5, 1984.

47. Associated Press, "Hospital Strains Oral Roberts' Purse Strings," *Hartford Courant*, March 29, 1987.

48. "Oral Roberts Plans to Close Hospital," *Business Chronicle* (Tulsa, OK), September 18, 1989.

49. Arnold Hamilton, "Oral Roberts to Shut Down Hospital and Medical School at Tulsa," *Washington Post*, September 16, 1989.

50. Garry Abrams, "Ebbing Empire," *Los Angeles Times*, October 20, 1989.

51. "Cancer Center Leases City of Faith," *Journal Record* (Oklahoma City, OK), January 25, 1990.

52. Robby Trammell, "Chicago Cancer Center Leases Tower at ORU's City of Faith," *Oklahoman*, January 25, 1990.

53. William Gaines and Bill Grady, "Hospital Reaping Huge Profits on Cancer Victim 'Guinea Pigs,'" *Chicago Tribune*, October 21, 1979.

54. Bill Grady, "Hospital's Cancer Care Called Danger to Public," *Chicago Tribune*, June 12, 1980.

55. William Gaines and Bill Grady, "Zion Hospital, Clinic Targets of Two Probes," *Chicago Tribune*, March 4, 1980.

56. William Gaines and Bill Grady, "Hospital Accused of 'Brain Washing'," *Chicago Tribune*, March 9, 1980.

57. Judy Klemesrud, "A Woman's Fight Against Breast Cancer," *New York Times*, August 5, 1985.

58. Klemesrud's *New York Times* story was picked up via syndication in "Personal Experience Furthers Woman's Fight Against Breast Cancer," *Tampa Bay Times*, August 14, 1985.

59. Klemesrud's syndicated piece also appeared in "Woman Declares War on Breast Cancer," *South Florida Sun-Sentinel*, October 15, 1985.

60. "Judy Klemesrud (1939–1985)," Iowa Women's Archives, University of Iowa Libraries, Iowa City, IA. An online biographical note provides some background on the *New York Times* reporter Judy Klemesrud, who died from cancer at forty-six in 1985 (shortly after publishing her story on Nancy Brinker), website accessed May 15, 2022, http://collguides .lib.uiowa.edu/?IWA0094.

    As we'll see, many journalists have been affected by cancer. Whether they need disclose a diagnosis as a source of potential bias is an open question.

61. Nancy Brinker, phone interview with the author, July 2, 2019.

62. Nancy G. Brinker and Joni Rodgers, *Promise Me* (New York: Three Rivers, 2010), [The journalists] "could call it 'female cancer' or 'a woman's cancer,'" 205.

63. Melva Weber, "Health: Breast-Health Groups Band Together," *Vogue*, September 1, 1986.

64. Amy Schiffman Langer, interview with the author, February 10, 2020.

65. "About NABCO," data from February 9, 2002, retrieved at *Internet Archive*, https://web .archive.org/web/20020209151734/http://www.nabco.org/index.php/12#cf.

66. Bill Stokes, "Breast Cancer's Biggest Foe May be Knowledge," *Chicago Tribune*, September 25, 1986.

67. Judy Foreman, "The War on Breast Cancer," *Ladies' Home Journal*, October 1988.

68. George Herbert W. Bush, *Proclamation 6202—National Breast Cancer Awareness Month, 1990* (Santa Barbara: American Presidency Project, University of California, Santa Barbara, 1990), https://www.presidency.ucsb.edu/node/268378.

69. "In the Slammer," *Pensacola News*, April 25, 1985.

70. "Jail-a-Thon to Aid Cancer Society," *Hartford Courant*, June 4, 1985.

71. "Wanted by the American Cancer Society" (advertisement), *Asheville Citizen-Times*, June 5, 1983.

72. "Don't Miss This Opportunity," (classified ads: "personals") *Daily Tar Heel* (Chapel Hill, NC) November 3, 1982.

73. "Roger O'Quinn Speaks at Annual Cancer Meeting," *Rocky Mount Telegram*, September 25, 1980.

74. "Civic Leader Nominees Announced (Rev. Joseph P. Traynor)," *Indiana Gazette* (Indiana, PA), November 1, 1978.

75. "On the Lighter Side," *Indiana Gazette*, October 16, 1980.

76. "Jail-a-Thon Aids Cancer Unit," *Morning Call* (Allentown, PA), August 8, 1985.

77. "Jail-a-Thon Will Benefit Cancer Society," *Arizona Daily Sun*, March 27, 1988.

78. "'Jail-a-Thon' Announced," *Casper Star-Tribune* (Casper, WY), December 5, 1985.

79. "Cancer Society Plans 'Jail-a-Thon' Fund-Raiser," *Atlanta Constitution*, March 22, 1984.

80. "Cancer Society to Kick Off Its Jail-a-Thon," *Atlanta Daily World*, June 20, 1986.

81. Benjamin Epstein, "Mock Jail Cells Used to Extract 'Bail' at Cancer Society Benefit," *Los Angeles Times*, August 7, 1986.

82. Philip M. Boffey, "After Years of Cancer Alarms, Progress Amid the Mistakes," *New York Times*, March 20, 1984.

83. Richard Doll and Richard Peto, "The Causes of Cancer: Quantitative Estimates of Avoidable Risks of Cancer in the United States Today," *Journal of the National Cancer Institute* 66, no. 6 (June 1981): 1192–308, https://doi.org/10.1093/jnci/66.6.1192.

84. Carol McGraw and Jay Sharbutt, "Rock Hudson's Battle with AIDS Gives Boost to Public Awareness," *Los Angeles Times*, July 27, 1985.

85. Scot Haller, "The Long Goodbye: Rock Hudson 1925–85," *People*, October 21, 1985.

86. Susan M. Chambré, *Fighting for Our Lives: New York's AIDS Community and the Politics of Disease* (New Brunswick, NJ: Rutgers University Press, 2006), Kramer spoke at the community center, 120–122; first ACT UP demonstration, 122–23.

87. Guy Trebay, "Into the Breach, Clad in Adolfo," *New York Times*, August 4, 2010.

88. "Dame Elizabeth Taylor," amfAR, accessed May 15, 2022, https://www.amfar.org/about-amfar/trustee-biographies/dame-elizabeth-taylor/.

89. Lou Cannon, "Reagan to Undergo Intestinal Surgery Today: Government to Be Run from President's Bedside," *Washington Post*, July 13, 1985.

90. Boyce Rensberger, "Reagan Tumor Removed; No Cancer Evident: President's Surgeons Optimistic Pending Malignancy Test Results" *Washington Post*, July 14, 1985.

91. "President, Recovering Well, Faces Weeks of Light Duty," *Washington Post*, July 15, 1985.

92. Reagan Tumor Found to be Cancerous"; Susan Okie and Cristine Russell, "Chances of a Full Cure Called Better Than 50–50"; Boyce Rensberger, "No Evidence of Spread to Other Organs Detected," *Washington Post*, July 16, 1985.

93.   "Reagan's Illness: Nation Is Informed; Explanations by 2 Cancer Surgeons at Bethesda News Parley," *New York Times*, July 16, 1985.

94.   "Doctors Have a Tense Debate: Reagan 'Has' or 'Had' Cancer?," *Los Angeles Times*, July 20, 1985.

95.   Thomas H. Maugh II, "Reagan's Surgery for Colon Cancer Breaks a Taboo, Brings a Floodtide of Calls," *Los Angeles Times*, July 27, 1985.

96.   Martin L. Brown and Arnold L. Potosky, "The Presidential Effect: The Public Health Response to Media Coverage About Ronald Reagan's Colon Cancer Episode," *Public Opinion Quarterly* 54, no. 3 (Fall 1990): 317–29, https://doi.org/10.1086/269209.

97.   Fitzhugh Mullan, *Vital Signs: A Young Doctor's Struggle with Cancer* (New York: Farrar Straus and Giroux, 1982).

98.   Fitzhugh Mullan, "Seasons of Survival: Reflections of a Physician with Cancer," *NEJM* 313, no. 4 (July 25, 1985): 270–3, https://doi.org/10.1056/nejm198507253130421.

99.   Kenneth Miller, Brian Merry, and Joan Miller, "Seasons of Survivorship Revisited," *Cancer Journal* 14, no. 6 (November 2008): 369–74, https://doi.org/10.1097/ppo.0b013e31818edf60.

100. Julia H. Rowland, "What Are Cancer Survivors Telling Us?," *Cancer Journal* 14, no. 6 (November/December): 361–68, https://doi.org/10.1097/ppo.0b013e31818ec48e.

101. Elaine Schattner, "Who's a Survivor?," *Slate*, October 5, 2010, https://slate.com/technology /2010/10/an-oncologist-who-s-had-breast-cancer-considers-the-problematic-phrase-cancer -survivor.html.

102. "Survivorship Terms," Office of Cancer Survivorship, Division of Cancer Control & Population Sciences," NCI, accessed May 15, 2022, https://cancercontrol.cancer.gov/ocs/definitions. "An individual is considered a cancer survivor from the time of diagnosis, through the balance of life."

103. Fitzhugh Mullan, "A Letter from the President of NCCS"; and group photo, in *NCCS Newsletter: A National Networking Publication* 1, no. 1 (March 1987): 2, 3.

104. "Founding Members," *NCCS Newsletter: A National Networking Publication* 1, no. 2 (Summer 1987): 6.

105. *NCCS Newsletter: A National Networking Publication* 2, no. 2 (Spring 1988).

106. Jane Erikson, "Richard Bloch, Cancer Advocate and Warrior, Dies of Heart Failure at 78," *Oncology Times* 26, no. 16 (August 25, 2004): 30–31, https://doi.org/10.1097/01.COT.0000292100 .92294.b1.

107. Annette Bloch and Richard Bloch, introduction to *Fighting Cancer* (Kansas City, MO: R. A. Bloch Cancer Foundation, 1985), 13–19.

108. Loni White, "Winners Address 'Pep Rally' for Cancer Fighters," *Kansas City Times*, June 2, 1986.

109. Associated Press, "Former Cancer Victim Tells Rally to Believe You Can Beat Disease," *Springfield Leader and Press* (Springfield, MO), June 2, 1986.

110. "Survivors' Day—Cancer Is Not a Death Sentence," *Asheville Citizen-Times* (Asheville, NC), November 1, 1987.

111. Jane Bryant, "Standing Out: I Really Don't Have Time for Cancer,'" *Pittsburgh Press*, May 24, 1988.

112. "On the Schedule: Cancer Survivors Celebrate," *Lincoln Star* (Lincoln, NE), June 2, 1988.

113. "Events," *Rapid City Journal* (Rapid City, SD), June 2, 1988.

114. Associated Press, "Balloons, Strawberries and a Star Send a Message on Beating Cancer," *Boston Globe*, June 6, 1988.

115. "About National Cancer Survivors Day," Official Website of National Cancer Survivors Day, accessed May 15, 2022, https://ncsd.org/about-us/.

116. William Robbins, "Kansas City Journal; Spreading the Word: Cancer Is Beatable," *New York Times*, June 4, 1990.

117. Irvin Molotsky, "U.S. Approves Drug to Prolong Lives of AIDS Patients," *New York Times*, March 21, 1987.

118. Mark H. Furstenberg, "AZT the First AIDS Drug," *Washington Post*, September 15, 1987.

119. Kent A. Sepkowitz, "AIDS—The First 20 Years," *NEJM* 344, no. 23 (June 7, 2001): 1764–72, https://www.nejm.org/doi/full/10.1056/NEJM200106073442306.

120. Marilyn Chase, "AIDS Drug Comes to a Market Worried About Its Cost—Limited Supply of AZT, Access to Treatment Poses Problems in U.S.," *Wall Street Journal*, March 23, 1987.

121. *The Normal Heart*, by Larry Kramer, directed by Michael Lindsay-Hogg, Public Theater, New York, NY, 1985. The 2011 production I attended ran at the John Golden Theater, 252 West 45th St., New York, NY.

122. Frank Rich, "Theater: 'The Normal Heart' by Larry Kramer," *New York Times*, April 22, 1985.

123. Larry Kramer, "The Beginning of ACTing UP," in *Reports from the Holocaust: The Story of an AIDS Activist* (New York: St. Martin's, 1994), 127–39.

124. Larry Kramer, "The F.D.A.'s Callous Response to AIDS," *New York Times*, March 23, 1987.

125. Jason Deparle, "Rude, Rash, Effective, Act-Up Shifts AIDS Policy," *New York Times*, January 3, 1990.

126. David Handelman, "Act Up in Anger: A Controversial Group Has Become the Catalyst for Innovations in the Way We Fight AIDS," *Rolling Stone*, March 8, 1990.

127. Elizabeth Fee, "The AIDS Memorial Quilt," *American Journal of Public Health* 96, no. 6 (June 2006): 979, https://doi.org/10.2105/ajph.2006.088575.

128. Theresa Machemer, "You Can Now Explore All 48,000 Panels of the AIDS Memorial Quilt Online," *Smithsonian Magazine*, July 21, 2020.

129. "The History of the Quilt," National AIDS Memorial, accessed May 15, 2022, https://www.aidsmemorial.org/quilt-history.

130. Gina Kolata, "Doctors Stretch Rules on AIDS Drug," *New York Times*, December 21, 1987.

131. "HIV and AIDS—United States, 1981–2000," *Morbidity and Mortality Weekly Report* 50, no. 21 (June 1, 2001): 430–34.

132. Howard Markel, "Remembering Ryan White, the Teen Who Fought Against the Stigma of AIDS," *PBS NewsHour*, PBS, April 8, 2016.

133. "Cancer Statistics, 1988," *CA: A Cancer Journal for Clinicians* 38, no. 1 (January/February 1988): 5–22, https://doi.org/10.3322/canjclin.38.1.5.

134. Gilda Radner, *It's Always Something* (New York: Simon & Schuster, 1989). "The Rotor" and humiliation, 47; "baldness like the mark on a house that was quarantined," 102; At the Wellness Community, "the most magic thing we have . . ." 126–27; on not "coping with cancer", she "was fighting," 199; doctor spoke to Gene, the "Alchemist," 69–70. Citations refer to 2009 paperback edition.

135.   John Kendall, "'Saturday Night Live' Star Gilda Radner Dies at 42," *Los Angeles Times*, May 21, 1989.

136.   Dennis Hevesi, "Gilda Radner, 42, Comic Original of 'Saturday Night Live' Zaniness," *New York Times*, May 21, 1989.

8. ENTHUSIASM (1990–2000)

1.   Paul Tsongas, *Heading Home* (New York: Alfred A. Knopf, 1984).

2.   "Tsongas, Paul Efthemios," History, Art & Archives, U.S. House of Representatives, accessed May 16, 2022, https://history.house.gov/People/Listing/T/TSONGAS,-Paul-Efthemios -(T000393)/.

3.   "Tsongas Said to Be 'Doing Well' After Bone Marrow Transplant," *Boston Globe*, September 5, 1986.

4.   Paul Richter, "'St. Paul' Against the Odds," *Los Angeles Times*, February 20, 1992.

5.   Bill McAllister, "Tsongas Is Gambling He'll Beat the Odds Again," *Washington Post*, February 4, 1992.

6.   Christopher B. Daly, "His Medical Story: After Beating a Rare Cancer, Paul Tsongas Sets His Sights on the Presidency," *Washington Post*, January 28, 1992.

7.   Dolores Kong, "Tsongas Overcame Odds with Transplant," *Boston Globe*, March 8, 1991.

8.   Steven Pearlstein, "Tsongas a Swim Against the Tide," *Washington Post*, April 11, 1991.

9.   Robin Toner, "Defying the Wisdom for '92, Ex-Senator Tsongas Dives In," *New York Times*, April 10, 1991.

10.   Dan Balz, Mark Stencel (Associated Press), "Tsongas Comes Up for Air," *Washington Post*, November 22, 1991.

11.   "Road to the White House 1992: Paul Tsongas Campaign Appearances," C-SPAN, April 29, 1991, accessed May 16, 2022, https://www.c-span.org/video/?17920-1/paul-tsongas-campaign -appearances.

12.   Renée Loth, "Fit for the Fight? Paul Tsongas Challenges Our Politics, and Our Attitudes About Cancer: A 'Survivor' Boldly Confronts Americans' Fear of the 'Big C,'" *Boston Globe*, April 28, 1991.

13.   Lawrence K. Altman, "The 1992 Campaign: Candidate's Health; Tsongas Doctors Say 2d Round of Cancer Was Treated in '87," *New York Times*, April 22, 1992.

14.   Lawrence K. Altman, "Preliminary Results of Biopsy Point to Return of Cancer in Tsongas," *New York Times*, November 26, 1992.

15.   Associated Press, "Tsongas Battling Cancer Again," *St. Louis Post-Dispatch*, December 1, 1992.

16.   Scot Lehigh, "Tsongas Is Said to Face New Battle with Cancer," *Boston Globe*, November 25, 1992.

17.   Richard A. Knox, "Tsongas Hospitalized for Rare Blood Disorder," *Boston Globe*, March 29, 1996.

18.   Dolores Kong, "Tsongas to Get Bone Marrow from Sister," *Boston Globe*, March 30, 1996.

19.   Karen de Witt, "Paul Tsongas, Who Made Presidential Bid, Dies at 55," *New York Times*, January 20, 1997.

20.   Gilles Salles, Martin Barrett, Robin Foà, Joerg Maurer, Susan O'Brien, Nancy Valente, Michael Wenger, and David G. Maloney, "Rituximab in B-Cell Hematologic Malignancies:

A Review of 20 Years of Clinical Experience," *Advances in Therapy* 34, no. 10 (October 5, 2017): 2232–73, https://doi.org/10.1007/s12325-017-0612-x.

21. A. J. Grillo-Lopez, C. A. White, B. K. Dallaire, C. L. Varns, C. D. Shen, A. Wei, J. E. Leonard, A. McClure, R. Weaver, S. Cairelli, and J. Rosenberg, "Rituximab: The First Monoclonal Antibody Approved for the Treatment of Lymphoma," *Current Pharmaceutical Biotechnology* 1, no. 1 (2000): 1–9, http://dx.doi.org/10.2174/1389201003379059.

22. Clifford A. Hudis, "Trastuzumab—Mechanism of Action and Use in Clinical Practice," *NEJM* 357, no. 1 (July 5, 2007): 39–51, https://doi.org/10.1056/NEJMra043186.

23. Sara A. Hurvitz, Karen A. Gelmon, and Sara M. Tolaney, "Optimal Management of Early and Advanced HER2 Breast Cancer," in *American Society of Clinical Oncology 2017 Educational Book* 37, ed. Don S. Dizon (Alexandria, VA: American Society of Clinical Oncology, 2017), 76–92, https://doi.org/10.1200/EDBK_175630.

24. Jane Lowe Meisel, Vyshak Alva Venur, Michael Gnant, and Lisa Carey, "Evolution of Targeted Therapy in Breast Cancer: Where Precision Medicine Began," in *American Society of Clinical Oncology 2018 Educational Book 38*, ed. Don S. Dizon (Alexandria, VA: American Society of Clinical Oncology, 2018), 78–86, https://doi.org/10.1200/EDBK_201037.

25. Nicholas Wade, "Scientist at Work: Judah Folkman; A Lonely Warrior Against Cancer," *New York Times*, December 9, 1997.

26. Nicholas Wade, "Progress Reported in Attacking Tumor Blood Supply," *New York Times*, March 16, 1999.

27. *Cancer Warrior*, directed by Nancy Linde (Boston: WGBH, February 27, 2001), 60 min.

28. Erika Check Hayden, "Cutting Off Cancer's Supply Lines," *Nature* 458, no. 7239 (April 9, 2009): 686–87, https://doi.org/10.1038/458686b.

29. Some doctors consider tamoxifen as the first targeted anticancer agent because it interferes specifically with estrogen receptors. The NCI publishes a fact sheet on targeted cancer treatments: "Targeted Cancer Therapies," accessed May 16, 2022, https://www.cancer.gov/about-cancer/treatment/types/targeted-therapies/targeted-therapies-fact-sheet.

30. Mark Jeffery, "Association of Cancer Online Resources," *Lancet Oncology* 2, no. 6 (June 2001): 391, https://doi.org/10.1016/s1470-2045(00)00398-3.

31. Matthew Holt, "ACOR, Health 2.0 in the US & Europe: Gilles Frydman Tells All," *Health Care Blog*, January 1, 2010, https://thehealthcareblog.com/blog/2010/01/01/acor-health-2-0-in-the-us-europe-gilles-frydman-tells-all/.

32. Barbara Lackritz, "Leukemia Links: Chronic Lymphocytic Leukemia—GrannyBarb's Story" and ACOR, "Multiple Myeloma Survivor's Stories," data from February 2, 1998 retrieved at *Internet Archive*, https://web.archive.org/web/19980202051059/http://www.acor.org/diseases/hematology/leukemia/ and https://web.archive.org/web/19980202051218/http://www.acor.org/diseases/hematology/MM/.

33. M. Teresa de la Morena and Richard A. Gatti, "A History of Bone Marrow Transplantation," *Hematology/Oncology Clinics of North America* 25, no. 1 (February 1, 2011): 1–15, https://doi.org/10.1016/j.hoc.2010.11.001.

34. J. Paul Eder, Karen Antman, William Peters, W. David Henner, Anthony Elias, Thomas Shea, Sue Schryber, et al., "High-Dose Combination Alkylating Agent Chemotherapy with Autologous Bone Marrow Support for Metastatic Breast Cancer," *Journal of*

Clinical Oncology 4, no. 11 (November 1, 1986): 1592–97, https://dx.doi.org/10.1200/jco .1986.4.11.1592.

35.   William P. Peters, R. Davis, Elizabeth J. Shpall, Roy B. Jones, Maureen Ross, Lawrence B. Marks, Larry Norton, and David D. Hurd, "Adjuvant Chemotherapy Involving High-Dose Combination Cyclophosphamide, Cisplatin, and Carmustine and Autologous Bone Marrow Support for Stage II/III Breast Cancer Involving Ten or More Lymph Nodes (CALGB 8782): A Preliminary Report" [Abstract], *Proceedings of the American Society of Clinical Oncology:* 9 (May, 1990).

36.   Michelle M. Mello and Troyen A. Brennan, "The Controversy Over High-Dose Chemotherapy with Autologous Bone Marrow Transplant for Breast Cancer," *Health Affairs* 20, no. 5 (September/October 2001): 101–17.

37.   Richard A. Rettig, Peter D. Jacobson, Cynthia M. Farquhar, and Wade M. Aubry, "Jumping the Gun," in *False Hope: Bone Marrow Transplantation for Breast Cancer* (New York: Oxford University Press, 2007), 35–69.

38.   Cheryl P. Weinstock, "Lawyers Debate the Insurability of Bone-Marrow Transplants," *New York Times*, March 20, 1994.

39.   Siddhartha Mukherjee, "The Map and the Parachute," in *The Emperor of All Maladies: A Biography of Cancer* (New York: Scribner, 2010), 321–29.

40.   Roberta Altman, *Waking Up, Fighting Back: The Politics of Breast Cancer* (Boston: Little, Brown, 1996), 212.

41.   Richard A. Rettig, Peter D. Jacobson, Cynthia M. Farquhar, and Wade M. Aubry, "Government Mandates," in *False Hope: Bone Marrow Transplantation for Breast Cancer* (New York: Oxford University Press, 2007), 152–77.

42.   Richard A. Rettig, Peter D. Jacobson, Cynthia M. Farquhar, and Wade M. Aubry, "Values in Conflict," in *False Hope: Bone Marrow Transplantation for Breast Cancer* (New York: Oxford University Press, 2007), 259–86.

43.   Kara Smigel, "Women Flock to ABMT for Breast Cancer Without Final Proof," *Journal of the National Cancer Institute* 87, no. 13 (July 5, 1995): 952–55, https://doi.org/10.1093 /jnci/87.13.952.

44.   Gina Kolata, "Women Resist Trials to Test Marrow Transplants," *New York Times*, February 15, 1995, https://www.nytimes.com/1995/02/15/us/women-resist-trials-to-test-marrow -transplants.html.

45.   Gina Kolata and Kurt Eichenwald, "Hope for Sale: A Special Report; Business Thrives on Unproven Care, Leaving Science Behind," *New York Times*, October 3, 1999.

46.   Denise Grady, "Breast Cancer Researcher Admits Falsifying Data," *New York Times*, February 5, 2000.

47.   Marc E. Lippman, "High-Dose Chemotherapy plus Autologous Bone Marrow Transplantation for Metastatic Breast Cancer," *NEJM* 342, no. 15 (April 13, 2000): 1119–20, https:// doi.org/10.1056/nejm200004133421508.

48.   Musa Mayer, "When Clinical Trials Are Compromised: A Perspective from a Patient Advocate," *PLoS Medicine* 2, no. 11 (October 18, 2005): E358, https://doi.org/10.1371/journal .pmed.0020358.

49.   Jim Lehrer, "Facing the Issue: Hope or Hype?," *NewsHour with Jim Lehrer*, PBS, May 13, 1999, 57:15, available at American Archive of Public Broadcasting, http://americanarchive .org/catalog/cpb-aacip-507-4j09w09m8k.

50. Fran Visco, "Lessons from Breast Cancer Advocacy," *Oncology Times* 25, no. 21 (November 10, 2003): 19, https://doi.org/10.1097/01.Cot.0000291049.00974.58.
51. Larry Kramer, "The F.D.A.'s Callous Response to AIDS," *New York Times*, March 23, 1987.
52. Gerald E. Parsons, "Yellow Ribbons: Ties with Tradition," *Folklife Center News* 4, no. 2 (Summer 1981), https://www.loc.gov/folklife/ribbons/ribbons_81.html.
53. Gerald E. Parsons, "How the Yellow Ribbon Became a National Folk Symbol," *Folklife Center News* 13, no. 3 (Summer 1991): 9–11, https://www.loc.gov/folklife/ribbons/ribbons.html.
54. Jesse Green, "The Year of the Ribbon," *New York Times*, May 3, 1992.
55. "The Red Ribbon Project," Visual AIDS, accessed May 17, 2022, https://visualaids.org/projects/the-red-ribbon-project#.UhoZ1bxgPCo.
56. "5K Run!," *Daily News*, August 25, 1991.
57. Nadine Brozan, "Chronicle," Richard Johnson, column: listing, *New York Times*, September 21, 1991.
58. Richard Johnson, listing under "Young-ian Psychology: Sean & Men," *Daily News*, October 13, 1991.
59. "News from the Greater New York City Affiliate of Susan G. Komen for the Cure," *Connection* (Susan G. Komen for the Cure Greater New York City (Winter 2010).
60. "History of Komen Greater New York City," data from January 21, 2019 retrieved at *Internet Archive*, https://web.archive.org/web/20190121160213/http://www.komennyc.org/site/PageServer?pagename=about_history.
61. "Surfacing," *New York Times*, September 27, 1992.
62. Liz Smith, "Is Perot a Comeback Kid?," *Newsday*, July 29, 1992.
63. Kathleen Hendrix, "Peach Corps: Activism: Breast Cancer Has Afflicted Her Grandmother, Sister and Daughter, so Charlotte Haley Is Urging People to Wear Ribbons to 'Wake Up' America," *Los Angeles Times*, August 20, 1992.
64. "In Memoriam: Charlotte Haley, Creator of the First (Peach) Breast Cancer Ribbon," Breast Cancer Action, accessed May 17, 2022, https://www.bcaction.org/2014/06/24/in-memoriam-charlotte-haley-creator-of-the-first-peach-breast-cancer-ribbon/.
65. "*Self* Announces National Breast Cancer Awareness Campaign: 'Activist' Magazine Teams with Estee Lauder to Distribute Pink Ribbons," PR Newswire, September 11, 1992.
66. Enid Nemy, "At Work With: Evelyn Lauder; From Pink Lipstick to Pink Ribbons," *New York Times*, February 2, 1995.
67. Alexandra Penney, *The Bag Lady Papers: The Priceless Experience of Losing It All* (New York: Hachette, 2010), 173–76.
68. Cathy Horyn, "Evelyn H. Lauder, Champion of Breast Cancer Research, Dies at 75," *New York Times*, November 13, 2011.
69. David W. Grogan, "Stricken with a Deadly Cancer, Michael Landon Vows He'll Fight Back with Medicine and Prayer," *People Weekly*, April 22, 1991.
70. "With Courage and Character," *People Weekly*, May 6, 1991.
71. Mark Goodman, "Goodbye, Little Joe," *People Weekly*, July 15, 1991.
72. Peter B. Flint, "Michael Landon, 54, Little Joe on 'Bonanza' for 14 Years, Dies," *New York Times*, July 2, 1991.
73. Marci A. Landsmann, "TV's Family Man," *Cancer Today*, March 17, 2017.
74. "Audrey Hepburn's Tumor Found to Be Cancerous," *Los Angeles Times*, November 4, 1992.

75.   Scott Harris, "Audrey Hepburn, Actress and Humanitarian, Dies," *Los Angeles Times*, January 21, 1993.

76.   Caryn James, "Audrey Hepburn, Actress, Is Dead at 63," *New York Times*, January 21, 1993.

77.   Paul Feldman, "Frank Zappa, Iconoclast of Rock, Dies at 52," *Los Angeles Times*, December 6, 1993.

78.   Jamie Gangel, "Interview with Frank Zappa," *Today*, NBC, May 14, 1993. Available at https://youtu.be/UDYzuwG-gOE.

79.   Robert D. McFadden, "Jacqueline Kennedy Onassis Has Lymphoma," *New York Times*, February 11, 1994.

80.   Malcolm Gladwell, "Jacqueline Kennedy Onassis Dies at 64: Non-Hodgkin's Lymphoma Kills Former First Lady Noted for Her Style, Grace," *Washington Post*, May 20, 1994.

81.   Associated Press, "Gravely Ill Onassis Goes Home After Halting Cancer Treatment," *Deseret News*, May 19, 1994.

82.   Robert D. McFadden, "Death of a First Lady; Jacqueline Kennedy Onassis Dies of Cancer at 64," *New York Times*, May 20, 1994.

83.   Fran Visco, interview with the author, July 24, 2019.

84.   Amy Schiffman Langer, interview with the author, February 10, 2020.

85.   Susan M. Love and Karen Lindsey, *Dr. Susan Love's Breast Book* (Reading, MA: Addison-Wesley, 1990).

86.   Fran Visco, "Preparing for a Seat at the Research Table: The National Breast Cancer Coalition Fund's Project LEAD," *Journal of Oncology Practice* 1, no. 3 (September 2005): 125, https://doi.org/10.1200/jop.2005.1.3.125.

87.   Maren Klawiter, *The Biopolitics of Breast Cancer* (Minneapolis: University of Minnesota Press, 2008). In this sociological analysis of breast cancer activism in 1990s San Francisco, the author describes three coexisting "cultures of action" with distinct priorities, advocacy styles, and attitudes toward science, 40–48.

88.   Susan Ferraro, "The Anguished Politics of Breast Cancer" *New York Times Magazine*, August 15, 1993.

89.   Pia Peterson, "The Times Magazine Cover That Beamed a Light on a Movement," *New York Times*, August 15, 2018.

90.   Catherine C. Boring, Teresa S. Squires, and Tony Tong, "Cancer Statistics, 1993," *CA: A Cancer Journal for Clinicians* 43, no. 1 (January/February 1993): 7–26, https://dx.doi.org/10.3322/canjclin.43.1.7.

91.   Table IV-5 "Female Breast Cancer (Invasive)" and Figure IV-3, "Breast Cancer Stage Distribution," in *SEER Cancer Statistics Review, 1973–1993* (Bethesda, MD: National Cancer Institute IV-3, accessed May 17, 2022, https://seer.cancer.gov/archive/csr/1973_1993/breast.pdf.

92.   Roxanne Roberts, "Milken's Rising Stock; Junk Bond King Spearheads Cancer Fight," *Washington Post*, November 6, 1993.

93.   William D. Cohan, "Michael Milken Invented the Modern Junk Bond, Went to Prison, and then Became One of the Most Respected People on Wall Street," *Business Insider*, May 2, 2017.

94.   "Michael Milken's Career," *New York Times*, October 26, 2019.

95.   Reis Thebault, "Who Is Michael Milken, the 'Junk Bond King' Trump Just Pardoned?," *Washington Post*, February 18, 2020.

96.   "PCF Timeline," Prostate Cancer Foundation, accessed May 17, 2022, https://www.pcf
       .org/timeline/.

97.   David Vise, "The Redemption of Michael Milken: The Former Junk Bond Giant, Feted by
       King, Cosby, Calvin and . . . Clinton?," *Washington Post*, April 22, 1994.

98.   "Rethinking the War on Cancer: Moving from a War of Attrition to a Plan of Attack:
       Remarks by Michael Milken, Founder and Chairman, The Prostate Cancer Foundation,
       National Cancer Summit, Washington, DC, November 14, 1995," Michael Milken, Novem-
       ber 14, 1995, https://www.mikemilken.com/articles.taf?page=23.

99.   Andrew Holtz, Lou Waters (host), "Cancer Research Can Benefit from Investment
       Credits," CNN, November 14, 1995.

100.   Daniel Q. Haney, "Prostate Cancer Spurs Milken Into Research: Diagnosis Prompts Him
       to Helm of an Unprecedented Effort," *San Francisco Examiner*, November 26, 1995.

101.   "Milken Calls for Renewed War on Cancer, $20 Billion a Year International Effort," *Can-
       cer Letter* 21, no. 45 (November 24, 1995): 1–7.

102.   Peter Monaghan, "Attack on Prostate Cancer," *Chronicle of Higher Education* 41, no. 39
       (June 9, 1995). A29–30.

103.   Cora Daniels, "The Man Who Changed Medicine," *Fortune*, November 29, 2004.

104.   *Seinfeld*, "The Scofflaw," season 6, episode 13, directed by Andy Ackerman, NBC, January
       26, 1996.

105.   Edward C. Kaps, "The Role of the Support Group, 'Us Too,'" *Cancer* 74, no. S7 (October
       1, 1994): 2188–89, https://doi.org/10.1002/1097-0142%2819941001%2974%3A7%2B%3C2188
       %3A%3AAID-CNCR2820741732%3E3.0.CO%3B2-9.

106.   Karen M. Kedrowski and Marilyn Stine Sarow, *Cancer Activism: Gender, Media, and Public
       Policy* (Champaign: University of Illinois Press, 2007), 29–36.

107.   Edward Kaps, John Moenck, and Gerald Chodak, "Us TOO International—How It All
       Started," Archive: Us TOO Website, https://zerocancer.org/ustoo/History-of-Us-TOO/.
       (Originally published as "The Origin of Support Groups for Prostate Cancer Survivors
       and Their Families," *Family Urology* 6, no. 4 [November 2001].)

108.   Claudette Krizek, Cleora Roberts, Robin Ragan, Jeffrey J. Ferrara, and Beth Lord, "Gen-
       der and Cancer Support Group Participation," *Cancer Practice* 7, no. 2 (March/April 1999):
       86–92, https://doi.org/10.1046/j.1523-5394.1999.07206.x.

109.   Darice Bailer, "Support Group for Men with Prostate Cancer," *New York Times*, June 7, 1998.

110.   Jeannine Coreil and Ravish Behal, "Man to Man Prostate Cancer Support Groups," *Cancer
       Practice* 7, no. 3 (May/June 1999): 122–29, https://doi.org/10.1046/j.1523-5394.1999.07307.x.

111.   Rick Davis, interview with the author, November 7, 2019.

112.   Leon Jaroff, "The Man's Cancer," *Time*, April 1, 1996.

113.   Christine Gorman, "The Politics of Bob Dole's Prostate Cancer," *Time*, April 1, 1996.

114.   Anatole Broyard, *Intoxicated by My Illness* (New York: Clarkson Potter, 1992).

115.   Roxanne Roberts, "The Message Hits Home: Support for Mayor Barry at Cancer
       Research Dinner," *Washington Post*, November 16, 1995.

116.   "Arnold Palmer Is Diagnosed with Prostate Cancer," *San Diego Union-Tribune*, January 12, 1997.

117.   Jeff Babineau, "Palmer Begins His Fight Today; Golfer Arnold Palmer, Diagnosed with
       Prostate Cancer, Will Undergo Tests to Determine How Best to Treat the Disease,"
       Orlando Sentinel, January 13, 1997.

118.   "I'll Be Back: Yank Skipper Vows He'll Beat Prostate Cancer," *New York Daily News*, March 11, 1999.

119.   Shaun Powell, "Count on Joe to Beat It/Torre's Too Tough for Cancer," *Newsday*, March 11, 1999.

120.   "Roger Moore Undergoes Prostate Surgery," *Associated Press*, November 8, 1993.

121.   Moira Petty, "You Only Live Twice . . . Unless You're Roger Moore, and You've Beaten Heart Disease, Cancer and Pneumonia," *Daily Mail*, April 10, 2007.

122.   Roger Moore and Owen Gareth, *My Word Is My Bond* (New York: Collins, 2008), 306.

123.   "Obituary: Sir Roger Moore," *BBC News*, May 23, 2017.

124.   Margaret Edson, *W;t* (New York: Faber and Faber, 1993). Early performances of this play, featuring Kathleen Chalfant as Vivian, took place in Los Angeles, off Broadway in New York, and in Houston. A 2001 film adaptation starred Emma Thompson. The 2012 Broadway production, by the Manhattan Theater Company, starred Cynthia Nixon.

125.   Elaine Schattner, "What We're Talking About When We're Talking About Cancer," *Atlantic*, February 28.

126.   Lorrie Moore, "People Like That Are the Only People Here," *New Yorker*, January 27, 1997. This short story also appears in Lorrie Moore's 1998 collection of fiction, *Birds of America* (Knopf).

127.   "Lorrie Moore: Flipping Death the Bird," *Publisher's Weekly*, August 24, 1998.

128.   "William Tipping Leads American Cancer Society Into 1990's," *Journal of the National Cancer Institute* 81, no. 5 (March 1, 1989): 327–30, https://doi.org/10.1093/jnci/81.5.327.

129.   "Cancer Society to Dedicate Building," *Atlanta Constitution*, June 8, 1989.

130.   "History," Ovarian Cancer Research Alliance, accessed May 17, 2022, https://ocrahope.org/about/history/; "History of the Lustgarten Foundation," Lustgarten Foundation for Pancreatic Cancer Research, accessed June 14, 2022, https://lustgarten.org/leadership/story/; "Our History—Allies from the Start," Colorectal Cancer Alliance, accessed May 17, 2022, https://www.ccalliance.org/about/our-history.

131.   Christopher Anderson, "Uncharitable Actions," *Nature* 347, no. 6295 (October 25, 1990): 702, http://dx.doi.org/10.1038/347702b0.

132.   Judy Ward, "Cancerous Growth," *Financial World*, September 1, 1994, 54.

133.   PR Newswire, "Olive Garden Celebrates 20th Anniversary," press release, December 17, 2002, https://s2.q4cdn.com/922937207/files/doc_news/news_2002/news_2002_general/DRI_News_2002_12_17_General.pdf.

134.   "Giving Pennies," *Fort Worth Star-Telegram*, March 27, 2002.

135.   Jennifer Huberdeau, "Change for Charity," *North Adams Transcript*, February 14, 2009.

136.   Herald Wire Services, "Another Reason to Root for Homers," *Miami Herald*, June 13, 1997.

137.   Christopher Snowbeck, "Raising Money to Cure Prostate Cancer," *Pittsburgh Post-Gazette*, June 16, 1998.

138.   Jennifer Mann Fuller, "Social Campaigns Are on the Rise," *Kansas City Star*, October 5, 1996.

139.   Deborah Cushman, "Don Denims, Help Fight Breast Cancer," *Des Moines Register*, September 16, 1997.

140.   Denise Gellene, "Breast Cancer Strikes Chord with Corporations," *Los Angeles Times*, October 30, 1997.

141. Leukemia & Lymphoma Society, *Relentless for the Cures: 2000 Annual Report* (White Plains, NY: Leukemia & Lymphoma Society, 2000), 14, https://www.lls.org/sites/default/files/National/USA/Pdf/LLS_AR_2000.pdf.

142. Roxanne Roberts, "The First Lady's Women's Crusade: Some Critics Say Hillary Clinton Has Taken On a 'Safe' Issue. To Her, Breast Cancer Is Anything But," *Washington Post*, May 6, 1995.

143. Lisa Belkin, "Charity Begins at . . . the Marketing Meeting, the Gala Event, the Product Tie-In," *New York Times Magazine*, December 22, 1996.

144. Andrew Longmore, "Cycling: Strong Rider Out of the Storm: First Night: Lance Armstrong: An American Hero Can Claim His First Major Victory Since Beating Cancer," *Independent* (London, UK), October 11, 1998.

145. Associated Press, "Winning an Uphill Battle: The Tour De France Enters the Alps Today, but Leader Lance Armstrong Has Already Traveled a More Difficult Road in His Fight Against Cancer," Cleveland *Plain Dealer*, July 13, 1999.

146. Daniel Zwerdling and David Kestenbaum, "Profile: Cyclist Lance Armstrong and His Bout with Testicular Cancer," *All Things Considered* radio broadcast, NPR, Washington, DC, July 24, 1999. Lance Armstrong and his oncologist, Dr. Lawrence Einhorn, were interviewed.

147. Christopher Clarey, "Cycling; Throng Applauds American in Paris," *New York Times*, July 26, 1999.

148. Philip Hersh, "Cyclist Rides to a Miracle Less Than Three Years After Being Gravely Ill with Cancer, Lance Armstrong Wins the Grueling Tour de France," *Chicago Tribune*, July 26, 1999.

149. Randy Harvey, "Success Story: Tour de Lance; Armstrong's Miraculous Comeback from Cancer to a Tour Victory Is Worthy of an Exclamation Point, not a Question Mark," *Los Angeles Times*, July 26, 1999.

150. "Lance Armstrong's Victory Over Cancer, Tour de France Course Inspires World," *Detroit Free Press*, July 26, 1999.

151. Richard Hoffer, "Tour de Lance," *Sports Illustrated*, July 26, 1999.

152. Lance Armstrong with Sally Jenkins, *It's Not About the Bike: My Journey Back to Life* (New York: Putnam, 2000), 288.

153. Lawrence H. Einhorn, "Treatment of Testicular Cancer: A New and Improved Model," *Journal of Clinical Oncology* 8, no. 11 (November 1, 1990): 1777–81, https://doi.org/10.1200/jco.1990.8.11.1777.

154. Matthew James Reilley and Lance C. Pagliaro, "Testicular Choriocarcinoma: A Rare Variant That Requires a Unique Treatment Approach," *Current Oncology Reports* 17, no. 2 (February 3, 2015): 2, https://doi.org/10.1007/s11912-014-0430-0.

155. Juliet Macur, "Details of Doping Scheme Paint Armstrong as Leader," *New York Times*, October 10, 2012.

156. Dave Harmon and Suzanne Halliburton, "Cycling Team Describes Doping Culture," *Austin American-Statesman*, November 18, 2012.

157. Elaine Schattner, "Reconciling Lance Armstrong's Story with the Realities of Cancer Survival," *Atlantic*, December 7, 2012.

158. B. J. Druker, et al., Abstract # 1639 *Blood* S94 (1999), presented at the 41st annual meeting of the American Society of Hematology, New Orleans LA, December 3–7, 1999.

159. Associated Press, "Experimental Leukemia Pill Shows Great Promise," *Minneapolis Star Tribune*, December 4, 1999.

160. Charles L. Sawyers, "Chronic Myeloid Leukemia," *NEJM* 340, no. 17 (April 29, 1999): 1330–40, https://www.nejm.org/doi/full/10.1056/NEJM199904293401706.

161. Hannah Bower, Magnus Björkholm, Paul W. Dickman, Martin Höglund, Paul C. Lambert, and Therese M. L. Andersson, "Life Expectancy of Patients with Chronic Myeloid Leukemia Approaches the Life Expectancy of the General Population," *Journal of Clinical Oncology* 34, no. 24 (August 20, 2016): 2851–57, https://doi.org/10.1200/jco.2015.66.2866.

162. *Fight Club*, directed by David Fincher (United States: Twentieth Century Fox, 1999), 139 min.

9. COMPLICATIONS (2000–2010)

1. *Today*, "Katie Couric Gets a Colonoscopy," produced by Jeff Zucker, NBC, March 7, 2000.

2. *The Daily Show with Jon Stewart*, "Other News: Public Enema," season 4, episode 106, Comedy Central, March 7, 2000, https://www.cc.com/video/u03wrn/the-daily-show-with-jon-stewart-other-news-public-enema.

3. Lisa de Moraes, "NBC Tests Viewers' Intestinal Fortitude on 'Today,'" *Washington Post*, March 8, 2000.

4. Biography, "Katie Couric—First Woman to Anchor the CBS Evening News Alone," YouTube video, 2:45, uploaded February 25, 2014, https://youtu.be/yTihJ52GBeE.

5. Howard Rosenberg, "Couric's Crusade Is a True TV Public Service," *Los Angeles Times*, March 10, 2000.

6. Christine Gorman "Katie's Crusade," *Time*, March 13, 2000.

7. Lloyd Grove, "The New Man of 'Today': Illness and Marriage Have Tempered Hotshot Producer Jeff Zucker," *Washington Post*, November 12, 1998.

8. Gabriel Sherman, "Jeff Zucker Has Endured Cancer, Hollywood, and Being TV's Wunderkind. So Why Not Take on CNN?," *New York*, October 5, 2014.

9. *Colon Cancer: Greater Use of Screenings Would Save Lives—Hearing Before the Special Committee on Aging*, 106th Cong., 2nd Sess. (March 6, 2000).

10. Peter Cram, A. Mark Fendrick, John Inadomi, Mark E. Cowen, Daniel Carpenter, and Sandeep Vijan, "The Impact of a Celebrity Promotional Campaign on the Use of Colon Cancer Screening: The Katie Couric Effect," *Archives of Internal Medicine* 163, no. 13 (July 14, 2003): 1601–5, https://doi.org/10.1001/archinte.163.13.1601.

11. Barbara Ehrenreich, "Welcome to Cancerland," *Harper's Magazine*, November 1, 2001. Ehrenreich refers to "Breast Cancer Talk Project," data from November 30, 2001 retrieved at *Internet Archive*, https://web.archive.org/web/20011130020705/http://breastcancertalk.org.

12. Larry McMurtry, *Terms of Endearment* (New York: Simon & Schuster, 1975).

13. *Terms of Endearment*, directed by James L. Brooks (Hollywood: Paramount Pictures, 1983), 132 min. The film is based on the 1975 novel of the same name by Larry McMurtry.

14. *Sex and the City*, "The Ick Factor," season 6, episode 14, directed by Wendey Stanzler, HBO, January 11, 2004.

15. *Sex and the City*, "Catch-38," season 6, episode 15, directed by Michael Engler, HBO, January 18, 2004.

16. *Sex and the City*, "Out of the Frying Pan," season 6, episode 16, directed by Michael Engler, HBO, January 25, 2004.

17. Greg Kot, "The Grammys," *Chicago Tribune*, February 14, 2005.

18. Lynette Rice, "Grammys Flashback: Melissa Etheridge Reflects on Her Powerful 2005 Performance," *Entertainment Weekly*, January 28, 2018, https://ew.com/grammys/2018/01/28/grammys-flashback-melissa-etheridge-reflects-on-her-powerful-2005-performance/.

19. Anne Cassidy, "'So Many Women Are Surviving This,'" *Good Housekeeping*, September 1993.

20. "At Home with Olivia Newton-John," *Ladies' Home Journal*, April 1994, 158–61.

21. George Rush, Joanna Molloy, Marcus Baram, and K. C. Baker, "Carly Simon Battles Back from Breast Cancer," *New York Daily News*, May 5, 1998.

22. "Carly Simon Fighting Breast Cancer," CNN.com, May 5, 1998, http://www.cnn.com/SHOWBIZ/9805/05/carly.simon/.

23. "Carly Simon Doesn't Want Sympathy," *St. Petersburg Times* (St. Petersburg, FL), May 6, 1998.

24. Associated Press, "Sheryl Crow Undergoes Surgery for Breast Cancer," *Los Angeles Times*, February 25, 2006.

25. Gary Marks, "Faithfull Has Breast Cancer," *Birmingham Mail*, September 14, 2006.

26. "Weekend Pop! Faithfull Diagnosed with Cancer," *Boston Globe*, September 15, 2006.

27. "Cynthia Nixon's 'Survival and the City,'" CBS News, October 29, 2008, https://www.cbsnews.com/news/cynthia-nixons-survival-and-the-city/.

28. Lena Huang, "Q&A with Cynthia Nixon," *Cure Today*, May 12, 2011.

29. Dan Fletcher, "A Brief History of Wikipedia," *Time*, August 18, 2009.

30. Bill Thompson, "What Is It with Wikipedia?," BBC News, December 16, 2005, http://news.bbc.co.uk/2/hi/technology/4534712.stm.

31. Jessica E. Slavin, "Court Holds That Wikipedia Entries Are 'Inherently Unreliable,'" *Marquette University Law School Faculty Blog*, November 24, 2008, https://law.marquette.edu/facultyblog/2008/11/court-holds-that-wikipedia-entries-are-inherently-unreliable/.

32. "List of People with Breast Cancer," accessed May 18, 2022, Wikipedia, https://en.wikipedia.org/wiki/List_of_people_with_breast_cancer. Wikipedia lists those affected by profession as follows: acting, business, miscellaneous, music, politics and government, royalty, science, sports, television and radio, visual arts, and writing. See also "List of Breast Cancer Patients by Survival Status," Wikipedia, accessed May 18, 2022, https://en.wikipedia.org/wiki/List_of_breast_cancer_patients_by_survival_status. This page lists those affected by breast cancer status as follows: alive, died due to breast cancer, death attributed to other causes.

33. Phil Wahba, "Former KISS drummer: Men Get Breast Cancer Too," Reuters, October 22, 2009, https://www.reuters.com/article/us-kiss-cancer/former-kiss-drummer-men-get-breast-cancer-too-idUSTRE59L3DO20091022.

34. Robin Roberts, "ABC's Robin Roberts: 'I Have Breast Cancer,'" ABC News, July 31, 2007, https://abcnews.go.com/GMA/CancerPreventionAndTreatment/abcs-robin-roberts-breast-cancer/story?id=3430554.

35. Ann Powers, "Joey Ramone, Punk's Influential Yelper, Dies at 49," *New York Times*, April 16, 2001.

36. Ben Sisario, "Johnny Ramone, Pioneer Punk Guitarist, Is Dead at 55," *New York Times*, September 17, 2004.

37. Charles M. Young, "The Last Days of Johnny Ramone," *Rolling Stone*, October 14, 2004.

38. Mikal Gilmore, "The Curse of the Ramones," *Rolling Stone*, April 21, 2016.

39. Allan Kozinn, "Linda McCartney, Photographer of Rock Stars, Dies at 56," *New York Times*, April 20, 1998.

40. Richard Skanse, "Linda McCartney Dies at 56," *Rolling Stone*, April 20, 1998.

41. Allan Kozinn, "George Harrison, Former Beatle, Dies at 58," *New York Times*, November 30, 2001.

42. Oliver Poole, Hugh Davies, and Amit Roy, "The World Gently Weeps for George," *Sun Herald*, December 2, 2001.

43. David Fricke, "Q&A: Charlie Watts—An Interview with the Famed Rolling Stones Drummer About Throat Cancer and Recovery," *Rolling Stone*, September 22, 2005.

44. Associated Press, "Grateful Dead Bassist Lesh Has Prostate Cancer," Today.com, November 1, 2006, https://www.today.com/popculture/grateful-dead-bassist-lesh-has-prostate-cancer-1C9428470.

45. Campbell Robertson, "Pavarotti Has Surgery for Pancreatic Cancer," *New York Times*, July 8, 2006.

46. Bernard Holland, "Luciano Pavarotti Is Dead at 71," *New York Times*, September 6, 2007.

47. Renee Montagne and Steve Inskeep, "Luciano Pavarotti Succumbs to Cancer at 71," *Morning Edition*, radio broadcast, NPR, Washington, DC, September 6, 2007, 1 min, https://www.npr.org/templates/story/story.php?storyId=14204611.

48. *The Farewell*, directed by Lulu Wang (New York: A24, 2019), 100 min.

49. Kenneth Miller, "Kathy Bates on Road Trips, Surviving Cancer and Being a Late Bloomer," *AARP The Magazine*, October/November 2013.

50. Gina Shaw, "Kathy Bates Reflects on Life with Lymphedema," WebMD, April 6, 2017. https://www.webmd.com/cancer/features/kathy-bates-life-with-lymphedema#5.

51. Mackenzie Brown and Jennifer Graham Kizer, "Edie Falco Talks About Her Breast Cancer Journey," Health.com, April 26, 2011, data from February 13, 2022 retrieved from *Internet Archive*, https://web.archive.org/web/20220213040602/https://www.health.com/celebrities/edie-falco-talks-about-her-breast-cancer-journey.

52. *Anderson Live*, "Edie Falco Explains Why She Kept Mum About Her Cancer," CNN, April 11, 2012, YouTube video, 1:15, uploaded April 11, 2012, https://youtu.be/v2x1mRIQnH4.

53. Jacob Bernstein, "Nora Ephron's Final Act," *New York Times Magazine*, March 10, 2013.

54. Geoff Berkshire, " 'Everything Is Copy': Jacob Bernstein Talks Nora Ephron's Legacy and His Documentary Debut," *Variety*, March 21, 2016.

55. Nora Ephron, *I Feel Bad About My Neck* (New York: Knopf, 2006).

56. Nora Ephron, "Considering the Alternative," in *I Feel Bad About My Neck* (New York: Knopf, 2006), 127–37.

57. Charles McGrath, "Nora Ephron Dies at 71; Writer and Filmmaker with a Genius for Humor," *New York Times*, June 27, 2012.

58. Dan Balz and Rob Stein, "Kerry to Have Surgery for Prostate Cancer: Doctors Give 90 Percent Chance of Full Recovery," *Washington Post*, February 12, 2003.

59. Dan Balz, "Kerry Surgery Called Success," *Washington Post*, February 13, 2003.

60. Lawrence K. Altman, "On Kerry's Journey to Health, Stops for Shrapnel and Cancer," *New York Times*, October 3, 2004.

61. Pui-Wing Tam, "Apple Computer CEO Jobs Undergoes Successful Surgery," *Wall Street Journal*, August 2, 2004 .

62. Nick Wingfield, "Jobs Struggled with Health Problems for Years," *Wall Street Journal*, August 25, 2011.

63. John Markoff, "Steven P. Jobs, 1955–2011: Apple's Visionary Redefined Digital Age," *New York Times*, October 5, 2011.

64. Jessica E. Vascellaro, "Steve Jobs Downplayed His Cancer, Biographer Says," *Wall Street Journal*, October 24, 2011.

65. Charles Ornstein, "UCLA Hospital Scandal Grows; Some 127 Employees Peeked at Celebrities' Records, State Says, Nearly Double the Number First Reported," *Los Angeles Times*, August 5, 2008.

66. Charles Ornstein, "No Hiding Her Illness; Farrah Fawcett Says Her Struggle with Cancer Was Worsened By Breaches of Privacy. She Hopes Her Fight Helps Future Patients," *Los Angeles Times*, May 11, 2009.

67. "Ryan O'Neal Has Leukemia," CNN.com, May 2, 2001, http://www.cnn.com/2001/SHOWBIZ /Movies/05/02/oneal.cancer/index.html.

68. Valerie J. Nelson, "Farrah Fawcett Dies at 62; Actress Soared with, then Went Beyond, 'Charlie's Angels,'" *Los Angeles Times*, June 26, 2009.

69. *Farrah's Story*, directed by Alana Stewart (Burbank, CA: NBC, May 15, 2009), 120 min.

70. Susan Stewart, "Farrah Fawcett Dies of Cancer at 62," *New York Times*, June 25, 2009.

71. Alessandra Stanley, "TV Watch: 'Farrah's Story,'" *New York Times*, May 16, 2009.

72. Leslie Bennetts, "Beautiful People, Ugly Choices," *Vanity Fair*, September 2009.

73. N. Howlader, A. M. Noone, M. Krapcho, D. Miller, A. Brest, M. Yu, J. Ruhl, et al., eds., *SEER Cancer Statistics Review, 1975–2016* (Bethesda, MD: National Cancer Institute, 2019): table 2.6, "All Cancer Sites (Invasive): Age-adjusted U.S. Death Rates by Year, Race and Sex https://seer.cancer.gov/csr/1975_2016/; https://seer.cancer.gov/archive/csr/1975_2016 /results_merged/sect_02_all_sites.pdf.

74. Rebecca L. Siegel, Kimberly D. Miller, Hannah E. Fuchs, and Ahmedin Jemal, "Cancer Statistics, 2021," *CA: A Cancer Journal for Clinicians* 71, no. 1 (January/February 2021): 7–33, https://doi.org/10.3322/caac.21654.

75. Jessica D. Albano, Elizabeth Ward, Ahmedin Jemal, Robert Anderson, Vilma E. Cokkinides, Taylor Murray, Jane Henley, Jonathan Liff, and Michael J. Thun, "Cancer Mortality in the United States by Education Level and Race," *Journal of the National Cancer Institute* 99, no. 18 (September 19, 2007): 1384–94, https://doi.org/10.1093/jnci/djm127.

76. Since 2010, development of next-generation DNA sequencing and other tools has lowered the cost of sequencing a human or cancer genome to around $1,000, and increased the speed; the sequencing process, which until recently took days or weeks, now takes hours in a lab.

77. Francis S. Collins, Eric D. Green, Alan E. Guttmacher, Mark S. Guyer, and U.S. National Human Genome Research Institute, "A Vision for the Future of Genomics Research," *Nature* 422, no. 6934 (April 24, 2003): 835–47, https://doi.org/10.1038/nature01626.

78. Martin H. Cohen, John R. Johnson, Yeh-Fong Chen, Rajeshwari Sridhara, and Richard Pazdur, "FDA Drug Approval Summary: Erlotinib (Tarceva®) Tablets," *Oncologist* 10, no. 7 (August 1, 2005): 461–66, https://doi.org/10.1634/theoncologist.10-7-461.

79. Harald Zur Hausen, "Viruses in Human Cancers," *Science* 254, no. 5035 (November 22, 1991): 1167–73, https://doi.org/10.1126/science.1659743.

80. Joanna M. Cain and Mary K. Howett, "Preventing Cervical Cancer," *Science* 288, no. 5472 (June 9, 2000): 1753–55, https://doi.org/10.1126/science.288.5472.1753.

81. Ingrid T. Katz and Alexi A. Wright, "Preventing Cervical Cancer in the Developing World," *NEJM* 354, no. 11 (March 16, 2006): 1110, https://doi.org/10.1056/nejmp068031.

82. Patricia Braly, "Preventing Cervical Cancer," *Nature Medicine* 2, no. 7 (July 1, 1996): 749–51, https://doi.org/10.1038/nm0796-749.

83. Eve Dubé, Maryline Vivion, and Noni E. MacDonald, "Vaccine Hesitancy, Vaccine Refusal and the Anti-vaccine Movement: Influence, Impact and Implications," *Expert Review of Vaccines* 14, no. 1 (January 2, 2015): 99–117, https://doi.org/10.1586/14760584.2015.964212.

84. Xiaoli Nan and Kelly Madden, "HPV Vaccine Information in the Blogosphere: How Positive and Negative Blogs Influence Vaccine-Related Risk Perceptions, Attitudes, and Behavioral Intentions," *Health Communication* 27, no. 8 (November 1, 2012): 829–36, https://doi.org/10.1080/10410236.2012.661348.

85. Jim Dwyer, "Ferraro Is Battling Blood Cancer with a Potent Ally: Thalidomide," *New York Times*, June 19, 2001.

86. Josh Getlin, "Ferraro Battles Cancer with Once-Barred Drug," *Los Angeles Times*, June 20, 2001.

87. Seema Singhal, Jayesh Mehta, Raman Desikan, Dan Ayers, Paula Roberson, Paul Eddlemon, Nikhil Munshi, et al., "Antitumor Activity of Thalidomide in Refractory Multiple Myeloma," *NEJM* 341, no. 21 (November 18, 1999): 1565–71, https://doi.org/10.1056/nejm199911183412102.

88. Mike Celizic, "Geraldine Ferraro on Surviving Cancer," Today, August 31, 2007, https://www.today.com/news/geraldine-ferraro-surviving-cancer-wbna20527638.

89. Douglas Martin, "Geraldine A. Ferraro, 1935–2011: "She Ended the Men's Club of National Politics" *New York Times*, March 26, 2011.

90. Dianne C. Witter and John LeBas, "Cancer as a Chronic Disease," *OncoLog* 53, no. 4, April 2008.

91. Jane Brody, "Cancer as a Disease, Not a Death Sentence," *New York Times*, June 17, 2008.

92. Karen Roberts McNamara, "Blogging Breast Cancer: Language and Subjectivity in Women's Online Illness Narratives," (master's thesis, Georgetown University, 2007), http://hdl.handle.net/10822/551596.

93. Deborah S. Chung and Sujin Kim, "Blogging Activity Among Cancer Patients and Their Companions: Uses, Gratifications, and Predictors of Outcomes," *Journal of the American Society for Information Science and Technology* 59, no. 2 (January 15, 2008): 297–306, https://doi.org/10.1002/asi.20751.

94. "The Social Life of Health Information," Pew Research Center, June 11, 2009, https://www.pewresearch.org/internet/2009/06/11/the-social-life-of-health-information/.

95. Virginia Heffernan, "Just Google It: A Short History of a Newfound Verb," *Wired*, November 15, 2017.

96. David Gorski, "On the Nature of 'Alternative' Medicine Cancer Cure Testimonials," Science-Based Medicine, January 14, 2008. https://sciencebasedmedicine.org/on-the-nature-of-alternative-medicine-cancer-cure-testimonials/.

97. David Gorski ("Orac"), "Cancer Quack Robert O. Young Is Arrested and Arraigned, but Will He Be Convicted?," *Respectful Insolence* (blog), January 27, 2014, https://respectfulinsolence.com/2014/01/27/cancer-quack-robert-o-young-is-arrested-and-arraigned-but-will-he-be-convicted/.

98. Teri Figueroa, "Trial Starts for pH Miracle Author," *San Diego Union-Tribune*, November 18, 2015.

99. Teri Figueroa, "Jury Awards $105M in Suit Against pH Miracle Author," *San Diego Union-Tribune*, November 2, 2018.

100. Lisa Stein, "Living with Cancer: Kris Carr's Story," *Scientific American*, July 16, 2008, https://www.scientificamerican.com/article/living-with-cancer-kris-carr/.

101. Mireille Silcoff, "Kris Carr: Crazy Sexy Entrepreneur," *New York Times* Magazine, August 14, 2011.

102. Elaine Schattner, "Notes on Kris Carr and Crazy Sexy Cancer," *Medical Lessons* (blog), August 15, 2011, http://www.medicallessons.net/2011/08/notes-on-kris-carr-and-crazy-sexy-cancer/.

103. Founded by Dr. Stephen Barrett, Quackwatch began in 1969 as the Lehigh Valley Committee Against Health Fraud in Allentown, Pennsylvania. The website (https://quackwatch.org) was created in 1997 and is maintained by the Center for Inquiry, which has headquarters in Amherst, New York, and an executive office in Washington, DC.

104. Paige Brown Jarreau, "All the Science That Is Fit to Blog: An Analysis of Science Blogging Practices" (PhD diss., Louisiana State University, 2015), 1051, https://digitalcommons.lsu.edu/gradschool_dissertations/1051.

105. Scienceblogs.com was an invitation-only blog network founded in 2006 by Seed Media. Since 2018, a website note indicates that "ScienceBlogs.com" is a registered trademark of Science 2.0, which on its website (https://www.science20.com) indicates ownership by ION Publications LLC.

106. Curtis Brainard, "National Geographic Taking the Wheel at Scienceblogs.com," *Columbia Journalism Review*, April 26, 2011.

107. Julie Gilgoff, "'Breast Friends Forever' Will Walk for the Cure in San Francisco," Patch.com (Albany, CA), August 10, 2010, https://patch.com/california/albany/breast-friends-forever-will-walk-for-the-cure-in-san-francisco.

108. Tésa Nicolanti, "My Top 10 Tips for the Susan G. Komen 3-Day for the Cure," *2Wired2Tired* (blog), 2010, http://www.2wired2tired.com/my-top-10-tips-for-the-susan-g-komen-3-day-for-the-cure.

109. Peter Shinkle, "More than 61,000 Fill Downtown in Fight Against Breast Cancer," *St. Louis Post-Dispatch*, June 19, 2005.

110. Connie Lauerman, "Avon 2-Day Walk May Split Support," *Chicago Tribune*, August 21, 2002.

111. "Putting Corporate Might Behind Cancer Fight," *Herald-News* (Passaic, NJ), advertising supplement, October 8, 2003.

112. "Making Strides Against Breast Cancer," press release, SouthJersey.com, October 20, 2006, https://www.southjersey.com/article/15731/Making-Strides-Against-Breast-Cancer/90/.

113. Jean Starr, "Hitting Streets to Fight Cancer," *Times* (Munster, IN), October 16, 2006.

114. These descriptions are drawn in part from awareness and fundraising events, including Komen "Races for the Cure" and ACS "Making Strides" walks, that I've witnessed first-hand, besides many newspaper accounts and social media posts; I have cited a representative few.

115. "Boeing 757 Pink Plane," Delta Flight Museum, accessed May 19, 2022, https://www.deltamuseum.org/exhibits/delta-history/delta-brand/aircraft-livery_group/special-livery.

116. PRNewswire-FirstCall, "Delta Doubles Fundraising Efforts for the Breast Cancer Research Foundation with $1 Million Donation," press release, Delta News Hub, April 28, 2010, https://news.delta.com/delta-doubles-fundraising-efforts-breast-cancer-research -foundation-1-million-donation.

117. PRNewswire,"American Airlines Plans Multi-City 'Pinkout' to Fight Breast Cancer," press release, American Airlines Newsroom, September 30, 2010, https://news.aa.com /news/news-details/2010/American-Airlines-Plans-Multi-City-Pink-out-to-Fight -Breast-Cancer/default.aspx

118. StyleWatch (courtesy the Estée Lauder Companies), "Think Pink! Estée Lauder Breaks a World Record for Breast Cancer Awareness," *People*, last updated October 1, 2010, https://people.com/style/think-pink-estee-lauder-breaks-a-world-record-for-breast-cancer -awareness/.

119. Kristen Stephenson, "Five Breast Cancer Awareness Records for the Month of October," Guinness World Records, October 25, 2016, data from September 16, 2021, retrieved from Internet Archive, https://web.archive.org/web/20210916115805/https://people.com /style/think-pink-estee-lauder-breaks-a-world-record-for-breast-cancer-awareness/.

120. "Breast Cancer Campaign Turns Planet Pink: Too Much?," CBS News, October 20, 2011.

121. "Mrs. Bush's Remarks at a Breast Cancer Awareness Month Event," press release, White House of President George W. Bush, October 7, 2008, https://georgewbush-whitehouse .archives.gov/news/releases/2008/10/20081007-11.html.

122. Barbara Brenner, "The Crazy Days of Autumn," in *So Much to Be Done: The Writings of Breast Cancer Activist Barbara Brenner*, ed. Barbara Sjoholm (Minneapolis: University of Minnesota Press, 2016), 89–92.

123. Daniel S. Levine, "Breast Cancer Group Questions Value of Pink Ribbon Campaigns," *San Francisco Business Times*, October 3, 2005.

124. Courtney Hutchison, "Fried Chicken for the Cure?," ABC News Medical Unit, April 23, 2010, https://abcnews.go.com/Health/Wellness/kfc-fights-breast-cancer-fried-chicken /story?id=10458830.

125. Gayle A. Sulik, *Pink Ribbon Blues: How Breast Cancer Culture Undermines Women's Health* (New York: Oxford University Press, 2010).

126. *Weeds*, "Fashion of the Christ," season 1, episode 4, directed by Burr Steers, Showtime, August 29, 2005.

127. *Weeds*, "The Two Mrs. Scottsons," season 3, episode 8, directed by Craig Zisk, Showtime, October 1, 2007.

128. Dodai Stewart, "SCAR Project Exposes the Realities of Breast Cancer," *Jezebel*, October 13, 2010, https://jezebel.com/scar-project-exposes-the-realities-of-breast-cancer-5663067.

129. Mary K. DeShazer, introduction to *Mammographies: The Cultural Discourses of Breast Cancer Narratives* (Ann Arbor: University of Michigan Press, 2013), 1–16, https://www.jstor .org/stable/j.ctv3znzfk.4.

130. Marisa Acocella Marchetto, *Cancer Vixen: A True Story* (New York: Knopf, 2006).

131. S. L. Wisenberg, *The Adventures of Cancer Bitch* (Iowa City: University of Iowa Press, 2009).

132. "Mission, Vision, and History," LUNGevity Foundation, accessed May 19, 2022, https:// lungevity.org/about-us/mission-vision-history.

133. Jill Feldman, email message to the author, March 23, 2020.

134. "History," Sarcoma Foundation of America, accessed May 19, 2022, https://www.cure sarcoma.org/history/.

135. "About Us," Sarcoma Alliance, accessed May 19, 2022, https://sarcomaalliance.org /about-us/.

136. "Good Works: Celebrate St. Baldrick at Cancer Fund-Raiser," *Atlanta Journal-Constitution*, March 6, 2002.

137. Denis Hamill, "Part with Tradition, and Hair, for Charity," *New York Daily News*, February 25, 2003.

138. Kathleen Ruddy, St. Baldrick's Foundation CEO, interview with the author, February 26, 2020.

139. Jon Saraceno, "Valvano's Words Still Reverberate," *USA Today*, August 25, 2000.

140. Larry Stewart, "TV-Radio; It's Not Just Joking Matter at ESPYs," *Los Angeles Times*, July 13, 2007.

141. Ginny Mason, email message to the author, March 22, 2020.

142. Jay Levin, "Her Fight Against Breast Cancer Inspired Charity," *Record* (Bergen County, NJ), August 7, 2007.

143. "Mayor's Office Declares October 13 as First Metastatic Breast Cancer Awareness Day for New York City," PR Newswire, October 10, 2007.

144. Amy Sacks, "Your Bod, Babe! New Lease on Life. Research Into a Disease That Used to Be a Death Sentence for Women May Help Erase It," *New York Daily News*, October 11, 2007.

145. Jim Carlton, "Dot-Com Decline Turns Into Lift for the Dot-Orgs," *Wall Street Journal* March 12, 2001.

146. "Breast Cancer News That Could Save Your Life," *Redbook*, October 2001, 33–42.

147. McClatchy-Tribune, "Survivor uses Pink Fund to help breast cancer patients pay bills," *Houston Chronicle*, October 2, 2006.

148. Melba Newsome, "Soul Survivors: The Doctor Says, 'We've Found a Lump.' And then the Battle Begins," *HealthQuest*, October 31, 1998.

149. JCPenney salutes CHAMPIONS of change," advertisement, *Cosmopolitan*, May 1999, 191–94

150. Sharony Green, " 'We Beat Breast Cancer,' " *Essence*, October 2007.

151. Marc Ramirez, "Sisters of Hope; A breast-Cancer Survivor Emboldens Other African-American Women in Their Own Battle," *Seattle Times*, September 27, 2002.

152. Aliza Phillips, "Linking Up for the Battle Against Cancer," *Forward*, March 1, 2002; and meeting of Adina Fleischmann, director of Support Programs, Sharsheret, with the author, June 18, 2019.

153. Bill Keveney, "Stars Line Up for 'Stand Up,' " *USA Today*, September 8, 2008.

154. Taylor Swift, "Ronan," performed for the Stand Up To Cancer telethon September 9, 2012. "Ronan" appears in Swift's 2021 recording of her album *Red (Taylor's Version)*, YouTube video, 4:40, uploaded November 12, 2021, https://youtu.be/kdiBc4ogW7s.

155. Stand Up To Cancer UK, "Samuel L. Jackson's Love the Glove," YouTube video, 1:29, uploaded October 17, 2014, https://youtu.be/Oe5NsCZddys.

156. *Breaking Bad*, Season 1 (Culver City, CA, AMC, 2008), created by Vince Gilligan. The talking pillow scene takes place in episode 5 ("Gray Matter"), which aired February 24, 2008.

10. CANCER EVERYWHERE (2010–2020)

1. cookie4monster4, "Nothing More Than Feelings," YouTube video, 3:32, uploaded August 8, 2010, https://youtu.be/fa3XHeMtY3s.

2. Bryan Marquard, "Esther Earl, 16; Built an Online Following of Friends as She Battled Thyroid Cancer," Boston.com, August 29, 2010, http://archive.boston.com/bostonglobe /obituaries/articles/2010/08/29/esther_earl_16_built_an_online_following_of_friends _as_she_battled_thyroid_cancer/.

3. John Green, *The Fault in Our Stars* (New York: Dutton, 2012), 3–4.

4. Meredith Goldstein, "Esther Earl, Quincy Teen, Is Inspiration for Two Books," *Boston Globe*, February 1, 2014.

5. Alexandra Alter, "John Green and His Nerdfighters Are Upending the Summer Block-buster Model," *Wall Street Journal*, May 14, 2014.

6. Zakiya Jamal, "Meet Esther Earl, the Brave Girl Who Inspired *The Fault in Our Stars*," *People*, June 7, 2014, data from January 11, 2017 retrieved at Internet Archive, https://web .archive.org/web/20170111164122/http://www.people.com/celebrity/meet-Esther-Earl -the-Brave-Girl-Who-Inspired-The-Fault-in-Our-Stars/.

7. *The Fault in Our Stars*, directed by Josh Boone (Los Angeles: 20th Century Fox, 2014), 126 min.

8. Margaret Talbot, "The Teen Whisperer," *New Yorker*, June 9 and 16, 2014.

9. Dave deBronkart, "My Cancer Story—Short Version," *The New Life of e-Patient Dave* (blog), June 18, 2008, http://patientdave.blogspot.com/2008/06/my-cancer-story-short-version .html.

10. Maura Lerner, "Patient's Prescription: Get Online, Get Smart, Be Your Own Advocate," *Minneapolis Star-Tribune*, May 14, 2010.

11. Deborah Becker and Lily Tyson, "A Doctor and Patient on Participatory Medicine," radio broadcast, *WBUR*, Boston, January 11, 2018, 8:30, https://www.wbur.org/radioboston /2018/01/11/participatory-medicine-cancer.

12. Liz Szabo, "Breast Cancer Survivor Group Is a Social Movement," *USA Today*, October 23, 2012.

13. Alicia Staley, Deanna J. Attai, Jody Schoger, and Xeni Jardin, "Community-Building: Better than Chemo," South by Southwest Festival schedule, Austin, TX, March 10, 2014, https://schedule.sxsw.com/2014/2014/events/event_IAP22053.

14. Matthew S. Katz, Alicia C. Staley, and Deanna J. Attai, "A History of #BCSM and Insights for Patient-Centered Online Interaction and Engagement," *Journal of Patient-Centered Research and Reviews* 7, no. 4 (October 23, 2020): 304–12, https://doi.org /10.17294/2330-0698.1753.

15. Xeni Jardin (@xeni), "I have breast cancer. I am in good hands. There is a long road ahead and it leads to happiness and a cancer-free, long, healthy life," Twitter, December 1, 2011, 9:58 p.m., https://twitter.com/xeni/status/142437402626105344.

16. Bill Chappell, "Xeni Jardin Tells Twitter Fans She Has Breast Cancer," NPR, Decem-ber 2, 2011, https://www.npr.org/sections/alltechconsidered/2011/12/02/143072567/xeni -jardin-tells-twitter-fans-she-has-breast-cancer.

17. Julia Louis-Dreyfus (@OfficialJLD), "Just when you thought . . . ," Twitter, September 28, 2017, 1:15 p.m., https://twitter.com/officialjld/status/913452227104202752?.

18. Meena Jang, "Julia Louis-Dreyfus Reveals Breast Cancer Diagnosis," *Hollywood Reporter*, September 28, 2017, https://www.hollywoodreporter.com/news/general-news/julia-louis -dreyfus-reveals-breast-cancer-diagnosis-1044054/.

19. Jeopardy! (@Jeopardy), "A Message from Alex Trebek" (video), Twitter, March 6, 2019, 5:05 p.m., https://twitter.com/Jeopardy/status/1103416223331569664.

20. Chadwick Boseman (@chadwickboseman), "It is with immeasurable grief that we con-firm the passing of Chadwick Boseman . . ." (photo), Twitter, August 28, 2020, 10:11 P.M., https://twitter.com/chadwickboseman/status/1299530165463199747/.

21. "Alex Trebek Says He Has Stage 4 Pancreatic Cancer: 'I'm Going to Fight This'," CBS News, March 6, 2019, https://www.cbsnews.com/news/alex-trebek-cancer-prognosis -announced-by-jeopardy-host-in-video-2019-03-06/.

22. Benjamin VanHoose, "Chadwick Boseman's Final Tweet Becomes Most-Liked Ever: 'A Tribute Fit for a King,'" *People*, August 31, 2020, https://people.com/movies/chadwick -bosemans-posthumous-tweet-announcing-his-death-is-most-liked-twitter-post-ever/.

23. AACR Press Office, "Twitter Chat 101," *Cancer Research Catalyst* (blog), September 12, 2014, https://www.aacr.org/blog/2014/09/12/twitter-chat-101/.

24. Merry Jennifer Markham, Danielle Gentile, and David L. Graham, "Social Media for Networking, Professional Development, and Patient Engagement," *American Society of Clinical Oncology 2017 Educational Book* 37 , ed. Don S. Dizon, 37 (Alexandria, VA: Ameri-can Society of Clinical Oncology, 2017), 782–87, https://doi.org/10.1200/edbk_180077.

25. Steven Cutbirth, "Exploring ASCO's Featured Voices," W2O Group, June 2, 2017, https:// www.w2ogroup.com/exploring-ascos-featured-voices/.

26. Naveen Pemmaraju, Michael A. Thompson, Ruben A. Mesa, and Tejas Desai, "Analysis of the Use and Impact of Twitter During American Society of Clinical Oncology Annual Meetings from 2011 to 2016: Focus on Advanced Metrics and User Trends," *Journal of Oncology Practice* 13, no. 7 (July 1, 2017): e623–31, https://doi.org/10.1200/jop.2017.021634.

27. Christopher Hitchens, *Mortality* (New York: Twelve, 2012), "campaign of denial," 2–3; "taunting the Reaper," 5; "on a website of 'the faithful,'" 12–13; "an exhilarating and a melancholy time," 30–31.

28. Graydon Carter, "Foreword" to *Mortality*, by Christopher Hitchens (New York: Twelve, 2012): xiv; Carol Blue, "Afterword" to Mortality, by Christopher Hitchens:102–3.

29. William Grimes, "Christopher Hitchens, Polemicist Who Slashed All, Freely, Dies at 62," *New York Times*, December 16, 2011.

30. Sharon Begley and Susan Roberts, "Komen Charity Under Microscope for Funding, Science," Reuters, February 8, 2012, https://www.reuters.com/article/us-usa-healthcare -komen-research/insight-komen-charity-under-microscope-for-funding-science -idUSTRE8171KW20120208.

31. Susan G. Komen for the Cure, *2010–2011 Annual Report* (Dallas, TX: Susan G. Komen for the Cure, 2012).

32. Tax forms (990) for Susan G. Komen for the Cure and the Breast Cancer Research Foun-dation (BCRF) reviewed for years 2005 through 2019. Accessed June 1, 2022 via "Nonprofit Explorer," ProPublica, https://projects.propublica.org/nonprofits/. Komen documents accessed through this page, https://projects.propublica.org/nonprofits/organizations /752462834; BCRF documents accessed through this page, https://projects.propublica .org/nonprofits/organizations/133727250.

33. Pam Belluck, "Cancer Group Halts Financing to Planned Parenthood," *New York Times*, February 1, 2012.

34. Nicholas Jackson, "Who Is Behind Susan G. Komen's Split from Planned Parenthood?," *Atlantic*, February 1, 2012.

35. Jeffrey Goldberg, "Top Susan G. Komen Official Resigned Over Planned Parenthood Cave-In," *Atlantic*, February 2, 2012.

36. Greg Sargent, "Two Dozen Senators Call on Komen to Reverse Planned Parenthood Decision," *Washington Post*, February 2, 2012.

37. Pam Belluck, Jennifer Preston, and Gardiner Harris, "Cancer Group Backs Down on Cutting Off Planned Parenthood," *New York Times*, February 3, 2012.

38. Katie Leslie, "Handel Hits Back as She Steps Down," *Atlanta Journal-Constitution*, February 8, 2012.

39. Elizabeth Flock, "Susan G. Komen's Funding Cut to Planned Parenthood Only Latest in String of Controversies," *Washington Post*. February 1, 2012.

40. Kate Pickert, *Radical: The Science, Culture, and History of Breast Cancer in America* (New York: Hachette, 2019), Pickert summarizes the 2012 Komen episode, 94–98.

41. H. Gilbert Welch, Lisa M. Schwartz, and Steven Woloshin, *Overdiagnosed: Making People Sick in the Pursuit of Health* (Boston: Beacon, 2011).

42. H. Gilbert Welch, "You Have to Gamble on Your Health," *New York Times*, October 10, 2011.

43. David H. Newman, "Ignoring the Science on Mammograms," *New York Times*, November 28, 2012.

44. Elaine Schattner, "Correcting a Decade of Negative News About Mammography," *Clinical Imaging* 60, no. 2 (April 1, 2020): 265–70, https://doi.org/10.1016/j.clinimag.2019.03.011.

45. Peggy Orenstein, "Our Feel-Good War on Breast Cancer," *New York Times Magazine*, April 25, 2013.

46. Peggy Orenstein, "35 and Mortal: A Breast Cancer Diary," *New York Times Magazine*, June 29, 1997.

47. Robin Roberts and Veronica Chambers, *Everybody's Got Something* (New York: Grand Central, 2014).

48. Amy Robach, *Better: How I Let Go of Control, Held On to Hope, and Found Joy in My Darkest Hour* (New York: Ballantine, 2015).

49. Joan Lunden, *Had I Known: A Memoir of Survival* (New York: Harper, 2015).

50. Hoda Kotb, *Hoda: How I Survived War Zones, Bad Hair, Cancer, and Kathie Lee* (New York: Simon & Schuster, 2010).

51. "NBC's Andrea Mitchell Reveals She Has Breast Cancer," NBC News, September 7, 2011, https://www.nbcnews.com/id/wbna44427588.

52. Lloyd Grove, "Cokie Roberts Reveals Her Cancer Diagnosis," *Washington Post*, August 6, 2002.

53. Nina Totenberg, "'The Personification Of Human Decency': Nina Totenberg Remembers Cokie Roberts," *All Things Considered*, radio broadcast, NPR, Washington, DC, September 17, 2019, 4 min.

54. Lisa de Moraes, "Robin Roberts Diagnosed with Rare Blood Disorder; Tells 'GMA' Viewers 'I'm Going to Beat This,'" *Washington Post*, June 11, 2012.

55. Deborah Kotz, "Robin Roberts's Blood Disorder Linked to Breast Cancer Treatment: How Big Is the Risk?," *Boston Globe*, June 18, 2012.

56. David Bauder, "Robin Roberts Returns to 'Good Morning America,'" Associated Press, February 20, 2013, https://apnews.com/article/33a7e808777b497698e7cd9a7727ef49.

57. Stephen M. Silverman, "Robin Roberts Welcomed Back to GMA by the Obamas, *People*, February 20, 2013, https://people.com/tv/robin-roberts-returns-to-good-morning-america/.

58. "Robin Roberts Teams Up with Be The Match to Help Save Lives," Be The Match, September 27, 2012, https://bethematch.org/news/news-releases/robin-roberts-teams-up -with-be-the-match-to-help-save-lives/.

59. Jacque Wilson, "Robin Roberts Found a Match, but Others Likely Won't Be as Lucky," CNN.com, June 12, 2012, https://www.cnn.com/2012/06/12/health/roberts-bone-marrow -minority-donation/index.html.

60. *Good Morning America*, "Valerie Harper Discusses Cancer Diagnosis on 'GMA,'" ABC News, March 12, 2013.

61. Valerie Harper, *I, Rhoda* (New York: Gallery, 2013).

62. Michelle Tauber and Johnny Dodd, "Valerie Harper Has Terminal Brain Cancer," *People*, March 06, 2013, https://people.com/celebrity/valerie-harper-has-brain-cancer -leptomeningeal-carcinomatosis/.

63. Randee Dawn, "Valerie Harper on Why She Joined 'Dancing With the Stars': 'Why Not?,'" Today.com, September 19, 2013, https://www.today.com/popculture/valerie-harper -why-she-joined-dancing-stars-why-not-4B11198179.

64. Meg Grant, "Valerie Harper: Fearless, Funny and Footloose," *AARP The Magazine*, October/November 2013.

65. Michael Rothman, "Valerie Harper 'Not Sad' About 'Dancing With the Stars' Loss," ABC News, October 8, 2013, https://abcnews.go.com/blogs/entertainment/2013/10/valerie-harper -not-sad-about-dancing-with-the-stars-loss.

66. Bruce Weber, "Valerie Harper, Who Won Fame and Emmys as 'Rhoda,' Dies at 80," *New York Times*, August 30, 2019.

67. Erin Jensen, "GoFundMe Created to Ease Valerie Harper's 'Unrelenting Medical Costs' Amid Cancer Fight," *USA Today*, July 18, 2019.

68. Rob Liefeld and Fabian Nicieza, *The Beginning of the End, Pt. 1* (New York: Marvel, 1991).

69. Sara Beth Lowe, "'Deadpool' Gets Cancer Right: Debunking the 'Hero' Survivor Myth, One Smart-Aleck Joke at a Time," *Salon*, February 21, 2016, https://www.salon.com/2016 /02/21/deadpool_gets_cancer_right_debunking_the_hero_survivor_myth_one_smart _aleck_joke_at_a_time/.

70. Arye Dworken, "Revisiting the Strange Cinematic Debut of Deadpool in *X-Men Origins: Wolverine*," *Vulture*, May 18, 2018, https://www.vulture.com/2018/05/revisiting-the-strange -cinematic-debut-of-deadpool.html.

71. *Deadpool*, directed by Tim Miller (Los Angeles: 20th Century Fox, 2016), 108 min.

72. *Deadpool 2*, directed by David Leitch (Los Angeles: 20th Century Fox, 2019), 119 min.

73. Ana Dumaraog, "Natalie Portman Hints at Jane Foster Cancer Storyline in *Thor 4*," ScreenRant, October 8, 2020, https://screenrant.com/thor-4-movie-jane-foster-cancer -natalie-portman/.

74. Spencer Perry, "Mighty Thor Creator Teases Natalie Portman's Role in *Thor: Love and Thunder*," Comicbook.com, May 20, 2021, https://comicbook.com/marvel/news/mighty -thor-creator-teases-natalie-portmans-role-thor-love-thunder/.

75. *Thor: Love and Thunder*, directed by Taika Waititi (Los Angeles: 20th Century Fox 118 min.), 2022.

76. *50/50*, directed by Jonathan Levine (Santa Monica, CA: Summit Entertainment, 2011), 100 min.

77. Elaine Schattner, "50–50, A Serious Film About a Young Man with a Rare Cancer," *Medical Lessons* (blog), February 17, 2012, http://www.medicallessons.net/2012/02/50-50-a -serious-film-about-a-young-man-with-a-malignant-schwannoma/.

78. *The Big C*, created by Darlene Hunt, Showtime, 2010–2013.

79. Alessandra Stanley, "It's Hello Cancer, Goodbye Inhibitions," *New York Times*, August 15, 2010.

80. Elaine Schattner, "Does Cathy Make the Right Cancer Treatment Decision in *The Big C*?," *Medical Lessons* (blog), November 22, 2010, http://www.medicallessons.net/2010/11/does -cathy-make-the-right-cancer-treatment-decision-in-the-big-c/. This is one of many posts by the author about seasons 1 and 2 of this series.

81. *Chasing Life*, developed by Susanna Fogel and Joni Lefkowitz, ABC Family, 2014–2015.

82. Elaine Schattner, " 'Chasing Life,' My Favorite Soap Opera About a Young Journalist with Leukemia," *Forbes*, January 20, 2015.

83. Mark Dagostino, "*Survivor*'s Ethan Zohn Has Cancer," *People*, May 18, 2009, https://people .com/celebrity/survivors-ethan-zohn-has-cancer/.

84. Mark Dagostino, "Ethan Zohn Begins New Treatment," *People*, October 1, 2009, https:// people.com/celebrity/ethan-zohn-begins-new-treatment/.

85. Cynthia Wang, "*Survivor*'s Ethan Zohn's Cancer Is in Remission," *People*, May 15, 2010, https://people.com/celebrity/survivors-ethan-zohns-cancer-is-in-remission/.

86. Julie Jordan, "Ethan Zohn's Cancer Returns," *People*, November 2, 2011, https://people .com/celebrity/ethan-zohns-cancer-is-back/.

87. Julie Jordan, "Ethan Zohn Undergoes Stem-Cell Transplant," *People*, February 29, 2012, https://people.com/celebrity/ethan-zohn-undergoes-stem-cell-transplant/.

88. Mike Bloom, "*Survivor* Legend Ethan Zohn Discusses His Journey Through Cancer and Back to the Island," *Parade*, December 20, 2020, https://parade.com/996584/mikebloom /survivor-ethan-zohn-interview/.

89. Tim Stack, " 'Survivor: Africa' Winner Ethan Zohn Battling Cancer," *Entertainment Weekly*, May 18, 2009, https://ew.com/article/2009/05/18/survivor-africa/.

90. Whitney Pastorek, " 'Survivor' Winner Ethan Zohn's Cancer Is in Remission," *Entertainment Weekly*, May 15, 2010, https://ew.com/article/2010/05/15/survivor-winner-ethan -zohn-cancer-is-in-remission/.

91. Kate Ward, "Ethan Zohn Has Cancer Relapse," *Entertainment Weekly*, November 2, 2011, https://ew.com/article/2011/11/02/ethan-zohn-cancer-returns/.

92. Dalton Ross, "An Emotional Ethan Zohn on 'a *Survivor* Moment I'll Never Forget,' " *Entertainment Weekly*, March 4, 2020, https://ew.com/tv/survivor-ethan-zohn-winners -at-war-interview-edge-extinction/.

93. Cristina Everett, " 'Real Housewives of Orange County' star Tamra Barney: I Had Cervical Cancer," *New York Daily News*, April 10, 2012.

94. Allison Takeda, " 'Real Housewives' Star Tamra Barney Reveals Cervical Cancer Battle," EverydayHealth, April 11, 2012, data from August 10, 2012 retrieved at *Internet Archive*, http://web.archive.org/web/20120810205358/https://www.everydayhealth.com/cervical -cancer/0411/real-housewives-star-tamra-barney-reveals-cervical-cancer-battle.aspx.

95. Nicol Natale, "RHOC's Tamra Judge Says the "Small Black Flat Freckle" on Her Butt Turned Out to Be Melanoma," *Prevention*, October 28, 2020.

96. Kathy Ehrich Dowd, "Camille Grammer Tells Dr. Oz: 'I'm Feeling Great' After Cancer Scare and Alleged Abuse," *People*, November 14, 2013, https://people.com/tv/camille-grammer-tells-dr-oz-im-feeling-great-after-cancer-scare-and-alleged-abuse/.

97. "Camille Grammer's Battle with Endometrial Cancer," *The Doctors*, January 15, 2015, https://www.thedoctorstv.com/articles/2888-camille-grammer-s-battle-with-endometrial-cancer.

98. Laura Rosenfeld, "The Real Housewives of Orange County's Peggy Sulahian Clarifies Her Cancer Scare," *Daily Dish*, BravoTV, September 28, 2017, https://www.bravotv.com/the-daily-dish/the-real-housewives-of-orange-countys-peggy-sulahian-breast-cancer-explained

99. "Why Are So Many of Bravo's 'Real Housewives' Facing Cancer? How Their Fierceness Helps Them Fight Back," SurvivorNet, May 28, 2019, https://www.survivornet.com/articles/real-housewives-cancer-awareness/.

100. *Late Show with David Letterman*, "Michael Douglas on Having Throat Cancer," CBS, August 31, 2010, YouTube video, 4:59, uploaded September 1, 2010, https://youtu.be/wEMkW1lu5Ps

101. Deborah Kotz, "Michael Douglas Cancer Diagnosis: What You Need to Know," *US News & World Report*, September 1, 2010.

102. Catherine Shoard, "Michael Douglas: I Actually Had Tongue Cancer," *Guardian*, October 10, 2013, https://www.theguardian.com/film/2013/oct/10/michael-douglas-tongue-cancer.

103. K.c. Blumm, "Michael Douglas: I Lied—I Actually Had Tongue Cancer," *People*, October 11, 2013, https://people.com/celebrity/michael-douglas-i-lied-i-actually-had-tongue-cancer/.

104. Xan Brooks, "Michael Douglas on Liberace, Cannes, Cancer and Cunnilingus," *Guardian*, June 2, 2013, https://www.theguardian.com/film/2013/jun/02/michael-douglas-liberace-cancer-cunnilingus.

105. Steven Reinberg, "Michael Douglas Blames His Cancer on Oral Sex," *WebMD*, June 3, 2013, https://www.webmd.com/sexual-conditions/news/20130603/michael-douglas-blames-his-throat-cancer-on-oral-sex#.

106. Tom Phillips and Virginia Lopez, "Hugo Chávez Tells of Cancer Diagnosis," *Guardian*, July 1, 2011, https://www.theguardian.com/world/2011/jul/01/hugo-chavez-cancer-diagnosis.

107. Simon Romero, "Chávez Says a Cancerous Tumor Was Removed," *New York Times*, July 1, 2011.

108. Simon Romero, "Hugo Chávez Says His Cancer Is Gone," *New York Times*, October 20, 2011.

109. William Neuman, "Venezuelan Official Confirms Chávez Receiving Cancer Treatments," *New York Times*, March 2, 2013.

110. The deceased Venezuelan leader's handle is @chavezcandanga.

111. William Neuman, "Venezuela: Panel Will Investigate Roots of Cancer That Killed Chávez," *New York Times*, March 12, 2013.

112. Angelina Jolie, "My Medical Choice," *New York Times*, May 14, 2013.

113. Angelina Jolie Pitt, "Angelina Jolie Pitt: Diary of a Surgery," *New York Times*, March 24, 2015.

114. Jyoti Nangalia and Peter J. Campbell, "Genome Sequencing During a Patient's Journey Through Cancer," *NEJM* 381, no. 22 (November 28, 2019): 2145–56, https://doi.org/10.1056/NEJMra1910138.

115. Robert Pilarski, "The Role of *BRCA* Testing in Hereditary Pancreatic and Prostate Cancer Families," *American Society of Clinical Oncology 2019 Educational Book* 39, ed. Don S.

Dizon (Alexandria, VA: American Society of Clinical Oncology, 2019) 79–86, https://doi.org/10.1200/edbk_238977.

116.   Marleah Dean, Courtney L. Scherr, Meredith Clements, Rachel Koruo, Jennifer Martinez, and Amy Ross, "'When Information Is Not Enough': A Model for Understanding BRCA-Positive Previvors' Information Needs Regarding Hereditary Breast and Ovarian Cancer Risk," *Patient Education and Counseling* 100, no. 9 (September 1, 2017): 1738–43, https://doi.org/10.1016/j.pec.2017.03.013.

117.   Hannah Getachew-Smith, Amy A. Ross, Courtney L. Scherr, Marleah Dean, and Meredith L. Clements, "Previving: How Unaffected Women with a BRCA1/2 Mutation Navigate Previvor Identity," *Health Communication* 35, no. 10 (2020): 1256–65, https://doi.org/10.1080/10410236.2019.1625002.

118.   "What Is the HEROIC Registry?," AliveAndKickn, accessed June 1, 2022, https://www.aliveandkickn.org/copy-of-the-heroic-patient-registry-1.

119.   Colon Cancer Coalition, "AliveAndKickn and the Colon Cancer Coalition Look to Empower Patients Living with Lynch on Lynch Syndrome Awareness Day, March 22, 2020," press release, GlobeNewswire, March 16, 2020, https://www.globenewswire.com/news-release/2020/03/16/2001108/19272/en/AliveAndKickn-and-the-Colon-Cancer-Coalition-look-to-empower-patients-LIVING-WITH-LYNCH-on-Lynch-Syndrome-Awareness-Day-March-22-2020.html.

120.   *Pink & Blue: Colors of Hereditary Cancer*, directed by Alan M. Blassberg (Los Angeles: Pink and Blue Inc., 2015), 85 min.

121.   Arlene Weintraub, "All in the Family: Discussing Screenings and Preventative Surgery for Inherited Cancers," *Cure* Spring 2017.

122.   Kayleigh McEnany (@kayleighmcenany), "I did it!!! I'm officially a Previvor! #PreventativeMastectomy," Twitter, May 1, 2018, 8:55 p.m., https://twitter.com/kayleighmcenany/status/991481323217981440.

123.   Kayleigh McEnany, "Kayleigh McEnany: It's One Year Since My Preventative Double Mastectomy at Age 30—Here's How I Am Doing," Fox News, May 1, 2019; updated the next year with this title: "Kayleigh McEnany: After my 2018 preventive double mastectomy, here's how I'm doing," August 26, 2020, https://www.foxnews.com/opinion/kayleigh-mcenany-preventative-double-mastectomy-age-30.

124.   Lisa Bonchek Adams, *Writings on Metastatic Breast Cancer, Grief & Loss, Life, and Family* (blog), http://lisabadams.com/blog/.

125.   Lisa Bonchek Adams (@AdamsLisa), "Okay, fine, you asked for it: I'm going for one million tweets. #itsyourfault #Iloveyou," Twitter, October 5, 2012, 3:18 p.m., https://twitter.com/AdamsLisa/status/254299569339379712?.

126.   Emma G. Keller, "Forget Funeral Selfies. What Are the Ethics of Tweeting a Terminal Illness?," *Guardian*, January 8, 2014, data from January 9, 2014 retrieved at *Internet Archive*, https://web.archive.org/web/20140109033020/http:/www.theguardian.com/commentisfree/2014/jan/08/lisa-adams-tweeting-cancer-ethics.

127.   The interaction between Adams and Keller reveals how hard it is for journalists to be objective about cancer with which they've been diagnosed: "It isn't easy to face someone with metastatic disease, especially if you've had cancer yourself," Peggy Orenstein observed after interviewing a woman whose early-stage breast cancer recurred after treatment. "[Her] trajectory is my worst fear; the night after we spoke, I was haunted by

dreams of cancer's return," Orenstein admitted in the *New York Times Magazine*, April 25, 2013.

128. Emma G. Keller, "Double Mastectomy: My brutal 40-day Breast Cancer Cure," *Guardian*, April 27, 2012, https://www.theguardian.com/lifeandstyle/2012/apr/27/my-40-day-breast -cancer-emma-gilbey-keller.

129. Bill Keller, "How to Die," *New York Times*, October 7, 2012.

130. Bill Keller, "Heroic Measures," *New York Times*, January 12, 2014.

131. Katie Halper, "Former NYT Editor Mansplains to Cancer Patient to Shut Up and Die the Right Way," Feministing, January 14, 2014, http://feministing.com/2014/01/14/former -nyt-editor-mansplains-to-cancer-patient-to-shut-up-and-die-the-right-way/.

132. Xeni Jardin (@xeni), "5) It is bizarrely tone-deaf, ghoulish, & lacking in empathy all at once. It mansplains breast cancer, but as if talking about a pork chop," Twitter, January 13, 2014, 12:11 a.m., https://twitter.com/xeni/status/422596754987446272.

133. Greg Mitchell, "No Shame: Bill Keller Bullies Cancer Patient," *Nation*, January 13, 2014, data from January 16, 2014 retrieved at *Internet Archive*, https://web.archive.org/web/20140116042054 /http://www.thenation.com:80/blog/177889/no-shame-bill-keller-bullies-cancer-victim.

134. Zeynep Tufekci, "Social Media Is a Conversation, Not a Press Release," *Medium*, January 13, 2014, https://medium.com/technology-and-society/social-media-is-a-conversation-not-a -press-release-4d811b45840d.

135. Margaret Sullivan, "Readers Lash Out About Bill Keller's Column on a Woman with Cancer," *New York Times*, January 13, 2014.

136. Jeremy Snyder, "Crowdfunding for Medical Care: Ethical Issues in an Emerging Health Care Funding Practice," *Hastings Center Report* 46, no. 6 (November 22, 2016): 36–42, https:// doi.org/10.1002/hast.645.

137. Caroline Mayer, "Turning To The Web To Help Pay Medical Bills," Kaiser Health News, July 2, 2013, https://khn.org/news/online-fundraising-to-help-pay-medical-bills-takes-hold/.

138. Stephen Marche, "Go Fund Yourself," *Mother Jones*, January/February 2018.

139. Meg Tirrell, "When Unapproved Drugs Are the Only Hope," CNBC, August 5, 2014, https://www.cnbc.com/2014/08/05/a-case-for-compassionate-use-when-unapproved -drugs-are-the-only-hope.html.

140. Anna Marum, "Remembering Nathalie Traller, a Fighter to the End," *Oregonian*, October 10, 2015.

141. Jules Montague, "Münchausen by Internet: The Sickness Bloggers Who Fake It Online," *Guardian*, April 29, 2015, https://www.theguardian.com/society/2015/apr/29/jules-gibson -munchausen-by-internet-sickness-bloggers-fake-it-whole-pantry.

142. Róisín Lanigan, "The Internet Has a Cancer-Faking Problem," *Atlantic*, May 6, 2019.

143. Josh Moon, "A Really Big Lie," *Alabama Political Reporter*, May 5, 2017.

144. Nathan Heller, "The Hidden Cost of GoFundMe Health Care," *New Yorker*, July 1, 2019.

145. "AG Yost Announces Settlement with Man Accused of Misrepresenting Cancer Diagnosis to Solicit Donations," press release, Ohio Attorney General's Office, Columbus, Ohio, July 29, 2019.

146. Abby Ellin, "He Was the Face of a Bike-a-thon to Fight Cancer. He Was Also a Fake," *New York Times*, August 1, 2019.

147. Sam Brodsky and Dante Kanter, "Pelotonia Cyclist John Looker Faked Cancer for Over a Decade," *Kenyon Collegian*, August 28, 2019.

148. Denise Grady, "Faking Pain and Suffering in Internet Support Groups," *New York Times*, April 23, 1998.

149. Ian Parker, "A Suspense Novelist's Trail of Deceptions," *New Yorker*, February 11, 2019.

150. *Sick Note*, seasons 1 and 2, directed by Matt Lipsey, Netflix, 2017, 2018.

151. *Mythomaniac*, season 1, created by Anne Berest and Fabrice Gobert, Netflix, 2019.

152. Elaine Schattner, "October with Metastatic Breast Cancer," *Atlantic*, October 17, 2012.

153. Elaine Schattner, "New, Metastatic Breast Cancer Alliance Sets a Cooperative Tone," *Huffington Post*, October 15, 2013, https://www.huffpost.com/entry/a-new-metastatic-breast-cancer-alliance_b_4098412.

154. Elaine Schattner, "Landscape Analysis Reveals How Little Is Known, or Said, About Metastatic Breast Cancer," *Forbes*, October 13, 2014.

155. Metastatic Breast Cancer Alliance, *Metastatic Breast Cancer Landscape Analysis: Research Report* (New York: Metastatic Breast Cancer Alliance, October 2014), https://www.mbcalliance.org/flipbook-landscape/.

156. Jennie Grimes, "Philadelphia Story," Putting the Grrrrr in Grimes," *Jennie Grimes* (blog), April 13, 2015, https://jenniegrimes.wordpress.com/2015/04/13/philadelphia-story/.

157. Elaine Schattner, "Notes from the 'Die-In,' a Demonstration for Metastatic Breast Cancer," *Forbes*, October 30, 2015.

158. Marie McCullough, "Fighting to Tame Metastatic Breast Cancer," *Philadelphia Inquirer*, May 1, 2016.

159. Sue Rochman, "Raising Their Voices," *Cancer Today*, Fall 2018.

160. Mary Engel, "Beth Caldwell's Impact on Metastatic Breast Cancer," Fred Hutch, November 3, 2017, https://www.fredhutch.org/en/news/center-news/2017/11/beth-caldwell-impact-metastatic-breast-cancer.html.

161. Audited financial statements for the years 2016 -2019 are available at METAvivor's website, Accessed June 1, 2022 https://www.metavivor.org/financials/.

162. "METAvivor Announces 2017 Grant Awards for Metastatic Cancer Research," *Cancer Letter* 44, no. 1 (January 5, 2018).

163. METAvivor Board Members, "METAvivor Announces 2019 Grant Awards for Metastatic Breast Cancer Research," METAvivor, December 30, 2019, https://www.metavivor.org/blog/metavivor-announces-2019-grant-awards-for-metastatic-breast-cancer-research/.

164. Anna Moeslein, "*Not Just One* Is Equal Parts Heartbreaking and Inspiring," *Glamour*, October 22, 2020.

165. Eisai Inc., "#ThisIsMBC Perseverance Campaign from Eisai and METAvivor Captures the Joys, Difficulties and Realities Faced by People Living with Metastatic Breast Cancer," press release, Cision PR Newswire, December 8, 2020, https://www.prnewswire.com/news-releases/thisismbc-perseverance-campaign-from-eisai-and-metavivor-captures-the-joys-difficulties-and-realities-faced-by-people-living-with-metastatic-breast-cancer-301188296.html.

166. "Breast Cancer: A Story Half Told," accessed June 1, 2022, https://www.storyhalftold.com/. This website is sponsored by Pfizer Inc.

167. "Pfizer Partners with Breast Cancer Leaders to Chronicle the Lives of Women with Metastatic Breast Cancer Through the Lenses of Prominent Photographers," press release, Pfizer, September 30, 2015, https://www.pfizer.com/news/press-release/press-release

-detail/pfizer_partners_with_breast_cancer_leaders_to_chronicle_the_lives_of_women
_with_metastatic_breast_cancer_through_the_lenses_of_prominent_photographers.

168.   Beth Snyder Bulik, "Picture This: Pfizer Advances Its Metastatic Breast Cancer Awareness
Campaign with Day-in-the-Life Photography," Fierce Pharma, October 26, 2015, https://
www.fiercepharma.com/marketing/picture-pfizer-advances-its-metastatic-breast-cancer
-awareness-campaign-day-life.

169.   Marissa Gold, "A Day in the Life of a 40-Year-Old Woman with Advanced Breast Cancer," Glamour, October 12, 2015.

170.   Alexia Fernández, "Mira Sorvino on Raising Awareness for Metastatic Breast Cancer After Losing Two Friends," People, October 11, 2018, data from October 11, 2018
retrieved at Internet Archive, https://web.archive.org/web/20181011194443/https://people
.com/health/mira-sorvino-raising-awareness-metastatic-breast-cancer/.

171.   Good Morning America, "How to Do the 'Thriver' Yoga Routine for Metastatic Breast
Cancer," ABC News, October 11, 2018, https://abcnews.go.com/GMA/GMA_Day/video
/thriver-yoga-routine-metastatic-breast-cancer-awareness-58437497.

172.   "Lilly and Metastatic Breast Cancer Advocates Launch Thriver Movement to Elevate
Understanding of the Daily Impact of the Disease, Encourage Public to do More for
MBC," press release, Lilly, October 12, 2018, https://investor.lilly.com/news-releases/news
-release-details/lilly-and-metastatic-breast-cancer-advocates-launch-thriver.

173.   "#ThisIsMBC Serenity Project" (2017), #ThisIsMBC Elements Project" (2018), #Thi-
sIsMBC Beneath the Breast Project" (2019), "#ThisIsMBC Perseverance Project" (2020),
"#ThisIsMBC FearLESS Project" (2021), accessed June 1, 2022, https://www.mbcinfocenter
.com/this-is-mbc. This website is sponsored by Eisai Inc.

174.   Merel Hennink, Geert Vandeweyer, Janet Freeman-Daily, and the ROSiders, "The Roles
of Patient Groups in Fostering Cancer Research," Nature Reviews Clinical Oncology 17, no.
2 (February 2020): 65–66, https://doi.org/10.1038/s41571-019-0314-1.

175.   ROSidersAccessed June 1, 2022, can be found at https://www.therosiders.org/.

176.   EGFR Resisters, Accessed June 1, 2022, https://egfrcancer.org/.

177.   Exon 20 Group, an initiative of the International Cancer Advocacy Network, Accessed
June 1, 2022, https://exon20group.org/.

178.   KRAS Kickers, Accessed June 1, 2022, https://www.kraskickers.org/.

179.   Nikhil Swaminathan, "Ted Kennedy Diagnosed with Malignant Brain Tumor," Scientific American, May 20, 2008, https://www.scientificamerican.com/article/ted-kennedy-diagnosed-wit/.

180.   John M. Broder, "Edward M. Kennedy, Senate Stalwart, Is Dead at 77," New York Times,
August 26, 2009.

181.   Karen Tumulty, "John McCain, 'Maverick' of the Senate and Former POW, Dies at 81,"
Washington Post, August 25, 2018.

182.   Duane Mitchell, "Why Is Glioblastoma, the Cancer That Killed John McCain, So
Deadly?," Scientific American, August 27, 2018, https://www.scientificamerican.com/article
/why-is-glioblastoma-the-cancer-that-killed-john-mccain-so-deadly/.

183.   Michael D. Shear, "Beau Biden, Vice President Joe Biden's Son, Dies at 46," New York
Times, May 30, 2015.

184.   "Full Text: Biden's Announcement That He Won't Run for President," Washington Post,
October 21, 2015.

185.   PBS NewsHour, "Obama: 'Let's Make America the Country That Cures Cancer,'" You-Tube video, 1:17, uploaded January 12, 2016, https://youtu.be/EJDyBBGncQc.

186.   Matthew Bin Han Ong, "Obama Announces Moonshot to Cure Cancer," *Cancer Letter* 42, no. 2 (January 16, 2016).

187.   Gardiner Harris, "$1 Billion Planned for Cancer 'Moonshot,'" *New York Times*, February 1, 2016.

188.   "Biden Time: The US Vice-President's Cancer Project Is Winning Hearts and Minds," *Nature* 532, no. 7600 (April 27, 2016): 414, https://doi.org/10.1038/532414a.

189.   Matthew Bin Han Ong, "House Passes 21st Century Cures Act, Slating $4.8 Billion for NIH, Moonshot," *Cancer Letter* 42, no. 44 (December 2, 2016).

190.   Elizabeth M. Jaffee, Chi Van Dang, David B. Agus, Brian M. Alexander, Kenneth C. Anderson, Alan Ashworth, Anna D. Barker, et al., "Future Cancer Research Priorities in the USA: A *Lancet Oncology* Commission," *Lancet Oncology* 18, no. 11 (November 1, 2017): e653–706, https://doi.org/10.1016/S1470-2045(17)30698-8.

191.   John Wagner, "Donald Trump Jr. Mocks Joe Biden for Vowing to Cure Cancer if Elected President," *Washington Post*, June 19, 2019.

192.   Stephen Braun, "Biden Anti-cancer Groups Could Pose Influence Concerns," AP News, June 19, 2019, https://apnews.com/article/joe-biden-technology-health-archive-health-care-industry-b38b45df035246cb9d2272a7ebb22752.

193.   Lev Facher and Matthew Herper, "Biden Cancer Initiative to Suspend Operations as 2020 Campaign Heats Up," *Stat News*, July 15, 2019, https://www.statnews.com/2019/07/15/biden-cancer-initiative-suspend-operations/.

194.   "President Carter Shares Cancer Diagnosis," press release, Emory Winship Cancer Institute, August 20, 2015, https://winshipcancer.emory.edu/about-us/newsroom/press-releases/2015/president-carter-shares-cancer-diagnosis.

195.   The Carter Center, "Excerpts from Former U.S. President Jimmy Carter's Aug. 20 News Conference," YouTube video, 5:55, uploaded August 21, 2015, https://www.youtube.com/watch?v=5Jt35IIjVSM.

196.   Abby Phillip, "Former President Jimmy Carter Says Cancer Has Spread to His Brain," *Washington Post*, August 20, 2015.

197.   President Obama (@POTUS44), "President Carter is as good a man as they come. Michelle and I are praying for him and Rosalynn. We're all pulling for you, Jimmy," Twitter, August 20, 2015, 1:14 p.m., https://twitter.com/POTUS44/status/634413305516412928?s=20.

198.   George H. W. Bush (@GeorgeHWBush), "I spoke with President Carter to wish him well, and he sounded strong. Bar and I are wishing him the very best as he fights the good fight," Twitter, August 20, 2015, 3:34 p.m., https://twitter.com/GeorgeHWBush/status/634448503322771456?s=20.

199.   Colleen Jenkins, "Former President Jimmy Carter Says He Is Cancer Free," Reuters, December 6, 2015, https://www.reuters.com/article/us-usa-carter-idUSKBN0TP0MC20151207.

200.   Kathleen Foody (Associated Press), "Jimmy Carter Says He No Longer Needs Cancer Treatment," *Stat News*, March 7, 2016, https://www.statnews.com/2016/03/07/jimmy-carter-cancer-treatment/.

201.   "President and Mrs. Carter Spend One Week Building Homes with Habitat for Humanity in Memphis, Tennessee," press release, Habitat for Humanity, August 22, 2016, https://www.habitat.org/newsroom/08-22-2016-Carter-Work-Project-kickoff.

202. Associated Press, "U.S. Watch (Tennessee: Carter Talks Fight with Cancer)," *Wall Street Journal*, August 23, 2016.

203. Leslie Salzillo, "Jimmy Carter Takes Interview, While Building Homes, to Discuss Controversial Issues—Because He Can," Daily Kos, August 30, 2016, https://www.dailykos.com/stories/2016/8/30/1565072/-Jimmy-Carter-takes-a-break-building-Habitat-homes-to-discuss-poverty-Israel-and-Citizens-United.

204. PRNewswire-USNewswire, "Taboo of the Black Eyed Peas Reveals Recent Testicular Cancer Battle, Releases 'The Fight' to Support the American Cancer Society," press release, American Cancer Society, November 16, 2016, http://pressroom.cancer.org/2016-11-16-Taboo-of-the-Black-Eyed-Peas-Reveals-Recent-Testicular-Cancer-Battle-Releases-The-Fight-to-Support-the-American-Cancer-Society.

205. Elaine Schattner, "Taboo of the Black Eyed Peas Has a Message for Cancer Patients," *Forbes*, November 17, 2016.

206. Beyoncé G. Knowles, *Lemonade*, visual album (New York: HBO, April 23, 2016), 65 min.

207. Lia Beck, "The 'Lemonade' Message You Probably Missed," *Bustle*, May 6, 2016, https://www.bustle.com/articles/159180-the-powerful-woman-in-beyonces-lemonade-you-probably-missed-but-need-to-know.

208. Jessica Ravitz, "The Naked Truth," CNN.com, March 31, 2017, https://edition.cnn.com/2017/03/31/health/hfr-paulette-leaphart-naked-truth/index.html.

209. Paul Kalanithi, "How Long Have I Got Left?," *New York Times*, January 24, 2014.

210. Paul Kalanithi, "My Last Day as a Surgeon," *New Yorker*, January 11, 2016.

211. Paul Kalanithi, *When Breath Becomes Air* (New York: Random House, 2016).

212. Trisha Greenhalgh and Liz O'Riordan, *The Complete Guide to Breast Cancer: How to Feel Empowered and Take Control* (London: Vermilion, 2018).

213. Beverly A. Zavaleta, *Braving Chemo: What to Expect, How to Prepare and How to Get Through It* (Brownsville, TX: Sugar Plum, 2019).

214. Uzma Yunus, *Left Boob Gone Rogue: My Life with Breast Cancer* (self-published, 2019).

215. Ruth Bader Ginsburg, "Remarks for Women's Health Research Dinner – May 7, 2001," Iowa State University Archives of Women's Political Communication, May 7, 2001, https://awpc.cattcenter.iastate.edu/2017/03/21/remarks-for-womens-health-research-dinner-may-7-2001/.

216. Press release, Supreme Court of the United States, February 5, 2009, https://www.supremecourt.gov/publicinfo/press/pressreleases/pr_02-05-09.

217. Robert Barnes and Laurie McGinley, "Ruth Bader Ginsburg Has Surgery for Malignant Nodules in Her Lung," *Washington Post*, December 21, 2018.

218. Press release, Supreme Court of the United States, August 23, 2019, https://www.supremecourt.gov/publicinfo/press/pressreleases/pr_08-23-19.

219. Ruth Bader Ginsburg, "Statement from Justice Ruth Bader Ginsburg," press release, Supreme Court of the United States, July 17, 2020, https://www.supremecourt.gov/publicinfo/press/pressreleases/pr_07-17-20.

220. Linda Greenhouse, "Ruth Bader Ginsburg, Supreme Court's Feminist Icon, Is Dead at 87," *New York Times*, September 18, 2020.

221. Nina Totenberg, "Justice Ruth Bader Ginsburg, Champion of Gender Equality, Dies at 87," *Weekend Edition Saturday*, radio broadcast, NPR, Washington, DC, September 18, 2020, 9 min.

222.   Jen Yamato, "Chadwick Boseman: Cancer claims portrayer of 'Black Panther,' Real Icons," *Los Angeles Times*, August 29, 2020.

223.   Reggie Ugwu and Michael Levenson, "'Black Panther' Star Chadwick Boseman Dies of Cancer at 43," *New York Times*, August 29, 2020.

224.   Kate Bowler, *Everything Happens for a Reason: And Other Lies I've Loved* (New York: Random House, 2018), "What if everything is random?" 113.

225.   Cristian Tomasetti and Bert Vogelstein, "Variation in Cancer Risk Among Tissues Can Be Explained by the Number of Stem Cell Divisions," *Science* 347, no. 6217 (January 2, 2015): 78–81, https://doi.org/10.1126/science.1260825.

226.   Jennifer Couzin-Frankel, "The Bad Luck of Cancer," *Science* 347, no. 6217 (January 2, 2015): 12, https://doi.org/10.1126/science.347.6217.12.

227.   Cristian Tomasetti, Lu Li, and Bert Vogelstein, "Stem Cell Divisions, Somatic Mutations, Cancer Etiology, and Cancer Prevention," *Science* 355, no. 6331 (March 24, 2017): 1330–34, https://doi.org/10.1126/science.aaf9011.

228.   James Gallagher, "Most Cancer Types 'Just Bad Luck,'" BBC News, January 2, 2015, https://www.bbc.com/news/health-30641833.

229.   Ben Brumfield, "Scientists: Random Gene Mutations Primary Cause of Most Cancer," CNN.com, January 3, 2015, https://www.cnn.com/2015/01/02/health/cancer-random-mutation/index.html.

230.   Denise Grady, "Cancer's Random Assault," *New York Times*, January 5, 2015.

231.   Jennifer Couzin-Frankel, "Backlash Greets 'Bad Luck' Cancer Study and Coverage," *Science* 347, no. 6219 (January 16, 2015): 224, https://doi.org/10.1126/science.347.6219.224.

232.   Sharon Begley (*Stat News*), "Most Cancer Cases Arise from 'Bad Luck,'" *Scientific American*, March 24, 2017, https://www.scientificamerican.com/article/most-cancer-cases-arise-from-bad-luck/.

233.   Sharon Begley, "Most Cancer Mutations Due to 'Bad Luck,' But Many Cases Still Preventable," *Stat News*, March 23, 2017, https://www.statnews.com/2017/03/23/cancer-mutations-prevention-bad-luck/.

234.   Ed Yong, "No, We Can't Say Whether Cancer Is Mostly Bad Luck," *Atlantic*, March 28, 2017.

235.   Harris Poll, *ASCO 2019 Cancer Opinions Survey* (New York: Harris Poll on behalf of the American Society of Clinical Oncology, 2019), https://www.asco.org/sites/new-www.asco.org/files/content-files/blog-release/pdf/2019-ASCO-Cancer-Opinion-Survey-Final-Report.pdf.

11. THE MODERN PATIENT'S BURDEN

1.   Samuel Hopkins Adams, "What Can We Do About Cancer?," *Ladies' Home Journal*, May 1913, 21–22.

2.   Elaine Schattner, "Can Cancer Truths Be Told? Challenges for Medical Journalism," *American Society of Clinical Oncology 2017 Educational Book* 37, ed. Don S. Dizon (Alexandria, VA: American Society of Clinical Oncology, 2017), 3–11, https://doi.org/10.1200/edbk_100011.

3.   Paul R. Johnson, "Patient Autonomy in Decision Making: Recent Trends in Medical Ethics," *Linacre Quarterly* 53, no. 2 (May 1, 1986): 37–46, https://doi.org/10.1080/00243639.1986.11877848.

4.   Ezekiel J. Emanuel and Linda L. Emanuel, "Four Models of the Physician-Patient Relationship," *JAMA* 267, no. 16 (April 22, 1992): 2221–26, https://doi.org/10.1001/jama.1992.03480160079038.

5. Barron H. Lerner, "Ill Patient, Public Activist: Rose Kushner's Attack on Breast Cancer Chemotherapy," *Bulletin of the History of Medicine* 81, no. 1 (Spring 2007): 224–40, https://doi.org/10.1353/bhm.2007.0006.

6. George W. Sledge, "Patients and Physicians in the Era of Modern Cancer Care," *JAMA* 321, no. 9 (February 15, 2019): 829–30, https://doi.org/10.1001/jama.2018.17334.

7. Domenico Montanaro, "There's a Stark Red-Blue Divide When It Comes to States' Vaccination Rates," NPR, June 9, 2021, https://www.npr.org/2021/06/09/1004430257/theres-a-stark-red-blue-divide-when-it-comes-to-states-vaccination-rates.

8. Cary Funk and John Gramlich, "10 Facts About Americans and Coronavirus Vaccines," Pew Research Center, September 20, 2021, https://www.pewresearch.org/fact-tank/2021/09/20/10-facts-about-americans-and-coronavirus-vaccines/.

9. David Leonhardt, "Red Covid," *New York Times*, September 27, 2021.

10. Daniel Wood and Geoff Brumfiel, "Pro-Trump Counties Now Have Far Higher COVID Death Rates. Misinformation Is to Blame," *Morning Edition*, radio broadcast, NPR, Washington, DC, December 5, 2021, 3 min., NPR, https://www.npr.org/sections/health-shots/2021/12/05/1059828993/data-vaccine-misinformation-trump-counties-covid-death-rate.

11. "Infodemic," World Health Organization, accessed June 1, 2022, https://www.who.int/health-topics/infodemic.

12. WHO, UN, UNICEF, UNDP, UNESCO, UNAIDS, ITU, UN Global Pulse, and IFRC (joint statement), "Managing the COVID-19 Infodemic: Promoting Healthy Behaviours and Mitigating the Harm from Misinformation and Disinformation," World Health Organization, September 23, 2020, https://www.who.int/news/item/23-09-2020-managing-the-covid-19-infodemic-promoting-healthy-behaviours-and-mitigating-the-harm-from-misinformation-and-disinformation.

13. Sarah Berry, Therese Jones, and Erin Lamb, "Editors' Introduction: Health Humanities: The Future of Pre-health Education Is Here," *Journal of Medical Humanities* 38 no. 4 (July 24, 2017): 353–60, https://doi.org/10.1007/s10912-017-9466-0.

14. Lisa Howley, Elizabeth Gaufberg, and Brandy King, *The Fundamental Role of the Arts and Humanities in Medical Education* (Washington, DC: Association of American Medical Colleges, 2020).

12. CANCER IS NOT AS IT USED TO BE

1. David M. Hyman, Barry S. Taylor, and José Baselga, "Implementing Genome-Driven Oncology," *Cell* 168, no. 4 (February 9, 2017): 584–99, https://dx.doi.org/10.1016/j.cell.2016.12.015.

2. Chandan Kumar-Sinha and Arul M. Chinnaiyan, "Precision Oncology in the Age of Integrative Genomics," *Nature Biotechnology* 36, no. 1 (January 2018): 46–60, https://doi.org/10.1038/nbt.4017.

3. Jason K. Sicklick, Shumei Kato, Ryosuke Okamura, Maria Schwaederle, Michael E. Hahn, Casey B. Williams, Pradip De, et al., "Molecular Profiling of Cancer Patients Enables Personalized Combination Therapy: The I-PREDICT Study," *Nature Medicine* 25, no. 5 (May 2019): 744–50, https://doi.org/10.1038/s41591-019-0407-5.

4. Murray Aitken and Alana Simorellis, *Supporting Precision Oncology: Targeted Therapies, Immuno-oncology, and Predictive Biomarker-Based Medicines* (Parsippany, NJ: IQVIA Institute for Human Data Science, 2020).

5.   Vinay Prasad, "Perspective: The Precision-Oncology Illusion," *Nature* 537, no. S63 (September 7, 2016), https://doi.org/doi:10.1038/537S63a.

6.   Richard Harris, "Tweeting Oncologist Draws Ire and Admiration for Calling Out Hype," *Weekend Edition Saturday*, radio broadcast, NPR, Washington, DC, June 4, 2018, 7 min. https://www.npr.org/sections/health-shots/2018/06/24/621068147/tweeting-oncologist-draws-ire-and-admiration-for-calling-out-hype.

7.   Rajesh R. Singh, Rajyalakshmi Luthra, Mark J. Routbort, Keyur P. Patel, and L. Jeffrey Medeiros, "Implementation of Next Generation Sequencing in Clinical Molecular Diagnostic Laboratories: Advantages, Challenges and Potential," *Expert Review of Precision Medicine and Drug Development* 1, no. 1: 109–20, https://doi.org/10.1080/23808993.2015.1120401.

8.   Michail Ignatiadis, George W. Sledge, and Stefanie S. Jeffrey, "Liquid Biopsy Enters the Clinic—Implementation Issues and Future Challenges," *Nature Reviews Clinical Oncology* 18 (May 2021): 297–312, https://doi.org/10.1038/s41571-020-00457-x.

9.   Elaine Kilgour, Dominic G. Rothwell, Ged Brady, and Caroline Dive, "Liquid Biopsy-Based Biomarkers of Treatment Response and Resistance," *Cancer Cell* 37, no. 4 (April 13, 2020): 485–95, https://doi.org/10.1016/j.ccell.2020.03.012.

10. Thierry André, Kai-Keen Shiu, Tae Won Kim, Benny Vittrup Jensen, Lars Henrik Jensen, Cornelis Punt, Denis Smith, et al., "Pembrolizumab in Microsatellite-Instability–High Advanced Colorectal Cancer," *NEJM* 383, no. 23 (December 3, 2020): 2207–18, https://doi.org/10.1056/NEJMoa2017699.

11. Ed S. Kheder and David S. Hong, "Emerging Targeted Therapy for Tumors with *NTRK* Fusion Proteins," *Clinical Cancer Research* 24, no. 23 (December 3, 2018): 5807–14, https://doi.org/10.1158/1078-0432.Ccr-18-1156.

12. Gideon M. Blumenthal and Richard Pazdur, "Approvals in 2018: A Histology-Agnostic New Molecular Entity, Novel End Points and Real-Time Review," *Nature Reviews Clinical Oncology* 16, no. 3 (March 2019): 139–41, https://doi.org/10.1038/s41571-019-0170-z.

13. Ann-Marie Looney, Khurram Nawaz, and Rachel M. Webster, "Tumour-Agnostic Therapies," *Nature Reviews Drug Discovery* 19, no. 6 (June 2020): 383–84, https://dx.doi.org/10.1038/d41573-020-00015-1.

14. Clifton Leaf, "The Little Orange Pill," in *The Truth in Small Doses: Why We're Losing the War on Cancer and How to Win It* (New York: Simon & Schuster, 2013), 89–112.

15. Apostolia M. Tsimberidou, Elena Fountzilas, Mina Nikanjam, and Razelle Kurzrock, "Review of Precision Cancer Medicine: Evolution of the Treatment Paradigm," *Cancer Treatment Reviews* 86 (June 1, 2020): 102019, https://doi.org/10.1016/j.ctrv.2020.102019.

16. Jennifer S. Temel, Joseph A. Greer, Alona Muzikansky, Emily R. Gallagher, Sonal Admane, Vicki A. Jackson, Constance M. Dahlin, et al., "Early Palliative Care for Patients with Metastatic Non–Small-Cell Lung Cancer," *NEJM* 363, no. 8 (August 19, 2010): 733–42, https://doi.org/10.1056/nejmoa1000678.

17. David Hui and Eduardo Bruera, "Integrating Palliative Care Into the Trajectory of Cancer Care," *Nature Reviews Clinical Oncology* 13, no. 3 (March 2016): 159–71, https://doi.org/10.1038/nrclinonc.2015.201.

18. Betty R. Ferrell, Jennifer S. Temel, Sarah Temin, Erin R. Alesi, Tracy A. Balboni, Ethan M. Basch, Janice I. Firn, et al., "Integration of Palliative Care Into Standard Oncology Care: American Society of Clinical Oncology Clinical Practice Guideline Update,"

Journal of Clinical Oncology 35, no. 1 (January 1, 2017): 96–112, https://doi.org/10.1200/jco .2016.70.1474.

19.   Francisco Martínez-Jiménez, Ferran Muiños, Inéz Sentís, Jordi Deu-Pons, Iker Reyes-Salazar, Claudia Arnedo-Pac, Loris Mularoni, et al., "A Compendium of Mutational Cancer Driver Genes," *Nature Reviews Cancer* 20, no. 10 (August 10, 2020): 555–72, https://doi.org /10.1038/s41568-020-0290-x.

20.   Michael F. Berger and Elaine R. Mardis, "The Emerging Clinical Relevance of Genomics in Cancer Medicine," *Nature Reviews Clinical Oncology* 15 (March 29, 2018): 353–65, https://doi.org/10.1038/s41571-018-0002-6.

13. IS CANCER TREATMENT A LUXURY?

1.   Beth Caldwell (@CultPerfectMoms), "12. I know the longer I live, the more I cost @ fepblue. But this is how insurance works: we pay premiums and we get health care. #Save Beth," Twitter, November 7, 2016, 3:21 p.m., https://twitter.com/CultPerfectMoms/status /795722832831356928.

2.   Beth Caldwell, "The Dakotans," *Cult of Perfect Motherhood* (blog), October 3, 2016, http:// cultofperfectmotherhood.com/the-dakotans/.

3.   Beth Caldwell, "Denial," *Cult of Perfect Motherhood* (blog), November 4, 2016, http://cult ofperfectmotherhood.com/denial/.

4.   Beth Caldwell, "Denial, Part 2," *Cult of Perfect Motherhood* (blog), November 19, 2016, http://cultofperfectmotherhood.com/denial-part-2/.

5.   Beth Caldwell, "Denial, Part 3: VICTORY!," *Cult of Perfect Motherhood* (blog), November 28, 2016, http://cultofperfectmotherhood.com/denial-part-3-victory/.

6.   Beth Caldwell, "Progression," *Cult of Perfect Motherhood* (blog), August 11, 2017, http:// cultofperfectmotherhood.com/progression/.

7.   Anne B. Martin, Micah Hartman, Benjamin Washington, Aaron Catlin, "National Health Spending: Faster Growth in 2015 as Coverage Expands and Utilization Increases," *Health Affairs* 36, no. 1 (January 2017): 166–76, https://doi.org/10.1377/hlthaff.2016.1330.

8.   Samuel J. Hong, Edward C. Li, Linda M. Matusiak, and Glen T. Schumock, "Spending on Antineoplastic Agents in the United States, 2011 to 2016," *Journal of Oncology Practice* 14, no. 11 (November 1, 2018): e683–91, https://ascopubs.org/doi/abs/10.1200/JOP.18.00069.

9.   Angela B. Mariotto, Lindsey Enewold, Jingxuan Zhao, Christopher A. Zeruto, and K. Robin Yabroff, "Medical Care Costs Associated with Cancer Survivorship in the United States," *Cancer Epidemiology Biomarkers & Prevention* 29, no. 7 (July 2020): 1304–12, https:// dx.doi.org/10.1158/1055-9965.epi-19-1534.

10.   With exception, information on prices of molecular profiling tests of tumor specimens and liquid biopsy samples is opaque. The list price for the FoundationOne test is $5,800 and for the FoundationOne Heme test is $7,200; See "Patient Information Guide," Foundation Medicine, accessed June 4, 2022, https://assets.ctfassets.net/vhribv12lmne /5BJHWaCe1Gwu8CaksomGS8/8169541f7d6a0ad110bccof228fbbe41/Patient_Information _Guide.pdf.

       A 2019 paper indicates the list price for Caris Molecular Intelligence multiplatform tumor profiling was £5,000 in the United Kingdom. See Gilbert Spizzo, Uwe Siebert,

Guenther Gastl, Andreas Voss, Klaus Schuster, Robert Leonard, and Andreas Seeber, "Cost-Comparison Analysis of a Multiplatform Tumour Profiling Service to Guide Advanced Cancer Treatment," *Cost Effectiveness and Resource Allocation* 17, no. 23 (October 21, 2019), https://doi.org/10.1186/s12962-019-0191-6.

Guardant offers a liquid (tumor profiling) test, Guardant360 CDx, that lists for $5,000; "Coverage Information for patients" pop-up note in: "Tests for Patients with Advanced Cancer," Guardant Health, accessed June 4, 2022, https://guardanthealth.com/products/tests-for-patients-with-advanced-cancer/.

11.   Murray Aitken and Michael Kleinrock, *Global Oncology Trends 2021: Outlook to 2025* (Parsippany, NJ: IQVIA Institute for Human Data Science, 2021), https://www.iqvia.com/-/media/iqvia/pdfs/institute-reports/global-oncology-trends-2021/global-oncology-trends-report-2021-05-21-forweb.pdf.

12.   Victoria S. Blinder, "Pain, Financial Hardship, and Employment in Cancer Survivors," *Journal of Clinical Oncology* 40, no. 1: 1–4, https://doi.org/10.1200/jco.21.01812.

13.   Pricivel M. Carrera, Hagop M. Kantarjian, and Victoria S. Blinder, "The Financial Burden and Distress of Patients with Cancer: Understanding and Stepping Up Action on the Financial Toxicity Of Cancer Treatment," *CA: A Cancer Journal for Clinicians* 68, no. 2 (March/April 2018): 153–65, https://dx.doi.org/10.3322/caac.21443.

14.   Robert Lentz, Al B. Benson III, and Sheetal Kircher, "Financial Toxicity in Cancer Care: Prevalence, Causes, Consequences, and Reduction Strategies," *Journal of Surgical Oncology* 120, no. 1 (July 1, 2019): 85–92, https://doi.org/10.1002/jso.25374.

15.   Albert Soiland, "Some Economic Aspects of the Cancer Problem," *Radiology* 14, no. 3 (March 1, 1930): 240–53, https://doi.org/10.1148/14.3.240.

16.   With coupons, discounts for generic cancer medications (sometimes available after the patent has expired) can be significant, ranging upwards of 75 percent and as high as 98 percent; how those immediate savings for patients affect payers' costs and, indirectly, insurance premiums, is not clear.

17.   Experts in Chronic Myeloid Leukemia, "The Price of Drugs for Chronic Myeloid Leukemia (CML) Is a Reflection of the Unsustainable Prices of Cancer Drugs: From the Perspective of a Large Group of CML Experts," *Blood* 121, no. 22 (May 30, 2013): 4439–42, https://dx.doi.org/10.1182/blood-2013-03-490003.

18.   Examples of prices for a month's worth of targeted oral cancer medications include Lumakras (sotorasib), Amgen's once-daily pill targeting particular *KRAS* mutations in lung cancer (over $18,000, with coupons); Rozlytrek (entrectinib), Roche's tumor-agnostic medication targeting some *ROS1*-positive and *NTRK*-rearranged tumors ($18,000, with coupons); and Xpovio (selinexor), Karyopharm's oral agent used in combination with other drugs for multiple myeloma and some types of lymphoma (around $25,000). Prices re-checked June 5, 2022, at the GoodRX website: https://www.goodrx.com/lumakras, https://www.goodrx.com/rozlytrek, https://www.goodrx.com/xpovio.

19.   John Wilkerson and Amy Lotven, "CMS Expected to Reject MassHealth Request for a Closed Drug Formulary," InsideHealthPolicy, March 27, 2018, https://insidehealthpolicy.com/share/102940.

20.   Nicholas Bagley and Rachel Sachs, "Massachusetts Wants to Drive Down Medicaid Drug Costs: Why Is the Administration So Nervous?," *Health Affairs* (blog, now *Forefront*) April 5, 2018, https://www.healthaffairs.org/do/10.1377/forefront.20180404.93363/full/.

21. Rachel Sachs, "Understanding Medicare's Aduhelm Coverage Decision," *Health Affairs Forefront*, January 12, 2022, https://www.healthaffairs.org/do/10.1377/forefront.20220112 .876687/.

22. Inmaculada Hernandez, Chester B. Good, David M. Cutler, Walid F. Gellad, Natasha Parekh, and William H. Shrank, "The Contribution of New Product Entry Versus Existing Product Inflation in the Rising Costs of Drugs," *Health Affairs* 38, no. 1 (January 2019): 76–83, https://doi.org/10.1377/hlthaff.2018.05147.

23. Alison Kodjak, "Prescription Drug Costs Driven by Manufacturer Price Hikes, Not Innovation," NPR Health News, January 7, 2019, https://www.npr.org/sections/health -shots/2019/01/07/682986630/prescription-drug-costs-driven-by-manufacturer-price -hikes-not-innovation.

24. Lisa S. Chen, Prithviraj Bose, Nichole D. Cruz, Yongying Jiang, Qi Wu, Philip A. Thompson, Shuju Feng, et al., "A Pilot Study of Lower Doses of Ibrutinib in Patients with Chronic Lymphocytic Leukemia," *Blood* 132, no. 21 (November 22, 2018): 2249–59, https://doi .org/10.1182/blood-2018-06-860593.

25. Gunjan Sinha, "Experts Push for New Cancer Drug Dosing Recommendations," *Undark*, December 9, 2020, https://undark.org/2020/12/09/cancer-drugs-less-might-be-more/.

26. Elaine Schattner, "Memo to Candidates: Support for U.S. Cancer Research Crosses Party Lines," *Forbes*, September 16, 2015.

27. Robert Pear, "Medical Research? Congress Cheers. Medical Care? Congress Brawls," *New York Times*, January 7, 2018.

28. Jeffrey M. Jones, "Americans Still Favor Private Healthcare System," Gallup, December 4, 2019, https://news.gallup.com/poll/268985/americans-favor-private-healthcare-system .aspx.

29. Jessica Wapner, "The Cancer Epidemic in Central Appalachia," *Newsweek*, July 31, 2015.

30. Ali H. Mokdad, Laura Dwyer-Lindgren, Christina Fitzmaurice, Rebecca W. Stubbs, Amelia Bertozzi-Villa, Chloe Morozoff, Raghid Charara, Christine Allen, Mohsen Naghavi, and Christopher J. L. Murray, "Trends and Patterns of Disparities in Cancer Mortality Among US Counties, 1980–2014," *JAMA* 317, no. 4 (January 24/31, 2017): 388–406, https://doi.org/10.1001/jama.2016.20324.

31. Otis Webb Brawley and Paul Goldberg, *How We Do Harm* (New York: St. Martin's, 2011). Brawley, an oncologist who is Black, was raised in Detroit and worked at Atlanta's Grady hospital, reflects: "Folks I grew up with were worried that the doctors who treated them had no idea what they were doing, that they were experimenting," 30.

32. Kristen Pallok, Fernando De Maio, and David A. Ansell, "Structural Racism—A 60-Year-Old Black Woman with Breast Cancer," *NEJM* 380, no. 16 (April 18, 2019): 1489–93, https://doi.org/10.1056/NEJMp1811499.

33. Katherine Reeder-Hayes, Sharon Peacock Hinton, Ke Meng, Lisa A. Carey, and Stacie B. Dusetzina, "Disparities in Use of Human Epidermal Growth Hormone Receptor 2–Targeted Therapy for Early-Stage Breast Cancer," *Journal of Clinical Oncology* 34, no. 17 (June 10, 2016): 2003–9, https://dx.doi.org/10.1200/jco.2015.65.8716.

34. Bobby Daly and Olufunmilayo I. Olopade, "A Perfect Storm: How Tumor Biology, Genomics, and Health Care Delivery Patterns Collide to Create a Racial Survival Disparity in Breast Cancer and Proposed Interventions for Change," *CA: A Cancer Journal for Clinicians* 65, no. 3 (May/June 2015): 221–38, https://doi.org/10.3322/caac.21271.

35.   Nancy Krieger, "Measures of Racism, Sexism, Heterosexism, and Gender Binarism for Health Equity Research: From Structural Injustice to Embodied Harm—An Ecosocial Analysis," *Annual Review of Public Health* 41 (April 2020): 37–62, https://www.annualreviews.org/doi/abs/10.1146/annurev-publhealth-040119-094017.

36.   Lauren L. Palazzo, Deirdre F. Sheehan, Angela C. Tramontano, and Chung Yin Kong, "Disparities and Trends in Genetic Testing and Erlotinib Treatment Among Metastatic Non–Small Cell Lung Cancer Patients," *Cancer Epidemiology Biomarkers & Prevention* 28, no. 5 (May 2019): 926–34, https://doi.org/10.1158/1055-9965.Epi-18-0917.

37.   Daniel M. Sheinson, William B. Wong, Craig S. Meyer, Stella Stergiopoulos, Katherine T. Lofgren, Carlos Flores, Devon V. Adams, and Mark E. Fleury, "Trends in Use of Next-Generation Sequencing in Patients with Solid Tumors by Race and Ethnicity After Implementation of the Medicare National Coverage Determination," *JAMA Network Open* 4, no. 12 (December 9, 2021): e2138219, https://doi.org/10.1001/jamanetworkopen.2021.38219.

38.   Anne Boyer, *The Undying* (New York: Farrar, Straus and Giroux, 2019), 86.

14. HAS AWARENESS BACKFIRED?

1.   Deborah A. Whippen and George P. Canellos, "Burnout Syndrome in the Practice of Oncology: Results of a Random Survey of 1,000 Oncologists," *Journal of Clinical Oncology* 9, no. 10 (October 1, 1991): 1916–20, https://doi.org/10.1200/jco.1991.9.10.1916.

2.   Allen C. Sherman, Donna Edwards, Stephanie Simonton, and Paulette Mehta, "Caregiver Stress and Burnout in an Oncology Unit," *Palliative and Supportive Care* 4 no., 1 (March 2006): 65–80, https://doi.org/10.1017/s1478951506060081.

3.   Guillermo A. Cañadas-De La Fuente, Jose L. Gómez-Urquiza, Elena M. Ortega-Campos, Gustavo R. Cañadas, Luis Albendín-García, and Emilia I. De La Fuente-Solana, "Prevalence of Burnout Syndrome in Oncology Nursing: A Meta-analytic Study," *Psycho-Oncology* 27, no. 5 (May 2018): 1426–33, https://doi.org/10.1002/pon.4632.

4.   Leslie Kane, *Medscape Oncologist Lifestyle, Happiness & Burnout Report 2019* (New York: Medscape, February 20, 2019), https://www.medscape.com/slideshow/2019-lifestyle-oncologist-6011132.

5.   Mary Lasker Papers, 1940–1993, box 96 (includes 1952), Columbia University Libraries, Special Collections, New York, NY. Correspondence with Marguerite Clark of *Newsweek*, itinerary of ACS tour for journalists.

6.   Mary Lasker Papers, 1940–1993, box 538, science writers (folder), Columbia University Libraries, Special Collections, New York, NY. National Association of Science Writers newsletter includes an amusing report by Victor Cohn on the ACS retreat for journalists in Excelsior Springs.

7.   Daniel S. Greenberg, "A Critical Look at Cancer Coverage," *Columbia Journalism Review* 13, no. 5 (January/February 1975): 40–45.

8.   Daniel S. Greenberg, "Cancer: Now, the Bad News," *Washington Post*, January 19, 1975.

9.   Daniel S. Greenberg and Judith E. Randal, "Waging the Wrong War on Cancer: How the American Cancer Society Focuses on Search for Cures Rather Than on the Environmental Causes," *Washington Post*, May 1, 1977.

10.   Samuel S. Epstein, *The Politics of Cancer* (Garden City, NY: Anchor, 1979), 628.

11. Samuel S. Epstein and Jay Feldman, "'Negligible Risk' Is Still Much Too Great," *Los Angeles Times*, November 16, 1989.

12. Samuel S. Epstein, "Mammography Radiates Doubts: An Activist Coalition Fighting Breast Cancer Needs to Question the Line Doled Out by the Cancer Establishment," *Los Angeles Times*, January 28, 1992.

13. Sam Roberts, "Dr. Samuel Epstein, 91, Cassandra of Cancer Prevention, Dies," *New York Times*, April 25, 2018.

14. John C. Bailar III and Elaine M. Smith, "Progress Against Cancer?," *NEJM* 314, no. 19 (May 8, 1986): 1226–32, https://dx.doi.org/10.1056/nejm198605083141905.

15. John C. Bailar III and Heather L. Gornik, "Cancer Undefeated," *NEJM* 336, no. 22 (May 29, 1997): 1569–74, https://doi.org/10.1056/NEJM199705293362206.

16. John Marquart, Emerson Y. Chen, and Vinay Prasad, "Estimation of the Percentage of US Patients with Cancer Who Benefit from Genome-Driven Oncology," *JAMA Oncology* 4, no. 8 (August 2018): 1093–98, https://doi.org/10.1001/jamaoncol.2018.1660.

17. Elizabeth M. Jaffee, Chi Van Dang, David B. Agus, Brian M. Alexander, Kenneth C. Anderson, Alan Ashworth, Anna D. Barker, et al., "Future Cancer Research Priorities in the USA: A Lancet Oncology Commission," *Lancet Oncology* 18, no. 11 (November 1, 2017): e653–706, https://doi.org/10.1016/S1470-2045(17)30698-8.

18. Nadia Howlader, Gonçalo Forjaz, Meghan J. Mooradian, Rafael Meza, Chung Yin Kong, Kathleen A. Cronin, Angela B. Mariotto, Douglas R. Lowy, and Eric J. Feuer, "The Effect of Advances in Lung-Cancer Treatment on Population Mortality," *NEJM* 383, no. 7 (August 13, 2020): 640–49, https://dx.doi.org/10.1056/nejmoa1916623.

19. Juliana Berk-Krauss, Jennifer A. Stein, Jeffrey Weber, David Polsky, and Alan C. Geller, "New Systematic Therapies and Trends in Cutaneous Melanoma Deaths Among US Whites, 1986–2016," *American Journal of Public Health* 110, no. 5 (May 1, 2020): 731–33, https://doi.org/10.2105/ajph.2020.305567.

20. S. Jane Henley, Elizabeth M. Ward, Susan Scott, Jiemin Ma, Robert N. Anderson, Albert U. Firth, Cheryll C. Thomas, et al., "Annual Report to the Nation on the Status of Cancer, Part I: National Cancer Statistics," *Cancer* 126, no. 10 (May 15, 2020): 2225–49, https://doi.org/10.1002/cncr.32802.

21. Rebecca L. Siegel, Kimberly D. Miller, Hannah E. Fuchs, and Ahmedin Jemal, "Cancer Statistics, 2021," *CA: A Cancer Journal for Clinicians* 71, no. 1 (January/February 2021): 7–33, https://doi.org/10.3322/caac.21654.

22. Elaine Schattner, "Correcting a Decade of Negative News About Mammography," *Clinical Imaging* 60, no. 2 (April 2020): 265–70, https://doi.org/10.1016/j.clinimag.2019.03.011.

23. Elaine Schattner, "Can Cancer Truths Be Told? Challenges for Medical Journalism," *American Society of Clinical Oncology Educational Book* 37 (May 25, 2017), 3–11, https://doi.org/10.1200/EDBK_100011.

24. "About Us," HealthNewsReview.org, accessed June 5, 2022, https://www.healthnewsreview.org/about-us/.

25. Susan Perry, "Confused by a Drumbeat of Health News 'Dreck?' A Minnesota-Based Website Aims to Help," *MinnPost*, May 1, 2015, https://www.minnpost.com/second-opinion/2015/05/confused-drumbeat-health-news-dreck-minnesota-based-website-aims-help/.

26. John Horgan, "Cancer Medicine Is Failing Us," *Scientific American*, *Cross-Check* (blog) August 1, 2019, https://blogs.scientificamerican.com/cross-check/cancer-medicine-is-failing-us/.

27.   "Richard Smith: Dying of Cancer Is the Best Death," *BMJ Opinion*, December 31, 2014, https://blogs.bmj.com/bmj/2014/12/31/richard-smith-dying-of-cancer-is-the-best-death. (At the time of the publication, the *BMJ* labeled this online platform as a blog.)

28.   Bill Keller, "Heroic Measures," *New York Times*, January 12, 2014.

29.   Vinay Prasad, "Perspective: The Precision-Oncology Illusion," *Nature* 537, no. S63 (September 7, 2016), https://doi.org/doi:10.1038/537S63a.

30.   Meghana Keshavan, "Did He Really Just Tweet That? Dr. Vinay Prasad Takes on Big Pharma, Big Medicine, and His Own Colleagues—with Glee," *Stat News*, September 15, 2017, https://www.statnews.com/2017/09/15/vinay-prasad-profile/.

31.   Richard Harris, "Tweeting Oncologist Draws Ire and Admiration for Calling Out Hype," *Weekend Edition Sunday*, radio broadcast, NPR, Washington, DC, June 4, 2018, 7 min, https://www.npr.org/sections/health-shots/2018/06/24/621068147/tweeting-oncologist-draws-ire-and-admiration-for-calling-out-hype.

32.   Gina Kolata and Gardiner Harris, "'Moonshot' to Cure Cancer, to Be Led by Biden, Relies on Outmoded View of Disease," *New York Times*, January 13, 2016.

33.   Jarle Breivik, "We Won't Cure Cancer," *New York Times*, May 27, 2016, https://www.nytimes.com/2016/05/27/opinion/obamas-pointless-cancer-moonshot.html.

34.   Vinay Prasad, "Why a Cancer 'Moonshot' Is Unlikely to Find Us a Cure," *Washington Post*, January 29, 2016.

35.   Ike Swetlitz, "Moonshot to Cure Cancer? We've Heard That Before. Many Times," *Stat News*, January 15, 2016, https://www.statnews.com/2016/01/15/cancer-moonshot-rhetoric/.

36.   Bishal Gyawali, Richard Sullivan, and Christopher M. Booth, "Cancer Groundshot: Going Global Before Going to the Moon," *Lancet Oncology* 19, no. 3 (March 2018): 288–90, https://doi.org/10.1016/S1470-2045(18)30076-7.

37.   Annie Alexander, Rohini Kaluve, Jyothi S. Prabhu, Aruna Korlimarla, B. S. Srinath, Suraj Manjunath, Shekar Patil, K. S. Gopinath, and T. S. Sridhar, "The Impact of Breast Cancer on the Patient and the Family in Indian Perspective," *Indian Journal of Palliative Care* 25, no. 1 (January–March 2019): 66–72.

38.   Sui-Lee Wee and Elsie Chen, "A Chinese Pharmacist Found Out He Had Cancer. Then He Vanished," *New York Times*, August 20, 2018.

39.   M. Wallace, A. Bos, and C. Noble, "Cancer-Related Stigma in South Africa: Exploring Beliefs and Experiences Among Cancer Patients and the General Public," *Journal of Global Oncology* 4, no. S2 (September 28, 2018): 112s, https://doi.org/10.1200/jgo.18.53700.

15. CAN WE PREVENT CANCER?

1.   Ewing, a professor of pathology at Cornell University Medical College, was renowned for his cancer expertise. His 1919 textbook, *Neoplastic Diseases*, was read by cancer specialists in Europe and elsewhere and was updated in four later editions. At the 1926 international conference on cancer in Mohonk, New York, Ewing spoke on cancer prevention and, among other remarks, emphasized tobacco as a frequent cause of lip cancer: James Ewing, "The Prevention of Cancer," in *Cancer Control: Report of an International Symposium Held Under the Auspices of the American Society for the Control of Cancer, Lake Mohonk, New York, U.S.A., September 20–24, 1926* (Chicago: Surgical Publishing, 1927), 165–84.

2. James Ewing, "Cancer as a Public Health Problem," *Public Health Reports* 44, no. 35 (August 30, 1929): 2093–101.

3. "What Is Public Health?," accessed June 5, 2022, American Public Health Association, https://www.apha.org/what-is-public-health.

4. Madeline Drexler, "The Cancer Miracle Isn't a Cure. It's Prevention," *Harvard Public Health Magazine*, Fall 2019.

5. Brian E. Henderson, Ronald K. Ross, and Malcolm C. Pike, "Toward the Primary Prevention of Cancer," *Science* 254, no. 5035 (November 22, 1991): 1131–38, https://doi.org/10.1126/science.1957166.

6. Daniel Krewski, Jay H. Lubin, Jan M. Zielinski, Michael Alavanja, Vanessa S. Catalan, R. William Field, Judith B. Klotz, et al., "A Combined Analysis of North American Case-Control Studies of Residential Radon and Lung Cancer," *Journal of Toxicology and Environmental Health A* 69, no. 7 (April 2006): 533–97, https://doi.org/10.1080/15287390500260945.

7. Catherine de Martel, Damien Georges, Freddie Bray, Jacques Ferlay, and Gary M. Clifford, "Global Burden of Cancer Attributable to Infections in 2018: A Worldwide Incidence Analysis," *Lancet Global Health* 8, no. 2 (February 1, 2020): e180–e90, https://doi.org/10.1016/S2214-109X(19)30488-7.

8. Farhad Islami, Ann Goding Sauer, Kimberly D. Miller, Rebecca L., Siegel Stacey A. Fedewa, Eric J. Jacobs, Marjorie L. McCullough, et al., "Proportion and Number of Cancer Cases and Deaths Attributable to Potentially Modifiable Risk Factors in the United States," *CA: A Cancer Journal for Clinicians* 68, no. 1 (January/February 2018): 31–54, https://doi.org/10.3322/caac.21440.

9. Rebecca L. Siegel, Kimberly D. Miller, Hannah E. Fuchs, and Ahmedin Jemal, "Cancer Statistics, 2021," *CA: A Cancer Journal for Clinicians* 71, no. 1 (January/February 2021): 7–33, https://doi.org/10.3322/caac.21654.

10. Fatiha El Ghissassi, Robert Baan, Kurt Straif, Yann Grosse, Béatrice Secretan, Véronique Bouvard, Lamia Benbrahim-Tallaa, et al., "A Review Of Human Carcinogens—Part D: Radiation," *Lancet Oncology* 10, no. 8 (August 2009): 751–52, https://dx.doi.org/10.1016/s1470-2045(09)70213-x.

11. Jennifer A. Ligibel and Dana Wollins, "American Society of Clinical Oncology Obesity Initiative: Rationale, Progress, and Future Directions," *Journal of Clinical Oncology* 34, no. 35 (December 10, 2016): 4256–60, https://doi.org/10.1200/jco.2016.67.4051.

12. Centers for Disease Control and Prevention, "Cancer and Obesity," Vital Signs, last updated October 3, 2017, https://www.cdc.gov/vitalsigns/obesity-cancer/index.html.

13. Hyuna Sung, Rebecca L. Siegel, Lindsey A. Torre, Jonathan Pearson-Stuttard, Farhad Islami, Stacey A. Fedewa, Ann Goding Sauer, et al., "Global Patterns in Excess Body Weight and the Associated Cancer Burden," *CA: A Cancer Journal for Clinicians* 69, no. 2 (March/April 2019): 88–112, https://doi.org/10.3322/caac.21499.

14. Farhad Islami, Rebecca L. Siegel, and Ahmedin Jemal, "The Changing Landscape of Cancer in the USA—Opportunities for Advancing Prevention and Treatment," *Nature Reviews Clinical Oncology* 17, no. 10 (October 2020): 631–49, https://doi.org/10.1038/s41571-020-0378-y.

15. "Alcohol and Cancer," Centers for Disease Control and Prevention, last reviewed January 31, 2022, https://www.cdc.gov/cancer/alcohol/index.htm.

16.   Noelle K. LoConte, Abenaa M. Brewster, Judith S. Kaur, Janette K. Merrill, and Anthony J. Alberg, "Alcohol and Cancer: A Statement of the American Society of Clinical Oncology," *Journal of Clinical Oncology* 36, no. 1 (January 1, 2018): 83–93, https://doi.org/10.1200/jco.2017.76.1155.

17.   Rachel Carson, "Silent Spring—III," *New Yorker*, June 30, 1962.

18.   Dr. Wilhelm C. Hueper was a German-born physician who emigrated to the United States, worked for DuPont, and wrote a significant 1942 text, *Occupational Tumors and Allied Diseases*, on chemical toxins. In 1948, Hueper became director of the NCI's Environmental Cancer Section. For discussion of Hueper's Nazi leanings and racism, see Robert N. Proctor, *The Nazi War on Cancer* (Princeton, NJ: Princeton University Press, 1999), "Hueper's Secret," 13–34; and 70–71; Hueper's life and work on carcinogens is also covered by Sam Apple in *Ravenous: Otto Warburg, the Nazis, and the Search for the Cancer–Diet Connection* (New York: Liveright, 2021), 210–19.

19.   Eric Boyland, "Difficulties in Assessing Carcinogenic Activity," *Nature* 274, no. 5669 (July 27, 1978): 308, https://doi.org/10.1038/274308a0.

20.   William H. Goodson III, Leroy Lowe, David O. Carpenter, Michael Gilbertson, Abdul Manaf Ali, Adela Lopez de Cerain Salsamendi, Ahmed Lasfar, et al., "Assessing the Carcinogenic Potential of Low-Dose Exposures to Chemical Mixtures in the Environment: The Challenge Ahead," *Carcinogenesis* 36, no. S1 (June 2015): S254–96, https://doi.org/10.1093/carcin/bgv039.

21.   Eric Letouzé, Jayendra Shinde, Victor Renault, Gabrielle Couchy, Jean-Frédéric Blanc, Emmanuel Tubacher, Quentin Bayard, et al., "Mutational Signatures Reveal the Dynamic Interplay of Risk Factors and Cellular Processes During Liver Tumorigenesis," *Nature Communications* 8 (November 3, 2017): 1315, https://doi.org/10.1038/s41467-017-01358-x.

22.   Nicola Davis, "Causes of Cancer May Leave 'Fingerprints' in DNA, Scientists Say," *Guardian*, April 15, 2019, https://www.theguardian.com/science/2019/apr/15/causes-of-cancer-may-leave-fingerprints-in-dna-scientists-say.

23.   Jill E. Kucab, Xueqing Zou, Sandro Morganella, Madeleine Joel, A. Scott Nanda, Eszter Nagy, Celine Gomez, et al., "A Compendium of Mutational Signatures of Environmental Agents," *Cell* 177, no. 4 (April 11, 2019): 821–36, https://doi.org/10.1016/j.cell.2019.03.001.

24.   Ludmil B. Alexandrov, Jaegil Kim, Nicholas J. Haradhvala, Mi Ni Huang, Alvin Wei Tian Ng, Yang Wu, Arnoud Boot, et al., "The Repertoire of Mutational Signatures in Human Cancer," *Nature* 578, no. 7793 (February 5, 2020): 94–101, https://doi.org/10.1038/s41586-020-1943-3.

25.   Elaine Schattner, "A Call for More Research on Cancer's Environmental Triggers," NPR Health, July 12, 2019, https://www.npr.org/sections/health-shots/2019/07/12/740817989/a-call-for-more-research-on-cancers-environmental-triggers.

26.   Stephen M. Rappaport and Martyn T. Smith, "Environment and Disease Risks," *Science*, 330, no. 6003 (October 22, 2010): 460–61, https://www.science.org/doi/10.1126/science.1192603.

27.   Ariane Mbemi, Sunali Khanna, Sylvianne Njiki, Clement G. Yedjou, and Paul B. Tchounwou, "Impact of Gene–Environment Interactions on Cancer Development," *International Journal of Environmental Research and Public Health* 17, no. 21: (November 3, 2020), 8089, https://doi.org/10.3390/ijerph17218089.

28. Karoline B. Kuchenbaecker, John L. Hopper, Daniel R. Barnes, Kelly-Anne Phillips, Thea M. Mooij, Marie-José Roos-Blom, Sarah Jervis, et al., "Risks of Breast, Ovarian, and Contralateral Breast Cancer for *BRCA1* and *BRCA2* Mutation Carriers," *JAMA* 317, no. 23 (June 20, 2017): 2402–16, https://doi.org/10.1001/jama.2017.7112.

29. Cristian Tomasetti and Bert Vogelstein, "Variation in Cancer Risk Among Tissues Can Be Explained by the Number of Stem Cell Divisions," *Science* 347, no. 6217 (January 2, 2015): 78–81, https://doi.org/10.1126/science.1260825.

30. Cristian Tomasetti, Lu Li, and Bert Vogelstein, "Stem Cell Divisions, Somatic Mutations, Cancer Etiology, and Cancer Prevention," *Science* 355, no. 6331 (March 24, 2017): 1330–34, https://doi.org/10.1126/science.aaf9011.

31. Azra Raza, *The First Cell and the Human Costs of Pursuing Cancer to the Last* (New York: Basic, 2019).

32. "Mycotoxins," World Health Organization, May 9, 2018, https://www.who.int/news-room/fact-sheets/detail/mycotoxins.

33. Lydia E. Wroblewski, Richard M. Peek, and Keith T. Wilson, "*Helicobacter pylori* and Gastric Cancer: Factors That Modulate Disease Risk," *Clinical Microbiology Reviews* 23, no. 4 (October 1, 2010): 713–39, https://dx.doi.org/10.1128/cmr.00011-10.

34. Emilio Palumbo, "Association Between Schistosomiasis and Cancer: A Review," *Infectious Diseases in Clinical Practice* 15, no. 3 (May 2007): 145–48, https://doi.org/10.1097/01.idc.0000269904.90155.ce.

35. M. H. Mostafa, S. A. Sheweita, and P. J. O'Connor, "Relationship Between Schistosomiasis and Bladder Cancer," *Clinical Microbiology Reviews* 12, no. 1 (January 1999): 97–111, https://doi.org/10.1128/CMR.12.1.97.

36. "Parasites - Opisthorchis Infection," Centers for Disease Control and Prevention, last reviewed July 28, 2021, https://www.cdc.gov/parasites/opisthorchis/index.html; "About Opisthorchis," Centers for Disease Control and Prevention, last reviewed August 25, 2020, https://www.cdc.gov/parasites/opisthorchis/faqs.html.

37. "Parasites - Clonorchis," Centers for Disease Control and Prevention, last reviewed July 28, 2021, https://www.cdc.gov/parasites/clonorchis/; "About Clonorchis," Centers for Disease Control and Prevention, last reviewed October 21, 2020, https://www.cdc.gov/parasites/clonorchis/faqs.html.

38. John D. Groopman, Thomas W. Kensler, and Christopher P. Wild, "Protective Interventions to Prevent Aflatoxin-Induced Carcinogenesis in Developing Countries," *Annual Review of Public Health* 29 (April 2008): 187–203, https://doi.org/10.1146/annurev.publhealth.29.020907.090859.

39. Marc Arbyn, Elisabete Weiderpass, Laia Bruni, Silvia de Sanjosé, Mona Saraiya, Jacques Ferlay, and Freddie Bray, "Estimates of Incidence and Mortality of Cervical Cancer in 2018: A Worldwide Analysis," *Lancet Global Health* 8, no. 2 (February 1, 2020): e191–203, https://doi.org/10.1016/S2214-109X(19)30482-6.

40. Milena Falcaro, Alejandra Castañon, Busani Ndlela, Marta Checchi, Kate Soldan, Jamie Lopez-Bernal, Lucy Elliss-Brookes, and Peter Sasieni, "The Effects of the National HPV Vaccination Programme in England, UK, on Cervical Cancer and Grade 3 Cervical Intraepithelial Neoplasia Incidence: A Register-Based Observational Study," *Lancet* 398, no. 10316 (November 3, 2021): 2084–92, https://doi.org/10.1016/S0140-6736(21)02178-4.

41. Eyal Press, "A Preventable Cancer Is on the Rise in Alabama," *New Yorker*, April 6, 2020.

42. David Barboza, "E.P.A. Says It Pressed 3M for Action on Scotchgard Chemical," *New York Times*, May 19, 2000.

43. "Perfluorooctanoic Acid (PFOA), Teflon, and Related Chemicals," American Cancer Society, data from April 12, 2022 retrieved from Internet Archive, https://web.archive .org/web/20220412163711/https://www.cancer.org/cancer/cancer-causes/teflon-and -perfluorooctanoic-acid-pfoa.html.

44. Abrahm Lustgarten, "How the EPA and the Pentagon Downplayed a Growing Toxic Threat," *ProPublica*, July 9, 2018, https://www.propublica.org/article/how-the-epa-and-the-pentagon -downplayed-toxic-pfas-chemicals?.

45. Evan Belanger (Associated Press), "3M Tells Alabama That It Underreported Chemicals in River," *Star Tribune* (Minnesota) December 1, 2017.

46. Tiffany Kary and Christopher Cannon, "Cancer-linked Chemicals Manufactured by 3M Are Turning Up in Drinking Water," Bloomberg, November 2, 2018, https://www .bloomberg.com/graphics/2018-3M-groundwater-pollution-problem/.

47. Robert Bilott, "The 20-Year Legal Battle with DuPont That Started with One West Virginia Farmer," Marketplace, October 16, 2019, https://www.marketplace.org/2019/10/16 /the-20-year-legal-battle-with-dupont-that-started-with-one-west-virginia-farmer/.

48. Tom Dart, "A Trail of Toxicity: The US Military Bases Making People Sick," *Guardian*, May 23, 2019, http://www.theguardian.com/us-news/2019/may/23/chemical-colorado -springs-military-communities-pfcs.

49. Ted Alcorn, "Extensive Contamination with Potential Carcinogen Prompts Regulation Across the USA," *Lancet Oncology* 21, no. 3 (February 14, 2020): 340, https://doi.org /10.1016/S1470-2045(20)30090-5.

50. Philippe Grandjean and Richard Clapp, "Changing Interpretation of Human Health Risks from Perfluorinated Compounds," *Public Health Reports* 129, no. 6 (November– December 2014): 482–85, https://doi.org/10.1177/003335491412900605.

51. Kurunthachalam Kannan, Simonetta Corsolini, Jerzy Falandysz, Gilberto Fillmann, Kurunthachalam Senthil Kumar, Bommanna G. Loganathan, Mustafa Ali Mohd, Jesus Olivero, et al., "Perfluorooctanesulfonate and Related Fluorochemicals in Human Blood from Several Countries," *Environmental Science & Technology* 38, no. 17 (September 1, 2004): 4489–95, https://doi.org/10.1021/es0493446.

52. "Perfluoroalkyl and Polyfluoroalkyl Substances (PFAS)," National Institute of Environmental Health Sciences, last reviewed March 7, 2022, https://www.niehs.nih.gov/health /topics/agents/pfc/.

53. Elizabeth Ward, Ahmedin Jemal, Vilma Cokkinides, Gopal K. Singh, Cheryll Cardinez, Asma Ghafoor, and Michael Thun, "Cancer Disparities by Race/Ethnicity and Socioeconomic Status," *CA: A Cancer Journal for Clinicians* 54, no. 2 (March/April 2004): 78–93, https://doi.org/10.3322/canjclin.54.2.78.

54. Frederick L. Tyson, Katsi Cook, James Gavin, Clarice E. Gaylord, Charles Lee, Valerie P. Setlow, and Samuel Wilson, "Cancer, the Environment, and Environmental Justice," *Cancer* 83, no. S8 (October 15, 1998): 1784–92, https://doi.org/10.1002/(SICI)1097-0142 (19981015)83:8+<1784::AID-CNCR22>3.0.CO;2-P.

55. "Milwaukee Estuary Area of Concern," Wisconsin Department of Natural Resources, accessed May 3, 2022, https://dnr.wisconsin.gov/topic/GreatLakes/Milwaukee.html.

56. *Milwaukee Estuary Remedial Action Plan: A Plan to Clean Up Milwaukee's Rivers and Harbor* (Madison, WI: Wisconsin Water Quality Management Program, 1991), https://www.epa .gov/sites/default/files/2013-12/documents/milwaukeeest-rap_stage-i.pdf.

57. Laura Schulte, "The Milwaukee Estuary Could Soon Be Cleaner, Thanks to Another Round of Dredging and a New Sediment Containment Facility," *Milwaukee Journal Sentinel*, July 6, 2021.

58. "Learn About Polychlorinated Biphenyls (PCBs)," U.S. Environmental Protection Agency, accessed May 3, 2022, https://www.epa.gov/pcbs/learn-about-polychlorinated-biphenyls -pcbs#. See sections "Health Effects of PCBs" and "Cancer."

59. For a recent in-depth consideration of industrial pollution affecting the St. Lawrence River and Mohawk tribal lands, see Elizabeth Hoover, *The River Is in Us: Fighting Toxics in a Mohawk Community* (Minneapolis: University of Minnesota Press, 2017).

60. Adrianna Quintero-Somaini, Mayra Quirindongo, Evelyn Arévalo, Daniel Lashof, Erik Olson, and Gina Solomon, *Hidden Danger: Environmental Health Threats in the Latino Community* (New York: Natural Resources Defense Council, October 2004), https://www .nrdc.org/sites/default/files/latino_en.pdf.

61. Tristan Baurick, Lylla Younes, and Joan Meiners, "Welcome to 'Cancer Alley,' Where Toxic Air Is About to Get Worse," *ProPublica*, October 30, 2019, https://www.propublica .org/article/welcome-to-cancer-alley-where-toxic-air-is-about-to-get-worse.

62. Idna G. Castellón, "Cancer Alley and the Fight Against Environmental Racism," *Villanova Environmental Law Journal* 32, no. 1 (February 12, 2021), https://digitalcommons.law .villanova.edu/cgi/viewcontent.cgi?article=1440&context=elj.

63. Antonia Juhasz, "Louisiana's 'Cancer Alley' Is Getting Even More Toxic—But Residents Are Fighting Back," *Rolling Stone*, October 30, 2019, https://www.rollingstone.com /politics/politics-features/louisiana-cancer-alley-getting-more-toxic-905534/.

64. "Environmental Racism in Louisiana's 'Cancer Alley,' Must End, Say UN Human Rights Experts," UN News, March 2, 2021, https://news.un.org/en/story/2021/03/1086172.

65. Oliver Laughland, "Multibillion-Dollar Louisiana Plastics Plant Put on Pause in a Win for Activists," *Guardian*, August 18, 2021, https://www.theguardian.com/us-news/2021 /aug/18/louisiana-plastics-plant-toxic-emissions-cancer-alley.

66. David J. Mitchell, "Massive Louisiana Plastics Plant Faces 2+ Year Delay for Tougher Environmental Review," *Baton Rouge Advocate*, November 1, 2021, https://www.theadvocate .com/baton_rouge/news/article_c58e7f22-3997-11ec-909f-9bdd7461a90c.html.

67. James D. Yager and Nancy E. Davidson, "Estrogen Carcinogenesis in Breast Cancer," *NEJM* 354, no. 3 (January 19, 2006): 270–82, https://dx.doi.org/10.1056/nejmra050776.

68. Helmut K. Seitz and Peter Becker, "Alcohol Metabolism and Cancer Risk," *Alcohol Research & Health* 30, no. 1 (2007): 38–47.

69. Ying Liu, Nhi Nguyen, and Graham A. Colditz, "Links Between Alcohol Consumption and Breast Cancer: A Look at the Evidence," *Women's Health* 11, no. 1 (January 1, 2015): 65–77, https://dx.doi.org/10.2217/whe.14.62.

70. *The Normal Heart*, written by Larry Kramer, directed by Michael Lindsay-Hogg, Public Theater, New York, NY, 1985. The 2011 production I attended ran at the John Golden Theater, 252 West Forty-Fifth St., New York, NY.

EPILOGUE

1. Rebecca L. Siegel, Kimberly D. Miller, Hannah E. Fuchs, and Ahmedin Jemal, "Cancer Statistics, 2022," *CA: A Cancer Journal for Clinicians* 72, no. 1 (January/February 2020): 7–33, https://doi.org/10.3322/caac.21708.

2. American Cancer Society, *Cancer Facts & Figures 2022* (Atlanta: American Cancer Society, 2022), https://www.cancer.org/content/dam/cancer-org/research/cancer-facts-and-statistics/annual-cancer-facts-and-figures/2022/2022-cancer-facts-and-figures.pdf.

3. "Survival," National Cancer Institute Cancer Trends Progress Report, accessed May 3, 2022, https://progressreport.cancer.gov/after/survival.

4. Farhad Islami, Carmen E. Guerra, Adair Minihan, K. Robin Yabroff, Stacey A. Fedewa, Kirsten Sloan, Tracy L. Wiedt, et al., "American Cancer Society's Report on the Status of Cancer Disparities in the United States, 2021," *CA: A Cancer Journal for Clinicians* 72, no. 2 (March/April 2022): 112–43, https://doi.org/10.3322/caac.21703.

5. Philip Ball, "The Lightning-Fast Quest for COVID Vaccines—and What It Means for Other Diseases," *Nature*, 589 (December 18, 2020; print 2021): 16–18, https://www.nature.com/articles/d41586-020-03626-1.

6. Elie Dolgin, "How COVID Unlocked the Power of RNA Vaccines," *Nature* 589 (January 12, 2021): 189–91, https://www.nature.com/articles/d41586-021-00019-w.

7. Jon Gertner, "Unlocking the Covid Code," *New York Times Magazine*, March 25, 2021.

8. Susan Sontag, *Illness as Metaphor* (New York: Farrar, Straus and Giroux, 1978): 86–88.

INDEX

Page numbers in *italics* indicate illustrations.